# WHIPLASH, HEADACHE, AND NECK PAIN

*Research-based directions for physical therapies*

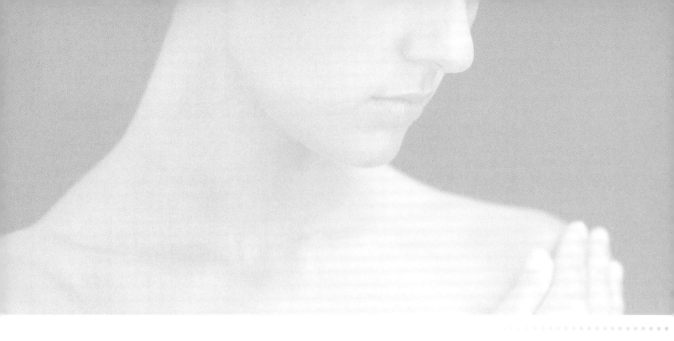

Publisher: *Sarena Wolfaard*
Commissioning Editor: *Claire Wilson*
Project Manager: *Jess Thompson*
Designer: *Stewart Larking*
Illustrator: *Precision Illustration*

# WHIPLASH, HEADACHE, AND NECK PAIN

*Research-based directions for physical therapies*

## Gwendolen Jull
PhD MPhty Grad Dip Manip Ther Dip Phty FACP
Professor of Physiotherapy, The University of Queensland, Australia;
Director, NHMRC Center of Clinical Research Excellence in Spinal Pain, Injury and Health, The University of Queensland, Australia;
Director of the Cervical Spine and Whiplash Research Unit, The University of Queensland, Australia;
Consultant Musculoskeletal Physiotherapist

## Michele Sterling
PhD MPhty Grad Dip Manip Ther B Phty
Associate Director, Centre for National Research on Disability and Rehabilitation Medicine (CONROD), The University of Queensland, Australia;
Director of the Cervical Spine and Whiplash Research Unit, The University of Queensland, Australia;
Senior Lecturer, Division of Physiotherapy, The University of Queensland, Australia

## Deborah Falla PhD B Phty (Hons)
NHMRC Research Fellow, NHMRC Center of Clinical Research Excellence in Spinal Pain, Injury and Health, The University of Queensland, Australia;
Associate Professor Center for Sensory-Motor Interaction,
Department of Health Science and Technology, Aalborg University, Denmark

## Julia Treleaven PhD B Phty
Clinical Manager of the Cervical Spine and Whiplash Research Unit, The University of Queensland, Australia;
Lecturer, Division of Physiotherapy, The University of Queensland, Australia

## Shaun O'Leary
PhD M Phty St (Manip Ther) B Phty (Hons)
Lecturer, Division of Physiotherapy, The University of Queensland, Australia;
Clinical Educator, Master of Musculoskeletal Physiotherapy Programme, The University of Queensland, Australia

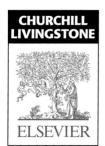

CHURCHILL LIVINGSTONE

ELSEVIER

Edinburgh  London  New York  Oxford  Philadelphia  St Louis  Sydney  Toronto  2008

CHURCHILL
LIVINGSTONE
ELSEVIER
An imprint of Elsevier Limited

First published 2008

ISBN: 978-0-443-10047-5

British Library Cataloguing in Publication Data
A catalogue record for this book is available from the British Library

Library of Congress Cataloging in Publication Data
A catalog record for this book is available from the Library of Congress

Notice
Neither the Publisher nor the Authors assume any responsibility for any loss or injury and/or damage to persons or property arising out of or related to any use of the material contained in this book. It is the responsibility of the treating practitioner, relying on independent expertise and knowledge of the patient, to determine the best treatment and method of application for the patient.

The Publisher

your source for books,
journals and multimedia
in the health sciences
**www.elsevierhealth.com**

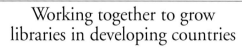

Working together to grow
libraries in developing countries

www.elsevier.com | www.bookaid.org | www.sabre.org

ELSEVIER    BOOK AID International    Sabre Foundation

Printed in China

# Contents

## Section 1 Introduction

## Section 2 Applied Clinical Sciences

## Section 3 Whiplash, Headache, and Cervicobrachial Pain

## Section 4 Therapeutics for Cervical Disorders

## Section 5 Conclusion

Research into cervical spine disorders played second fiddle to low-back pain for a large part of the 20th century. However, in the last two decades in particular, there has been a rapid increase in interest and research into cervical musculoskeletal disorders, which is well warranted.

Neck pain is beginning to rival low-back pain in its frequency and the economic and social costs for neck pain have increased leading into the 21st century. The seeming increase in the incidence of neck pain may be related to many factors, including advances in technologies in the workplace and thus the changing nature of work, the increased use of motor vehicles throughout the world, and the rapid rise of information technology and computer use which occupies many hours in sedentary, sustained postures.

Neck pain is now rapidly developing its own body of science. There are many examples in the literature of the 1980s and 1990s where knowledge gained for low-back pain was merely extrapolated and applied to cervical musculoskeletal disorders in both diagnostics and management. This was clearly inadequate, as more contemporary research is revealing. The cervical spine is anatomically and biomechanically very different from the lumbar spine, in accordance with the different functional roles of these regions. While the muscle systems in the two regions have some similarities, they also have vast differences, as could be expected with their different functions. In addition, cervical structures have unique neurophysiological connections to the vestibular and oculomotor systems. The structures of the cervical spine are vulnerable to trauma, as occurs, for example, in a motor vehicle crash in ways not experienced in the low back. The psychological reactions that can accompany neck pain are often quite different from those found with chronic low-back pain. In consequence, neck pain disorders can present with some unique problems. Fortunately the era of trying to force the application of knowledge from the low back to neck pain is gradually disappearing.

The diagnosis and management of cervical musculoskeletal disorders are assuming new directions. The focus on pathoanatomical diagnoses is gradually shifting towards a more processes or pathophysiological approach in the recognition that in the majority of neck disorders a definitive pathoanatomical cause may not be able to be readily identified in up to 80% of neck pain patients. This shift in focus has also been assisted by major advances in knowledge and technology. There have been dramatic advances in knowledge of pain mechanisms over recent decades. Technologies are assisting in bridging the gap between animal research and pain presentations in humans. Advances in electromyographic techniques have allowed a more comprehensive exploration of the cervical muscle system and motor control. There is more to explore and learn in all fields before we will fully understand neck pain. Nevertheless the rapid advances of the past two decades have laid a foundation for improvements in the understanding and management of cervical disorders which will benefit the neck pain patient and clinician alike.

This text emanates from the research and clinical interests of the authors over the past 10 years in particular. Collectively, we have particular interests in whiplash-associated disorders, cervicogenic headache, cervicobrachial, and idiopathic neck pain. As physiotherapists, we have researched towards developing enhanced clinical diagnoses of neck disorders as well as developing the foundations for specific rehabilitation and prevention strategies for neck pain. The research has developed from an applied clinical perspective. Our philosophy is that if we understand, identify, and quantify the abnormal features involved in neck disorders from a broad multisystems pathophysiological perspective, this will lay the foundation for better differential diagnosis and rehabilitation. It is our contention that understanding the underlying processes of cervical disorders as well as their development over time will assist in developing clinically meaningful subcategories of neck disorders and most importantly will direct the development of specific and relevant rehabilitation and prevention strategies. We have developed and tested new rehabilitation strategies for neck disorders and this process, like all research, is ongoing.

This text presents the applied sciences, assessment, and rehabilitation protocols for the management of cervical disorders. In writing the text, we have used the available international body of knowledge. However the text has principally been developed and guided by the outcomes of our research and its translation to clinical practice. Research is an ongoing process and we look forward to developments in the field over the next 10 years.

GJ
MS
DF
JT
and
S O'L
2008

*Whiplash, Headache, and Neck Pain* is a unique text presenting the examination, interpretation and the conservative management of specific disorders related to the cervical spine and neck. The disorders covered in the text are whiplash associated disorders both acute and chronic, cervicogenic headache and cervicobrachial pain. These specific disorders can be perplexing and as a result difficult to manage. However the disorders are dealt with by the authors in a manner which is enlightening. They provide a detailed clinical understanding and as a result a greater ability for the clinical prescription of more appropriate management strategies. This clinical understanding takes into account the individual with the complaint and the associated sensory, muscular and articular systems. Management is detailed by way of a multimodal approach. Hence the authors have provided a systematic approach towards a better understanding of the complexities of clinical investigation and management related to disorders of the cervical spine and neck.

*Whiplash, Headache, and Neck Pain* represents extensive research influenced by extensive clinical experience. The text is the culmination of many decades of combined work by the five authors. In particular, the senior author, Gwen Jull, has dedicated much of her time to developing an understanding of particular disorders of the cervical spine and neck based upon her clinical experience and extensive research. Her enthusiasm for research has been infectious, as is evident in the post graduate physiotherapy programs at the University of Queensland, Australia. In her position as Professor of Physiotherapy at the University of Queensland she has influenced the research of many post graduate students. This is evident in the academic development of the other authors. However

it must be said that all authors contributing to this text have developed and carried out their own individual research topics. Each author's individual and specific academic and clinical work has contributed towards the development and completion of the text. With extensive academic qualifications, research positions and teaching positions held by each author they have all been well qualified to contribute to *Whiplash, Headache, and Neck Pain*.

In support of the research which forms the structure of *Whiplash, Headache, and Neck Pain* has been the granting of considerable funding. This has been granted by the National Health and Medical Research Centre, Australia, the Australian Research Council, the Motor Accident's Research Council along with a number of other funding bodies. The granting of funding from these high profile bodies is an indication of the outstanding and competitive research proposals presented by the authors to the funding bodies. In addition to funding, as a guide to the academic level of the text, the authors attracted the attention of many national and international experts in similar fields of investigation. This attention led towards collaborative work with different aspects of the text's presentation.

For decades musculoskeletal physiotherapy and the conservative treatment for neck pain and associated disorders has been based upon the interpretation of signs and symptoms. These signs and symptoms were assumed to be specific to the articular system. In addition a diagnosis was purposely avoided. As a result, treatment, was based upon the presumption that the application of passive 'techniques' consisting of applied intermittent pressure to an anatomical site of pain over a spinal segment, resulted in the passive mobilization of the articulation. Should there have been a perceived improvement of mobility it was considered that the 'technique' was beneficial towards the resolution of the disorder. While this approach had merit towards the early development of musculoskeletal physiotherapy in the 1960s and 1970s its blind acceptance ultimately retarded the scientific development of the profession. As a result, the progressive development of more appropriate conservative managements for disorders of the cervical spine and neck were lacking.

Without intent, this approach is at last been challenged by the authors of *Whiplash, Headache, and Neck Pain*. They have questioned and researched, in depth, certain disorders of the cervical spine and neck resulting in the presentation of a much wider range of impairments additional to those of the articular system. As a natural progression to the description of a wide range of impairments associated with these disorders they also describe multimodal systems of management which are more appropriate to the nature of disorders of the cervical spine and neck. Within this multimodal approach are included not only physical managements but consideration of the psychological and psychosocial effects of the disorders.

The authors of *Whiplash, Headache, and Neck Pain* have advanced the status and credibility of musculoskeletal physiotherapy and the conservative management of specific disorders of the cervical spine and neck. They are congratulated on producing a text which clearly promotes a much greater understanding of the investigation and management of such disorders. They are also congratulated on enhancing future developments of musculoskeletal physiotherapy.

Bob Elvey
Dunsborough, Western Australia
2008

# Acknowledgments

Neck pain is a multifaceted disorder and the skills and knowledge required to research in the field require the assistance and collaboration of many people who have shared their expertise with us in collaborative research in the Cervical Spine and Whiplash Research Unit at the University of Queensland.

We would particularly like to acknowledge and thank firstly those at the University of Queensland – Professor Justin Kenardy, who has contributed to the research into psychological features, Professor Bill Vicenzino, Professor Paul Hodges, Dr Tina Souvlis and Ms Nancy LowChoy from the Division of Physiotherapy, and Associate Professor Luke Connelly for his health economics expertise.

We would also like to acknowledge the collaborations of Professor Roberto Merletti and Dr Alberto Rainoldi from the Laboratory of Neuromuscular System Engineering and Motor Rehabilitation, Politecnico di Torino, Italy; Professor Dario Farina, Professor Thomas Graven-Nielsen and Professor Lars Arendt-Nielsen, Aalborg University, Denmark; Associate Professor Eli Eliav, University of Medicine and Dentistry, New Jersey, USA; Professor Michele Curatolo, University of Bern, Switzerland; and Dr John Quintner, Consultant Physician in Rheumatology and Pain Medicine, Perth, WA.

Our PhD and Honours students have all contributed to the research of the Unit presented within this book and we thank them. Likewise, research cannot proceed without financial support and we acknowledge the research support we have received from the National Health and Medical Research Council, The Australian Research Council, The Physiotherapy Research Foundation, the Motor Accidents Insurance Commission (Qld), Suncorp General Insurance, and the Centre of National Research on Disability and Rehabilitation Medicine (CONROD).

We also acknowledge the patients we treat who challenge our clinical reasoning and technical skills. We especially thank all the people with neck pain who have volunteered to participate in our research projects. Without their contribution the research program could not occur.

Finally we would like to acknowledge Mr Chris Stacey of Marketing and Communications, The University of Queensland, for the photography and our models for the photographs, Karina O'Leary and Sabine Giesbrecht.

1

# Introduction

Neck pain is a relatively common complaint and affects some 70% of individuals at some time in their lives. International epidemiological data suggest that 40% of the population will suffer neck pain in any one year with a point prevalence of between 10 and 20%.[1] No age group or occupation appears immune and neck pain is second only to low-back pain in annual workers' compensation costs.[2] Furthermore neck pain tends to be a persistent and recurrent disorder and up to 60% of persons can expect some degree of ongoing pain for many years after their first episode.[3] This has substantial effects on quality of life. These statistics challenge clinicians of all disciplines to improve the worth of preventive and rehabilitative programs for cervical disorders.

Neck pain can be present in inflammatory arthropathies such as rheumatoid arthritis and ankylosing spondylitis, but by far the most common origins of neck pain are benign and relate to disorders originating in the cervical musculoskeletal system. An anatomical source of the condition may be evident on radiological imaging in some cases. Nevertheless, in relation to a definitive diagnosis, most neck pain presentations share a similar destiny to those of the low back in that for the majority of patients there can be no absolute certainty of the pathoanatomical cause of the pain. As a result, it has been recommended that neck pain is classified only as either idiopathic (that is, there is no apparent evident cause of the pain) or resulting from trauma such as whiplash-associated neck pain.[4] The major drawbacks of such generic categorizations are that they falsely assume some homogeneity within each category of neck pain. Such categorization offers little assistance or direction for management for the individual sufferer of neck pain.

A plethora of treatments have been described or tested for neck pain. They have been diverse and one approach can seemingly be the antithesis of another. This is probably symptomatic of the absence of clear diagnoses and directions for management. The current scientific status of conservative physical therapy treatments for neck pain is somewhat equivocal but evidence is growing. Systematic reviews are pointing to the evidence of benefit of multimodal approaches to management inclusive of activity, manual therapy, and exercise, with exercise being a key element of any combination of treatments.[5–7] Nevertheless it is apparent from clinical trials of neck pain patients that there are individual differences in responsiveness to the therapy under investigation, with some patients gaining excellent outcomes while, at the other extreme, others achieve no relevant benefits.[8–10] Heterogeneity in the complaints and treatment responsiveness, as is evident clinically, is the reality in neck pain patients.

This equivocal picture of neck pain realizes the importance of moving in new directions for the diagnosis and management of the neck pain patient. The neck is an intricate structure anatomically, neurophysiologically, and biomechanically. Neck pain patients may complain of a myriad of symptoms with and without attendant psychological features or reactions. We have taken what could be termed a pathophysiologically based approach to identify better the processes in the sensory and motor systems, in sensorimotor function, as well as the psychological features that are associated with neck pain and other associated symptoms. Understanding and quantifying what is happening to the person and to the sensory, articular, and muscle systems with neck pain have the potential to provide

definitive directions for precise interventions. We have conducted research into neck pain, with a particular interest in cervicogenic headache and whiplash-associated neck pain in the acute and chronic states.

The purpose of this book is to enhance understanding of neck pain and its management from an impairment/pathophysiological point of view. This will not be foreign to physiotherapists and other practitioners who provide conservative management for cervical disorders. Their methods of assessment rely on an interpretive analysis of presenting symptoms and signs in the articular, muscular, and neural systems in the psychosocial context of the patient to guide treatment and set management goals. What we aim to offer in this book is a strengthening research base for the examination and management plan through quantification of the impairments. In support of this approach, relatively close correlations exist between measures of impairment, functional limitations, and pain and disability in persons with cervical spine disorders.[11] A precise understanding of the problems presenting in the various systems gained from research provides the directives and rationale for treatment methods.

## Structure of the book

This book emanates directly from our research and clinical interests in neck pain and does not pretend to be a comprehensive dissertation on cervical musculoskeletal disorders. Rather the initial section presents the basic and applied clinical research that we and others have undertaken into neck pain disorders. Pain mechanisms and measurement of sensory disturbances will be highlighted, providing insight into neck pain for both assessment and management purposes. Comparisons will be made between whiplash-associated disorders and idiopathic neck pain throughout the text as, although there are many similarities in underlying processes in these categories of neck pain, there are differences, especially in relation to pain and changes in the sensory system as well as sensorimotor control.

The evidence supports the important role of exercise in the rehabilitation of the neck pain patient. This field has been one of our particular interests and will be emphasized in management of persons with cervical disorders. In a lead-up to the therapeutics, the anatomy of the cervical and axioscapular muscles and related biomechanics and pathomechanics will be presented. There will be an emphasis on applied anatomy of the articular system and the muscles' role in movement as well as support for the cervical and axioscapular regions. Our research into the nature of impairments in the muscle system associated with neck pain has highlighted the properties of muscle disturbances that have been determined in neck pain patients, including, importantly, alterations in muscle coordination, muscle fatigability as well as loss of strength and endurance. We will present original evidence of disturbances in patterns of muscle control, which implicate regular disturbances in the deep pre- and postvertebral muscles. This research provides the basis for the design of therapeutic exercise interventions presented in this text.

Other elements of disturbed sensorimotor control will be explored. The case for the role of disturbances in cervical somato-sensory information to the sensorimotor system as well as the resultant disturbances in cervical joint position sense, eye movement control, and balance will be presented in association with other elements such as the vestibular system. The neurophysiological basis for symptoms associated with neck pain such as dizziness, light-headedness, and unsteadiness, as well as attendant physical impairments which are particularly common in chronic whiplash-associated disorders will be explored. Assessment methods that can be used to depict the

deficits in a clinical situation will be described, as will be the implications for management and the research base for the design of therapeutic exercise interventions.

Current knowledge of the role that psychosocial factors play in neck pain, especially in whiplash-induced pain, will be explored. It seems that the psychosocial factors involved in neck pain may differ somewhat from those in low-back pain, which flaws automatic extrapolation of chronic low-back pain data to neck pain for the purposes of diagnosis and treatment.

In the next major section of the book, we present three common conditions that have been our particular interests in research. These are whiplash-associated disorders, cervicogenic headache, and cervicobrachial pain. Whiplash-associated disorders continue to present major challenges to all those involved in its management. The mechanisms of injury will be reviewed in relation to their possible injury sequelae. Whiplash-associated disorders are marked by their heterogeneity in presentation, which realizes the importance of understanding the variety of impairments that may present as well as indicators of prognosis. A classification system will be provided for whiplash-associated disorders based on identified physical and psychological disturbances shown to be present soon after the injury. It provides directions for the early diagnosis and management of the whiplash injury. The chapter on cervicogenic headache will have a focus on the differential diagnosis of cervicogenic headache from other frequent intermittent headaches, notably migraine without aura and tension-type headache. It will present research investigating the role of musculoskeletal impairment in frequent intermittent headache as well as a comprehensive description of the impairments in the cervical musculoskeletal system which characterizes cervicogenic headache. In discussing cervicobrachial pain, processes involved in somatic referred and neuropathic pain will be presented. The differential diagnosis of arm and neck pain and the effectiveness of current management strategies will be presented.

The final major section of this book draws together the basic and applied sciences. These are applied to the examination and management of patients with cervical disorders. In line with the evidence from systematic reviews, a multimodal program of management will be presented. It will highlight treatment in the context of a multisystems model, and emphasize a pathophysiological or processes-based approach. There will be a particular emphasis on therapeutic exercise and a detailed description of an exercise approach developed from our research will be provided.

The concluding section will draw together the main themes of the book. Although knowledge of cervical spine disorders has increased markedly in the last two decades, it is incomplete and future directions in research and clinical practice that are important in the conservative management of neck disorders will be discussed.

# References

1. *Fejer R, Kyvik K, Hartvigsen J*. The prevalence of neck pain in the world population: a systematic critical review of the literature. Eur Spine J 2006;15:834–848.

2. *Wright A, Mayer T, Gatchel R*. Outcomes of disabling cervical spine disorders in compensation injuries. A prospective comparison to tertiary rehabilitation response for chronic lumbar spinal disorders. Spine 1999;24:178–183.

3. *Gore D, Sepic S, Gardner G, et al*. Neck pain: a long-term follow-up of 205 patients. Spine 1987;12:1–5.

4. *Australian Acute Musculoskeletal Pain Guidelines Group*. Evidence Based Management of Acute Musculoskeletal Pain. Brisbane: Australian Academic Press, 2004.

5. *Gross A, Hoving J, Haines T, et al*. A Cochrane review of manipulation and mobilization for mechanical neck disorders. Spine 2004;29: 1541–1548.

6. *Kjellman GV, Skargren EI, Oberg BE*. A critical analysis of randomised clinical trials on neck pain and treatment efficacy. A review of the literature. Scand J Rehabil Med 1999;31:139–152.

7. *Verhagen A, Peeters G, de Bie R, et al*. Conservative treatments for whiplash. Cochrane Database Syst Rev 2004;1:CD003338.

8. *Bronfort G, Evans R, Nelson B, et al*. A randomised clinical trial of exercise and spinal manipulation for patients with chronic neck pain. Spine 2001;26:788–797.

9. *Hoving JL, Koes BW, deVet HC, et al*. Manual therapy, physical therapy or continued care by a general practitioner for patients with neck pain. Ann Intern Med 2002;136:713–722.

10. *Jull G, Trott P, Potter H, et al*. A randomized controlled trial of exercise and manipulative therapy for cervicogenic headache. Spine 2002;27:1835–1843.

11. *Hermann K, Reese C*. Relationships among selected measures of impairment, functional limitation, and disability in patients with cervical spine disorders. Phys Ther 2001;81: 903–914.

# 2

# Sensory Manifestations of Neck Pain

## Introduction

Pain and disability levels which are reported by people with neck pain are varied and range from low levels of pain and little disability to high levels of pain with a marked influence on daily life function. The reasons for such varied presentations are likely to be associated with different mechanisms underlying the various and heterogeneous neck pain conditions. Much of the past research and certainly the clinical diagnosis of neck pain have aimed to identify the pathoanatomical sources of the patient's reported symptoms. This approach has had limited success as a pathoanatomical diagnosis is not possible in the vast majority of neck pain patients. As a consequence, the focus has shifted in recent years more towards attempting to identify the underlying mechanisms or processes of the patient's pain syndrome.[1, 2] The purpose of this more specific diagnosis and classification of musculoskeletal pain syndromes is to help tailor interventions toward identifiable underlying processes to try to improve treatment success, particularly in some of the more recalcitrant neck pain disorders.

The presence of injury and inflammation, either as a consequence of frank injury as occurs following a whiplash injury or as a result of more insidious-onset microtrauma, is known to have profound effects on both peripheral and central pain-processing mechanisms. The explosive growth in the understanding of mechanisms responsible for pain and nociception has been as a result of investigation in animal models. Direct extrapolation to humans should be made with caution. However, by using quantitative sensory testing that utilizes a variety of stimuli to detect changes in sensory function, an appreciation of underlying disturbances in pain processing can be made.[3] Using such methods, advances have been made in the understanding of disturbances in pain-processing mechanisms in conditions such as fibromyalgia, osteoarthritis, and lateral epicondylalgia.[4–6] More recently, this process has commenced in the investigation of neck pain and as such has provided improved understanding of these conditions.

Following injury and ensuing inflammation, a cascade of events occurs in the periphery, spinal cord, and supraspinal centers leading to upregulation of nociceptive processes (readers are referred to Wright[7] for a detailed review). These changes have the potential to amplify the patient's pain as well as exert influences on the motor, sensori-motor, and autonomic nervous systems. This chapter will present findings of sensory changes demonstrated in patients with neck pain. It will also attempt to infer possible underlying mechanisms that may explain these sensory phenomena. For clarity, the sections will differentiate findings local to the cervical spine from those of a more widespread nature and those suggestive of a neuropathic condition. However it should be recognized that the neuroplastic nature of the nervous system dictates that there will be a close interrelationship between the local and remote sensory disturbances and clear differentiation is not always possible.

## Local cervical spine hyperalgesia – a peripheral nociceptive source of pain?

Local hyperalgesia within the cervical spine has been demonstrated in both idiopathic neck pain and neck pain following a whiplash injury. Sheather-Reid and Cohen[8] were the first to demonstrate the presence of hyperalgesic responses (decreased pain threshold and pain tolerance to electrocutaneous stimulation) within the cervical spines of subjects with chronic neck pain, predominantly of an idiopathic nature. Scott et al.[9] showed that local mechanical hyperalgesia (decreased pressure pain thresholds) was a feature of both chronic idiopathic neck pain and chronic whiplash-associated disorders (WAD). With respect to cervicogenic headache alone, lowered pressure pain thresholds have been demonstrated at numerous sites in the head and neck.[10]

In addition to its presence in the chronic stages of neck pain conditions, local mechanical hyperalgesia is evident in the acute stages following a whiplash injury irrespective of the symptom intensity and disability levels reported by the patient.[11, 12] Local mechanical hyperalgesia was shown to resolve over time (2–3 months) in those who recovered or reported continuing milder symptoms. However the local mechanical hyperalgesia persisted unchanged in whiplash patients reporting persistent symptoms of a moderate/severe nature at 6 months and 2 years postinjury (Figure 2.1).[13]

The presence of local mechanical hyperalgesia may represent areas of primary hyperalgesia resulting from sensitized peripheral nociceptors within injured cervical spine structures.[13] In the clinical environment, mechanical hyperalgesia in the cervical spine is usually detected via manual examination and this method shows some agreement to more quantifiable measures such as algometry, at least in idiopathic neck pain.[14]

There is an alternative hypothesis to that which proposes local mechanical hyperalgesia as a result of sensitized peripheral nociceptors. Sheather-Reid and Cohen[8] argue that the local hyperalgesic responses are examples of secondary hyperalgesia as a consequence of central sensitization of nociceptive pathways. They base this argument on the observation that neck pain patients are usually not

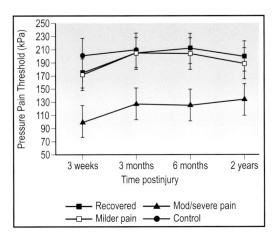

**Figure 2.1** Means (SEM) for pressure pain threshold at the cervical spine (C5–6) at 3 weeks, 3 months, 6 months, and 2 years post whiplash injury. Participants classified at 2 years postinjury: recovered, NDI < 8; milder pain, NDI 10–28; moderate/severe, NDI > 30. NDI, Neck Disability Index.

diagnosed with a specific musculoskeletal or neurological disease process that is clearly discernible with radiological imaging or other techniques. Negating this proposal is the substantial body of research suggesting that injuries to peripheral cervical structures do occur, at least following whiplash injury, and moreover persist unhealed into the chronic stage of the condition. Cadaveric studies have demonstrated injuries to numerous cervical structures that are not identifiable with radiological imaging techniques.[15-17] Placebo-controlled zygapophyseal joint blocks have demonstrated that the zygapophyseal joint is a continuing source of pain in a proportion of chronic whiplash subjects.[18] Furthermore recent studies using magnetic resonance imaging have shown unresolved lesions of the alar ligaments and tectorial membranes of whiplash-injured subjects with long-standing pain and disability.[19,20] These findings collectively indicate the importance of not overlooking the potential contribution of injured cervical spine structures to persistent pain and disability in WAD.

Whilst the search for dysfunction or pathology in cervical structures of those with neck pain has focused on radiological imaging or invasive anesthetic blocks of

relevant joints and nerves, the potential usefulness of manual examination of cervical segments has often been overlooked. When used as a test to identify the presence or absence of painful cervical segmental dysfunction in various population groups, it demonstrates good sensitivity and specificity as well as intertester reliability.[21-25] Those experienced in the use of manual examination in the diagnosis of neck pain should be assured by these findings and be confident in their skill to determine the presence or not of a possible continued peripheral (cervical) source of ongoing symptoms.

# Referred pain

Dysfunction of cervical structures such as the zygapophyseal joints, intervertebral disks, ligaments, or muscles may lead to referred pain[26] with the upper cervical segments (C0–3) referring into the head and the lower segments (C5–T1) into the upper limb.[27,28]

The mechanisms for somatic referred pain are not well understood but it is acknowledged that central mechanisms are at play and several models have been proposed. Pain may be referred to areas having the same segmental innervation and which converge on the same second-order neurons within the dorsal horn.[29] For example, in the case of cervicogenic headache, trigeminal and cervical afferents converge on the same second-order neurons, resulting in the perception of pain in the head arising from cervical structures.[30] It has been argued that the convergence model may not fully explain referred pain and that central sensitization processes such as the expansion and development of new receptive fields of dorsal horn neurons by noxious stimuli are involved.[31] Supraspinal mechanisms may also play a role but it is felt that, if they exist, they do so in parallel with spinal or brainstem mechanisms.[31]

Many patients with cervical spine pain will also report areas of referred pain to the head, shoulder region, and/or the arm. Whilst these conditions will likely involve sensitized peripheral nociceptors, it should be noted that central pain-processing mechanisms contribute to the patient's pain presentation.

# Generalized sensory hypersensitivity – evidence of augmented central pain-processing mechanisms

In addition to local areas of hyperalgesia, sensory disturbances may also occur in more widespread areas of the body, including the upper and lower limbs, even though the patient reports no symptoms in these distant body regions. These manifestations should not be confused with referred pain, where the patient reports pain in the upper limb or head in association with neck pain. The widespread sensory hypersensitivity found in some neck pain patients occurs in areas where, as mentioned, the patient does not necessarily report spontaneous pain. Local mechanical hyperalgesia in the cervical spine may be an indication of a peripheral nociceptive sensitization as a consequence of dysfunction in peripheral structures. However these more generalized responses are believed to be indicative of alterations in the neurobiological processing of nociception within the central nervous system.[13, 32]

Mechanical hyperalgesia locally within the cervical spine is a feature of both idiopathic neck pain and whiplash. The presence and extent of more widespread sensory disturbances may be a feature that differentiates whiplash from less severe neck pain conditions. Scott et al.[9] showed that people with chronic WAD had a more complex picture involving lowered pain thresholds for pressure, heat, and cold stimuli in areas remote to the cervical spine which were not present in those with idiopathic neck pain (Figure 2.2). The reasons for these differences between the conditions

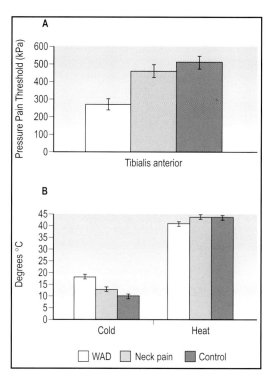

**Figure 2.2** Means (SEM). (A) Pressure pain thresholds at a remote site – tibialis anterior. (B) Heat and cold pain thresholds at the cervical spine for chronic whiplash (WAD, whiplash-associated disorder), idiopathic neck pain, and control groups.

are not clear but it has been demonstrated that conditions with more severe and widespread pain show greater degrees of sensory hypersensitivity.[33] Patients with WAD generally report higher levels of pain and disability[9, 34] and, at least clinically, tend to have more widespread pain. Interestingly, it has recently been shown that patients with chronic WAD and chronic cervical radiculopathy share a similar sensory presentation, with both conditions showing features of sensory hypersensitivity in association with higher pain and disability levels.[35] This suggests that these cervical spine conditions may have similar underlying mechanisms. It seems that both WAD and cervical radiculopathy are conditions involving more complex changes in the neurobiological processing of pain most likely occurring within the central nervous system.

Evidence for the presence of sensory hypersensitivity in chronic WAD is substantial. Koelbaek-Johansen et al.[36] demonstrated muscle hyperalgesia and larger areas of referred pain following intramuscular saline injection into both local (infraspinatus) and remote (tibialis anterior) areas to the site of pain in patients with chronic WAD. Hyperalgesic responses have also been found using electrical stimuli, via both transcutaneous and intramuscular applications.[37] These authors, in an attempt to modulate the sensory hypersensitivity, demonstrated that hypersensitivity was not decreased following local anesthesia of tender neck muscles, which they interpreted as reinforcing the role of central nervous system mechanisms.[37, 38] It should be noted that anesthesia of deeper tissues such as articular structures was not performed so that ongoing nociceptive input from such tissues could not be ruled out as contributing to the hypersensitivity. It is not known whether the blocking of nociceptive input from deeper structures (for example, using radiofrequency neurotomy of the median branch of the dorsal ramus to block pain from a zygapophyseal joint) has the capacity to modulate central hypersensitivity; however it appears that it is not a static state but one that may be potentially attenuated via peripheral input.

In a larger study, Sterling et al.[39] found widespread areas of lowered pain thresholds to mechanical stimuli using pressure algometry in 150 subjects with chronic WAD. Hypersensitivity was found over the posterior cervical region, over nerve tissue in the upper limbs, and over a remote site in the lower limb (muscle belly of tibialis anterior). None of the subjects experienced injury or pain in their lower limbs. Furthermore, whilst 50% of the subjects reported arm pain, there was no difference in pressure pain thresholds between those with and without arm symptoms, again demonstrating that the sensory changes are generalized in nature and lack a specific pattern of response.

Allodynia is defined as pain to a stimulus that is normally not painful (such as light touch or brushing). It is believed to be mediated by phenotypic change in Aβ fibers with low-threshold mechanoreceptors, such that these fibers now convey pain.[40] Although anecdotally this has been reported to be present in whiplash patients, it is yet to be extensively investigated. Preliminary evidence for the presence of allodynia comes from a study by Moog et al.[41] who demonstrated that pain was produced with vibration (a nonpainful stimulus) in 28 of 43 patients with chronic whiplash. Recently Chien et al.[35] demonstrated the potential presence of Aβ fiber dysfunction as contributing to ongoing pain in whiplash using electrical stimulation.

These widespread, generalized areas of mechanical hyperalgesia and allodynia probably reflect central nervous system hyperexcitability either as a consequence of spinal cord sensitization[36] or as a result of a loss of endogenous pain control mechanisms.[42,43] Treede and colleagues[43] argue that central sensitization leads to enlargement of mechanical receptive fields, which may explain local spreading of tenderness, but that widespread mechanical hypersensitivity is more likely to be due to alterations in descending pathways from the brainstem.

In addition to sensory disturbances illustrating the probable presence of alterations in the central nervous system processing of nociceptive pathways, motor correlates of this phenomenon have also been provided. Banic et al.[44] and Sterling et al.[45] have demonstrated facilitated nociceptor withdrawal reflexes (using electromyogram of biceps femoris muscle) in the lower limbs of people with chronic WAD following electrical stimulation of the sural nerve (Figure 2.3). The advantage of

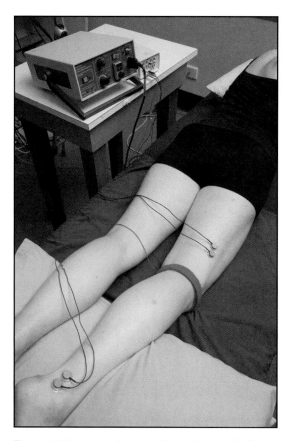

**Figure 2.3** Nociceptor withdrawal reflex test. Nociceptive flexion reflex is a spinal reflex where threshold muscle reflex activity is measured following electrical stimulation (Digitimer DS7A, Hertfordshire, UK) to the sural nerve at the ankle. The intensity of the current is progressively increased until reflex muscle activity is elicited in biceps femoris.

using the nociceptive withdrawal reflex is that it is a measure of spinal cord hyperexcitability[44] that does not rely on a cognitive response from the patient, as is required with pain threshold testing. These findings support our previous data of generalized hypersensitive responses (decreased elbow extension at pain threshold) to the brachial plexus provocation test (BPPT) in a chronic whiplash cohort. This was suggested to be a manifestation of heightened motor responses to a mechanical provocation.[46] The BPPT has been proposed to be a clinical correlate of the nociceptive flexor withdrawal response.[4] Whilst chronic whiplash subjects with clinical signs of mechanosensitive nerve tissue (25% of the cohort) demonstrated a greater loss of elbow extension at pain threshold, all whiplash subjects demonstrated significantly less elbow extension than the control group. Furthermore these responses occurred bilaterally in both groups (Figure 2.4). These findings of generalized hypersensitive motor responses to the BPPT may be another representation of motor correlates of central sensitization.[46]

Few studies have investigated the phenomenon of widespread sensory hypersensitivity in cervicogenic headache in isolation. Becser et al.[47] found decreased thermal detection thresholds in the face, neck, and hands of cervicogenic headache participants. Whilst this is a different measure than those more commonly used in investigation of WAD (detection, not pain thresholds, was measured), these generalized responses led the authors to propose that abnormal central processes may be at play. However it is not clear whether the cervicogenic headaches of the participants in this study were of a traumatic or nontraumatic origin. In view of findings of differences in the sensory presentation of idiopathic neck pain versus whiplash, it would seem that similar differentiation in cervicogenic headache will also be necessary.

## The development of sensory disturbances following whiplash injury

Most investigation of sensory disturbances in neck pain has focused on the chronic stage of the condition. However recent data demonstrate that the sensory disturbances observed in chronic WAD are in fact present from soon after the injury. In the acute stage of whiplash injury, local mechanical

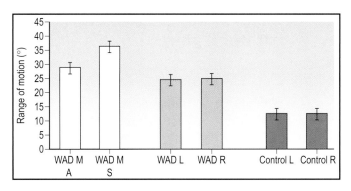

**Figure 2.4** Estimated marginal means (SEM) for range of movement (elbow extension) during the brachial plexus provocation test in the two whiplash groups and controls. WAD M, whiplash-associated disorder subjects with clinical signs of mechanosensitive nerve tissue; A, asymptomatic side; S, symptomatic side; WAD, whiplash-associated disorder subjects without signs of mechanosensitive nerve tissue; L, left side; R, right side.

hyperalgesia (decreased pressure pain thresholds) is present within the cervical spine irrespective of symptom intensity.[11, 12, 48] This local mechanical hyperalgesia tends to resolve over time (2–3 months) in those who recover or report continuing milder symptoms, but persists unchanged in whiplash patients who report persistent (6 months–2 years postinjury) symptoms of a moderate/severe nature (Figure 2.1).[13, 49]

Mechanical hyperalgesia is also present in the acute phase of the injury at sites other than the cervical spine.[11, 13] In contrast to local hyperalgesia, which appears to occur irrespective of levels of pain and disability, the presence of generalized hyperalgesia at this stage of the injury is apparent only in those individuals reporting much higher levels of pain and disability.[13] Kasch et al.[11] disputed that these more generalized sensory changes persisted into the period of chronicity. However these authors did not subgroup their whiplash cohort. Where classification of whiplash, based on pain and disability levels, is undertaken, it has been demonstrated that sensory hypersensitivity, including widespread mechanical and thermal (heat and cold) hyperalgesia as well as heightened responses to the BPPT, is present soon after injury in whiplash patients who develop persistent moderate/severe

symptoms.[13] Furthermore such sensory disturbances persist unchanged into the chronic phase of the condition (Figure 2.5). Generalized sensory hypersensitivity does not appear to be a feature of those with persistent milder symptoms or those who recover from the injury, at any stage of the condition.[13]

Psychological distress and anxiety can influence pain threshold responses in patients with musculoskeletal pain.[50] Certainly whiplash-injured patients in particular are psychologically distressed, both in the acute and chronic stages of the condition and those individuals with higher levels of pain and disability show greater distress.[51, 52] It is tempting to argue that the complex sensory changes seen in whiplash are due solely to the psychological influences on the reporting of pain responses by the whiplash patients.[53] However this argument is without basis. It has been shown that the differences in sensory presentation between whiplash and asymptomatic controls are not associated with higher distress levels in the whiplash group.[13] It is of interest that similar findings are emerging for fibromyalgia. Here it has been shown that enhanced sensitivity to pain is not an artifact of response bias as a consequence of psychological factors, but appears to be a

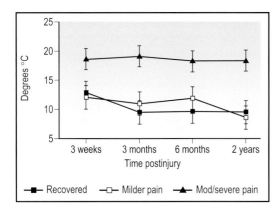

**Figure 2.5** Means (SEM) for cold pain threshold at 3 weeks, 3 months, 6 months and 2 years post whiplash injury. Participants classified at 2 years postinjury: recovered, NDI < 8; milder pain, NDI 10–28; moderate/severe, NDI > 30. NDI, Neck Disability Index.

correlate of central sensitization.[54] This is not to say that psychological distress does not play a role in the pain and disability experienced by patients with whiplash and other neck pain conditions. Additionally, it should be noted that supraspinal processes such as psychological factors (cognitions, emotions) can enhance central sensitization[55] and thus play a role in the complex physiological mechanisms underlying augmented central pain processing. Certainly it would appear that some sensory measures, particularly hyperalgesic responses away from the site of pain (for example in the leg), show an association with distress levels and catastrophization, although this relationship is inconsistent.[45] In contrast, spinal cord hyperexcitability measured with the nociceptive withdrawal reflex showed no correlation with these psychological substrates.[45] Although relationships between physical and psychological factors are extremely complex, it appears that psychological factors alone are unlikely to be solely responsible for the sensory disturbances and pain and disability seen in whiplash patients.

# Neuropathic features of neck pain

In addition to findings of local and generalized mechanical hyperalgesia, cold hyperalgesia and altered sympathetic nervous system activity have been demonstrated to occur in WAD. The longitudinal study by Sterling et al.[13] showed that a subgroup of whiplash patients who develop persistent moderate/severe symptoms (about 20–25% of the cohort) had additional changes in sensory function, including cold hyperalgesia and, in some cases, altered peripheral vasoconstrictor responses indicative of sympathetic nervous system dysfunction. These changes were present soon after injury and persisted unchanged throughout the study period (6-month follow-up). Cold hyperalgesia is a common feature of neuropathic pain due to peripheral nerve injury[56, 57] and sympathetic nervous system disturbances also occur in association with neuropathic pain.[58] The presence of these features in those with poor recovery following whiplash injury, together with findings from clinical studies where evidence of nerve tissue irritation and ensuing mechanosensitivity has been shown to be present in WAD,[46, 59] could be an indication that nerve injury is a contributor to persistent symptoms seen in this condition. This proposal is supported by cadaveric studies where injury to nerve tissue such as nerve roots and dorsal root ganglia has been demonstrated following motor vehicle crashes.[17]

Investigation of the presence of neuropathic-like sensory changes in idiopathic neck pain is scant. Irritation and/or compression of nerve tissue have been demonstrated in some patients with cervicogenic headache[60] and clinical tests of nerve tissue provocation also suggest the involvement of nerve tissue pathology in a small proportion of these patients.[25, 61] Cervicobrachial pain may, of course, be idiopathic in nature and this clinical entity will be discussed in Chapter 10. However, only one study to date has used psychophysical methods to investigate the presence of hypersensitivity to cold in idiopathic neck pain (without arm pain). Scott et al.[9] found that, whereas cold hyperalgesia was a feature of chronic WAD, it was not present in patients with idiopathic neck pain when compared to the responses of control subjects. In contrast, cold hyperalgesia (as well as other sensory features) is a characteristic of cervical radiculopathy,[35] suggesting that this condition and whiplash share similar underlying mechanisms (presumably neuropathic). Both conditions also demonstrated hypoesthetic changes (loss of sensitivity or increased detection thresholds) to a variety of modalities, including vibration, electrical and thermal stimuli, possibly indicating dysfunction of Aβ and C fibres.[35] Whilst these findings may not be unexpected in cervical radiculopathy where clinical signs of nerve conduction loss are apparent (decreased tendon reflexes, muscle power), their presence in patients with WAD II injuries (by definition no obvious conduction loss) may indicate the presence of a minor nerve injury or, in other words, a peripheral neuropathic pain condition. Preliminary data indicate that idiopathic neck pain may be spared from the hypoesthetic changes, reinforcing the proposal that whiplash is a distinct clinical entity.

These findings point to differences in pain-processing mechanisms between whiplash-induced neck pain and that of insidious-onset neck pain but similarities in the mechanisms between whiplash and cervical radiculopathy. The presence of altered sympathetic vasoconstrictive responses is yet to be investigated in idiopathic neck pain and this is an area that requires further research, particularly in view of the presence of sympathetic disturbances in other common musculoskeletal pain conditions, including lateral epicondylalgia and frozen shoulder.[62, 63]

# Influence of sensory changes on patient outcome

Recognition of sensory disturbances as outlined in this chapter is important for several reasons. In addition to the implications for assessment and management, sensory disturbances have been shown to have prognostic capacity for outcome following whiplash injury. The early presence of cold hyperalgesia and impaired peripheral vasoconstriction in addition to other higher levels of pain and disability, older age, range of movement loss, and posttraumatic stress symptoms have been shown to be predictive of a poor outcome at 6 months post motor vehicle crash.[64] These features, with the exception of sympathetic nervous system changes, continue to be significant prognostic indicators at 2 years postaccident.[49] Kasch et al.[65] have also found decreased cold pain tolerance to be a predictor of outcome at 12 months postinjury. The optimal management for these sensory disturbances is yet to be identified but their prognostic capacity indicates that early evaluation of whiplash should include assessment of sensory function.

# Implications for the assessment of neck pain patients

As has been outlined, there are profound differences in the sensory responses manifested within whiplash and idiopathic neck pain that likely reflect differences in the underlying physiological processes involved in nociceptive processing associated with these conditions. Even in consideration of whiplash alone, the presence of varying degrees of sensory change is evident and is a manifestation of the heterogeneity of WAD in both the acute and chronic stages of the condition. It is apparent that a thorough and detailed evaluation of such sensory changes is required with examination of each individual neck pain patient's condition.

Recent calls have been made to direct clinical examination toward the recognition and identification of processes involved in the patient's pain syndrome.[1, 43] At present sensory examination such as that required to detect the variety of sensory disturbances outlined above is rarely performed and, if it is performed, is usually limited to rudimentary assessment of muscle power, deep tendon reflexes, and light touch sensation. More detailed assessment of sensory changes in neck pain patients is necessary. The first stage of this assessment would be thorough recording of the patient's symptoms, including the nature of the pain. Although the usefulness of symptom classification as a way of clarifying pain mechanisms is debatable, it is a necessary part of the patient's assessment.[3] In recent times questionnaires have been developed that aim to identify specifically neuropathic-like pain.[66] Using the self-report version of the Leeds Assessment of Neuropathic Symptoms and Signs (S-LANSS) questionnaire,[67] Sterling[68] recently demonstrated that 30% of an acute whiplash cohort have a likely neuropathic condition, with certain items being particularly associated with higher levels of pain and disability. These were "electric shock"-type pain that comes in bursts, burning pain in the neck, and hyperalgesia to manual pressure. Inclusion of this questionnaire with particular attention to these items should be included in the clinical assessment of acute whiplash.

Quantitative sensory testing can also be utilized. This could include the measurement of mechanical pain thresholds with pressure algometry (Figure 2.6) and determination of

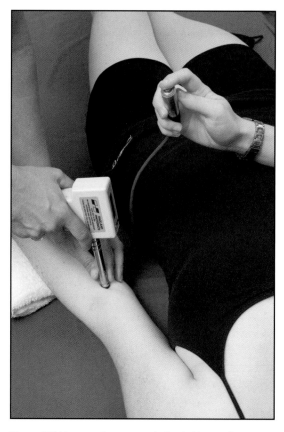

**Figure 2.6** Measure of pressure pain thresholds over the median nerve site with a pressure algometer (Somedic, Sweden).

the presence of allodynia with light tactile stimulation. Cold hyperalgesia is emerging as an important factor in both the prediction of outcome[49] and for gauging treatment responsiveness.[69] It is more difficult to measure clinically but options may include the use of thermorollers set at predetermined temperatures.[3] Recently we have shown that item four of the S-LANSS questionnaire ("electric shock"-type pain that comes in bursts) is strongly correlated to cold hyperalgesia in acute whiplash and this may be useful to include in the patient examination.[68]

However it should be noted that, whilst such sensory assessments can provide useful information, at present there is no consensus about the most appropriate method to use and with what to compare findings.[3] The development of the most appropriate sensory examination of whiplash-injured patients is at an early stage. Moves toward further development into clinically valid and useful measures are of vital importance.

Whilst we have discussed various ways of attempting to quantify sensory disturbance clinically, it is essential that clinicians also integrate information from the overall examination of the patient. For example, the patient whose neck is allodynic such that it precludes manual examination is certainly displaying signs of central hyperexcitability. A neck pain condition that the patient reports to be highly "irritable" (that is, the pain is easily provoked and does not settle easily) is displaying sensitivity to mechanical stimulation, in this case movement. Again this is likely to be indicative of augmented central pain-processing mechanisms. Thoughtful use of the BPPT may also be a useful clinical test of central hyperexcitability. Sterling[68] has recently shown that a bilateral loss of elbow extension (> 30° from 180°) strongly correlates with S-LANSS scores in patients with whiplash. If being used for this purpose, it is important that the BPPT is performed gently, with respect to symptoms. The elbow should be extended only to the first onset of pain (pain threshold). The clinician is looking for a bilateral loss of elbow extension, often in patients who do not report the presence of arm pain or other peripheral symptoms. In other words, there will be a generalized hypersensitive response to this test when such a response may not be expected.

# Implications for the management of neck pain

The presence or not and the nature of sensory disturbances in neck pain patients will have important ramifications for the management of these conditions. Findings of local mechanical hyperalgesia in the neck in isolation, with little evidence of more generalized widespread hyperalgesia, allodynia or cold hyperalgesia may be a manifestation of peripheral sensitization from injured cervical spine structures. Manual therapy to the cervical spine has been shown to decrease cervical mechanical hyperalgesia in the short term[14, 70] as well as having more long term effects on pain and disability.[71] This suggests its usefulness in managing neck pain. Exercise including specific exercise aimed at restoring cervical muscle recruitment patterns has been shown to be effective in managing neck pain[61, 71] with some evidence available to indicate that exercise may be able to influence mechanical hyperalgesia.[72]

Patients with additional features of widespread sensory hypersensitivity, allodynia and/or cold hyperalgesia will need to be managed with care. It is likely that any treatment leading to provocation and exacerbation of pain will facilitate hypersensitive sensory disturbances. It is thought that central sensitization is maintained by ongoing peripheral nociceptive afferent input,[73, 74] which could include the nonjudicious application of pain producing manipulative therapy or exercise. Gentle manual therapy techniques have been shown to produce effects (sympathetic nervous system changes, mechanical hypoalgesia and motor responses) that suggest the involvement of descending pain inhibitory control mechanisms as a mode of action. Since it has been suggested that widespread mechanical hypersensitivity may be, at least in part, due to loss of endogenous pain control mechanisms,[43] then it could be hypothesized that gentle manual therapy may be of some benefit in the management of patients with these sensory changes. Whilst the efficaciousness of manual therapy alone for widespread sensory hypersensitivity is not known, a physiotherapy approach including manual therapy, specific exercise and advice has been shown to be efficacious in whiplash patients with generalized mechanical hyperalgesia.[69] Interestingly, patients with additional changes of cold hyperalgesia failed to respond as well to this form of treatment. It has been proposed that these patients may require appropriate medication in addition to physiotherapy management.[69] Liaison between the musculoskeletal clinician and the medical practitioner will be necessary to ensure effective treatment of these patients.

Patients with sensory responses suggestive of sensitized nerve tissue involvement will also require careful management. These patients may be detected by responses to the BPPT, symptoms suggestive of sympathetic nervous system dysfunction, hyperalgesia to cold stimuli, and allodynia. Patients with these features tend to report significantly higher levels of pain and disability[13] as well as often describing their pain as burning and/or paroxysmal in nature.[3] The optimal management for patients with these characteristics is unclear. Pharmacological intervention is helpful in only one-third of patients with neuropathic pain regardless of underlying pathology or disease process.[75] Manual therapy of gentle lateral glide techniques has been shown to decrease pain and improve function in subjects with a specific diagnosis of cervicobrachial pain syndrome[76] but the efficacy of such techniques in whiplash patients with a more diverse sensory presentation is not known. It will be essential to provide non pain-provocative treatment for patients with signs suggestive of a neuropathic component to their pain in order to avoid exacerbation of their condition.

It is important to recognize that, in whiplash-injured subjects, sensory changes are present soon after injury. Our longitudinal study showed that all sensory changes, whether locally in the cervical spine or more widespread, and regardless of the type of stimuli, were in situ within a few weeks of injury and could occur even earlier than this time.[13] These findings demonstrate that appropriate intervention should be instituted at an early stage of the condition, most optimally as soon after the injury as possible. This approach is more likely to prevent the transition into chronicity for those whiplash patients at risk rather than delaying treatment.[77]

## Conclusion

Mechanical hyperalgesia of the cervical spine is a feature of both idiopathic and whiplash-induced neck pain and likely indicates peripheral sensitization as a consequence of injured cervical spine structures. Some whiplash-injured persons show additional sensory changes, including widespread sensory hypersensitivity to a variety of stimuli, cold hyperalgesia, and sympathetic nervous system disturbances that are likely manifestations of alterations in the neurobiological processing of pain, including central sensitization and loss of endogenous control mechanisms. Sensory responses suggestive of neuropathic-like pain are also a feature of this group of whiplash patients. Physical assessment of neck pain patients should extend to include more detailed sensory examination in order to detect such changes. Patients with sensory changes confined to the cervical spine and those with mechanical hyperalgesia only tend to respond well to physical therapy interventions of manual therapy and specific exercise. In contrast, those with more complex sensory disturbances are more recalcitrant to physical treatments and may require additional pharmacological management. It is vitally important that patients with these sensory changes are carefully managed and treatment must remain nonpain-provocative in nature.

# References

1. *Max M*. Is mechanism-based pain treatment attainable? Clinical trial issues. J Pain 2000;1: 2–9.

2. *Baron R*. Mechanisms of disease: neuropathic pain – a clinical perspective. Nat Clin Pract Neurol 2006;2:95–107.

3. *Jensen T, Baron R*. Translation of symptoms and signs into mechanisms in neuropathic pain. Pain 2003;102:1–8.

4. *Wright A, Thurnwald P, O'Callaghan J, et al*. Hyperalgesia in tennis elbow patients. J Musculoskel Pain 1994;2:83–97.

5. *Kosek E, Ekholm J, Hansson P*. Sensory dysfunction in fibromyalgia patients with implications for pathogenic mechanisms. Pain 1996;68:375–383.

6. *Farrell M, Gibson S, McMeeken J, et al*. Pain and hyperalgesia in osteoarthritis of the hands. J Rheum 2000;27:441–447.

7. *Wright A*. Neurophysiology of pain and pain modulation. In: Strong J, Unruh A, Wright A, et al. (eds) Pain: A Textbook for Therapists. London: Elsevier, 2002:43–64.

8. *Sheather-Reid R, Cohen M*. Psychophysical evidence for a neuropathic component of chronic neck pain. Pain 1998;75:341–347.

9. *Scott D, Jull G, Sterling M*. Sensory hypersensitivity is a feature of chronic whiplash-associated disorders but not chronic idiopathic neck pain. Clin J Pain 2005;21:175–181.

10. *Bovim G*. Cervicogenic headache, migraine and tension-type headace. Pressure pain threshold measurements. Pain 1992;51:169–173.

11. *Kasch H, Stengaard-Pedersen K, Arendt-Nielsen L, et al*. Pain thresholds and tenderness in neck and head following acute whiplash injury: a prospective study. Cephalalgia 2001;21:189–197.

12. *Sterling M, Jull G, Vicenzino B, et al*. Characterisation of acute whiplash-associated disorders. Spine 2004;29:182–188.

13. *Sterling M, Jull G, Vicenzino B, et al*. Sensory hypersensitivity occurs soon after whiplash injury and is associated with poor recovery. Pain 2003;104:509–517.

14. *Sterling M, Jull G, Wright A*. Cervical mobilisation: concurrent effects on pain, sympathetic nervous system activity and motor activity. Man Ther 2001;6:72–81.

15. *Jonsson H, Bring G, Rauschning W, et al*. Hidden cervical spine injuries in traffic accident victims with skull fractures. J Spinal Disord 1991;4:251–263.

16. *Jonsson H, Cesarini K, Sahlstedt B, et al*. Findings and outcome in whiplash-type neck distortions. Spine 1994;19:2733–2743.

17. *Taylor J, Taylor M*. Cervical spinal injuries: an autopsy study of 109 blunt injuries. J Musculoskel Pain 1996;4:61–79.

18. *Lord S, Barnsley L, Wallis B, et al*. Chronic cervical zygapophysial joint pain after whiplash: a placebo-controlled prevalence study. Spine 1996;21:1737–1745.

19. *Krakenes J, Kaale B, Moen G, et al*. MRI assessment of the alar ligaments in the late stage of whiplash injury – a study of structural abnormalities and observer agreement. Neuroradiol 2002;44:617–624.

20. *Krakenes J, Kaale B, Moen G, et al*. MRI of the tectorial and posterior atlanto-occipital membranes in the late stage of whiplash injury. Neuroradiol 2003;44:637–644.

21. *Jull GA, Bogduk N, Marsland A*. The accuracy of manual diagnosis for cervical zygapophysial joint pain syndromes. Med J Aust 1988;148:233–236.

22. *Jull G, Zito G, Trott PH, et al*. Inter-examiner reliability to detect painful upper cervical joint dysfunction. Aust J Physiother 1997;32:125–129.

23. *Gijsberts T, Duquet W, Stoekart R, et al*. Impaired mobility of the cervical spine as a tool in the diagnosis of cervicogenic headache. Cephalalgia 1999;19:436.

24. *Sandmark H, Nisell R*. Validity of five common manual neck pain provoking tests. Scand J Rehabil Med 1995;27:131–136.

25. *Zito G, Jull G, Story I*. Clinical tests of musculoskeletal dysfunction in the diagnosis of cervicogenic headache. Man Ther 2006;11:118–129.

26. *Bogduk N, April C*. On the nature of neck pain, discography and cervical zygapophyseal joint blocks. Pain 1993;54:213–217.

27. *Bogduk N*. The anatomical basis for spinal pain syndromes. J Manipul Physiol Ther 1995;18:603–605.

28. *Fukui S, Ohseto K, Shiotani M, et al*. Referred pain distribution of the cervical zygapophyseal joints and cervical dorsal rami. Pain 1996;68:79–83.

29. *Hoheisel U, Mense S, Simons D, et al*. Appearance of new receptive fields in rat dorsal horn neurons following noxius stimulation of skeletal muscle – a model for referral of muscle pain. Neurosci Lett 1993;153:9–12.

30. *Bogduk N*. Anatomy and physiology of headache. Biomed Pharmacother 1995;49:435–445.

31. *Graven-Nielsen T*. Fundamentals of muscle pain, referred pain and deep tissue hyperalgesia. Scand J Rheumatol 2006;35:1–43.

32. *Curatolo M, Arendt-Nielsen L, Petersen-Felix S*. Evidence, mechanisms and clinical implications of central hypersensitivity in chronic pain after whiplash injury. Clin J Pain 2004;20:469–476.

33. *Carli G, Suman A, Biasi G, et al*. Reactivity to superficial and deep stimuli in patients with chronic musculoskeletal pain. Pain 2002;100:259–269.

34. *Jull G, Kristjansson E, Dall'Alba P*. Impairment in the cervical flexors: a comparison of whiplash and insidious onset neck pain patients. Man Ther 2004;9:89–94.

35. *Chien A, Eliav E, Sterling M.* Hypoaesthesia occurs with sensory hypersensitivity in chronic whiplash: indication of a minor peripheral neuropathy? 2008; Man Ther in press.

36. *Koelbaek-Johansen M, Graven-Nielsen T, Schou-Olesen A, et al.* Muscular hyperalgesia and referred pain in chronic whiplash syndrome. Pain 1999;83:229–234.

37. *Curatolo M, Petersen-Felix S, Arendt-Nielsen L, et al.* Central hypersensitivity in chronic pain after whiplash injury. Clin J Pain 2001;17:306–315.

38. *Herren-Gerber R, Weiss D, Arendt-Nielsen L, et al.* Modulation of central hypersensitivity by nociceptive input in chronic neck pain after whiplash injury. Pain Med 2004;5:366–376.

39. *Sterling M, Treleaven J, Edwards S, et al.* Pressure pain thresholds in chronic whiplash-associated disorder: further evidence of altered central pain processing. J Musculoskel Pain 2002;10:69–81.

40. *Koltzenburg M, Torebjork H, Wahren L.* Nociceptor modulated central sensitization causes mechanical hyperalgesia in acute chemogenic and chronic neuropathic pain. Brain 1994;117:579–591.

41. *Moog M, Quintner J, Hall T, et al.* The late whiplash syndrome: a psychophysical study. Eur J Pain 2002;6:283–294.

42. *Ren K, Zhuo M, Willis W.* Multiplicity and plasticity of descending modulation of nociception: implications for persistent pain. In: Devor M, Rowbotham M, Wiesnfeld-Hallin Z (eds) IXth World Congress on Pain. Vienna: IASP, 2000.

43. *Treede R-D, Rolke R, Andrews K, et al.* Pain elicited by blunt pressure: neurobiological basis and clinical relevance. Pain 2002;98:235–240.

44. *Banic B, Petersen-Felix S, Andersen O, et al.* Evidence for spinal cord hypersensitivity in chronic pain after whiplash injury and in fibromyalgia. Pain 2004;107:7–15.

45. *Sterling M, Pettiford C, Hodkinson E, et al.* Psychological factors are related to some sensory pain thresholds but not nociceptive flexion reflex threshold in chronic whiplash. 2008; Clin J Pain in press.

46. *Sterling M, Treleaven J, Jull G.* Responses to a clinical test of mechanical provocation of nerve tissue in whiplash-associated disorders. Man Ther 2002;7:89–94.

47. *Becser N, Sand T, Pareja J, et al.* Thermal sensitivity in unilateral headaches. Cephalalgia 1998;18:675–683.

48. *Sterner Y, Toolanen G, Knibestol M, et al.* Prospective study of trigeminal sensibility after whiplash trauma. J Spinal Disord 2001;14:479–486.

49. *Sterling M, Jull G, Kenardy J.* Physical and psychological predictors of outcome following whiplash injury maintain predictive capacity at long term follow-up. Pain 2006;122:102–108.

50. *Rhudy J, Meagher M.* Fear and anxiety: divergent effects on human pain thresholds. Pain 2000;84:65–75.

51. *Radanov B, Begre S, Sturzenegger M, et al.* Course of psychological variables in whiplash injury – a 2-year follow-up with age, gender and education pair-matched patients. Pain 1996;64:429–434.

52. *Sterling M, Kenardy J, Jull G, et al.* The development of psychological changes following whiplash injury. Pain 2003;106:481–489.

53. *Ferrari R.* The clinical relevance of symptom amplification. Pain 2004;107:276.

54. *Petzke F, Gracely R, Park K, et al.* What do tender points measure? Influence of distress on four measures of tenderness. J Rheumatol 2003;30:567–574.

55. *Zusman M.* Forebrain mediated sensitisation of central pain pathways: 'non-specific' pain and a new image for MT. Man Ther 2002;7:80–88.

56. *Hatem S, Attal N, Willer J-C, et al.* Psychophysical study of the effects of topical application of menthol in healthy volunteers. Pain 2006;122:190–196.

57. *Bennett G.* Can we distinguish between inflammatory and neuropathic pain? Pain Res Manage 2006;11(Suppl. A):11–15.

58. *Baron R.* Peripheral Neuropathic Pain: From mechanisms to symptoms. Clin J Pain 2000; 16:512–520.

59. *Ide M, Ide J, Yamaga M, et al.* Symptoms and signs of irritation of the brachial plexus in whiplash injuries. J Bone Joint Surg (Br) 2001;83:226–229.

60. *Pikus H, Phillips J.* Characteristics of patients successfully treated for cervicogenic headache by surgical decompression of the second cervical root. Headache 1995;35:621–629.

61. *Jull G, Trott P, Potter H, et al.* A randomised controlled trial of physiotherapy management for cervicogenic headache. Spine 2002;27:1835–1843.

62. *Mani R, Cooper C, Kidd B, et al.* Use of laser Doppler flowmetry and transcutaneous oxygen tension electrodes to assess local autonomic dysfunction in patients with frozen shoulder. J R Soc Med 1989;82:536–538.

63. *Smith R, Papadopolous E, Mani R, et al.* Abnormal microvascular responses in lateral epicondylitis. Br J Rheumatol 1994;33:1166–1168.

64. *Sterling M, Jull G, Vicenzino B, et al.* Physical and psychological factors predict outcome following whiplash injury. Pain 2005;114:141–148.

65. *Kasch H, Qerama E, Bach F, et al.* Reduced cold pressor pain tolerance in non-recovered whiplash patients: a 1 year prospective study. Eur J Pain 2005;9:561–569.

66. *Bennett M, Attal N, Backonja M, et al.* Using screening tools to identify neuropathic pain. Pain 2007;127:199–203.

67. *Bennett M, Smith B, Torrance N, et al.* The S-LANSS score for identifying pain of predominantly neuropathic origin: validation for use in clinical and postal research. J Pain 2005;6:149–158.

68. *Sterling M, Pedlar A*. A neuropathic component is common in acute whiplash and associated with a more complex clinical presentation; submitted.

69. *Jull G, Sterling M, Kenardy J, et al*. Does the presence of sensory hypersensitivity influence outcomes of physical rehabilitation for chronic whiplash? A preliminary RCT. Pain 2007;129:28–34.

70. *Vicenzino B, Collins D, Benson H, et al*. An investigation of the interrelationship between manipulative therapy induced hypoalgesia and sympathoexcitation. J Manipul Physiol Ther 1998;21:448–453.

71. *Hoving J, Koes B, de Vet H, et al*. Manual therapy, physical therapy or continued care by a general practitioner for patients with neck pain. Ann Intern Med 2002;136:713–722.

72. *Ylinen J, Takala E, Kautianen H, et al*. Effect of long-term neck muscle training on pressure pain threshold: a randomised controlled trial. Eur J Pain 2005;9:673–681.

73. *Gracely R, Lynch S, Bennett G*. Painful neuropathy: altered central processing maintained dynamically by peripheral input. Pain 1992;51:175–194.

74. *Devor M*. Central versus peripheral substrates of persistent pain: which contributes more? Behav Brain Sci 1997;20:446–447.

75. *Sindrup S, Jensen T*. Efficacy of pharmacological treatments of neuropathic pain: an update and effect related to mechanism of drug action. Pain 1999;83:389–400.

76. *Allison G, Nagy B, Hall T*. A randomised clinical trial of manual therapy for cervicobrachial pain. Man Ther 2002;7:95–102.

77. *Siddall P, Cousins M*. Persistent pain as a disease entity: implications for clinical management. Anesth Analg 2004;510–520.

# 3

# Structure and Function of the Cervical Region

## Introduction

The cervical spine supports and orients the head in space relative to the thorax to serve the sensory systems. As such, sophisticated mobility and stability are demanded of the cervical musculoskeletal system. The mechanisms by which this is achieved and the consequences of impairment are of interest to those treating cervical disorders. This chapter reviews pertinent and applied clinical anatomy of the cervical spine.

## Structure and function of the cervical spine

Within the cervical spine there is an anatomical and functional division between the craniocervical and typical cervical regions with the transition occurring at the C2–3 motion segment. These regions have distinct differences in motion segment and muscular anatomy and have some autonomy of function. Cervical spine function is also intimately related to the workings of the thorax, shoulder girdles, and the temporomandibular region.

### Craniocervical region

The craniocervical region comprises the atlanto-occipital and atlantoaxial articulations. The configuration of the atlanto-occipital (C0–1) articulations permits generous motion in the sagittal plane, but lends itself to minimal motion in the frontal and transverse planes due to the steepness of the lateral walls of the atlas sockets and the tension of the joint capsules.[1] The structure of the atlantoaxial (C1–2) articulations combined with its relatively lax capsular ligaments permits a large excursion of motion, particularly in the transverse plane. Overall the craniocervical region accounts for approximately one-third of the sagittal plane motion and one-half of transverse plane motion of the cervical spine. This potential for motion is crucial for the sensory functions of the head. As such these motion segments have specific muscles dedicated to providing orientation[2,3] and specific craniovertebral ligaments that enhance their stability.[1,4]

The C2–3 motion segment provides the junction between the craniocervical and typical cervical regions. The configuration of this motion segment is somewhat unique and provides what Bogduk and Mercer[1] describe as an anchor for the apparatus that holds and moves the head on the typical cervical spine. The superior elements of the C3 vertebra possess large uncinate processes[5] and superior articular processes that not only face backwards and upwards, but also are medially inclined.[6] Thus, the bony configuration of the superior aspect of C3 forms a deep socket for its articulation with C2.[1] Such an enhancement of bony stability appears appropriate considering the abundance of converging muscles that attach particularly to the posterior elements of the axis. The axis forms a junction for the superior and inferior attachments of the deep posterior muscles of the typical cervical and craniocervical regions, respectively (Figure 3.1). In this manner the deep muscles of the typical cervical region may further anchor the atlas, providing a stable base for craniocervical muscle function.

### Typical cervical region

Typical cervical motion segments have characteristics unique to other spinal regions. The adult typical cervical motion segment is characterized by the presence of uncovertebral joints and a transverse fissure that divides the posterior aspect of the intervertebral disk.[7-9] Fissuring of the intervertebral disk appears to be a normal response to the formation of the uncinate processes and the repeated translational and torsional strain imposed by daily movement of these motion segments. The annulus of the adult intervertebral disk is crescent-shaped and relatively absent posteriorly (replaced by a fibrocartilage structure) except for a thin vertically oriented layer.[8] Anteriorly the annulus is horizontally oriented and interwoven and contains high concentrations of collagen consistent with torsional demands.[8,10,11]

Typical cervical spine zygapophyseal joints are oriented in the vicinity of 40° to the vertical, with the exception of the facets at C3 and C7 that have a steeper orientation.[12] When viewed in the plane of the cervical facet joints, the structure of the fissured intervertebral disk and uncovertebral joints provide the typical cervical motion segments with the structure of an ellipsoid joint.[1,5,13] This joint structure permits flexion–extension and strongly coupled ipsilateral axial rotation and lateral flexion motions, with the exception of the C2–3 motion segment, where both ipsilateral and contralateral coupled motion has been observed.[1,5,14]

## Muscles of the cervical spine

Within the cervical muscle system there is a division between the muscles that primarily span the craniocervical region, those that span the typical cervical region, and those that span both regions. The differentiation of these craniocervical and typical cervical muscles is most obvious in the deeper muscle layers (Figures 3.1 and 3.2). The trapezius and levator scapulae muscles also have attachments to the cranium and

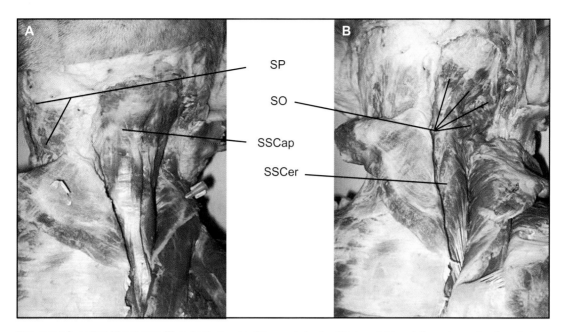

**Figure 3.1** Superficial (A) and deep (B) posterior muscles of the cervical spine. The superficial posterior neck muscles, the splenius capitis and cervicis (SP) and the semispinalis capitis (SSCap) muscles, span both craniocervical and typical cervical motion segments. In contrast the deeper muscles tend to be more discrete to either the craniocervical (suboccipital (SO)) or typical cervical (semispinalis cervicis (SSCer), cervical multifidus) regions.

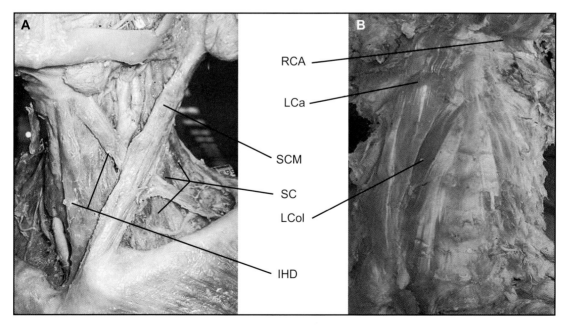

**Figure 3.2** Superficial (A) and deep (B) anterolateral muscles of the cervical spine. The superficial anterior neck muscles such as the sternocleidomastoid (SCM) and the infrahyoid (IHD) muscle group span both craniocervical and typical cervical motion segments. In contrast the deeper muscles tend to be more discrete to either the craniocervical (longus capitis (LCa), rectus capitis anterior (RCA)) or typical cervical regions (longus colli (LCol), scalene (SC)) muscles.

cervical spine, but are primarily considered muscles of the shoulder girdle.

## Muscles of the craniocervical region

Posteriorly, the craniocervical muscles consist of the deep suboccipital group, including the rectus capitis posterior major and minor, obliquus capitis inferior and superior muscles. These muscles are important proprioceptive monitors with connections to the vestibular and visual systems (Chapter 5).[15, 16] The longus capitis, rectus capitis anterior, and rectus capitis lateralis form the anterolateral craniocervical group. The longus capitis has attachments as far caudad as C6; however its fibers span the craniocervical spine.[17]

## Muscles of the typical cervical region

Posteriorly the cervical muscles consist of the semispinalis cervicis and the cervical multifidus muscles. Their attachments to the axis represent the junction of the typical cervical and craniocervical deep posterior neck muscles. Anteriorly the longus colli muscle has extensive attachments along the entire length of the typical cervical region and attaches as far cephalad as C1. Laterally the typical cervical region is covered by the three portions of the scalene muscles.

## Muscles spanning both craniocervical and typical cervical regions

Superficial cervical muscles such as the splenius capitis and cervicis, semispinalis capitis, and the longissimus capitis span both the craniocervical and typical cervical regions posteriorly. Anterolaterally the suprahyoid and infrahyoid muscle groups and the sternocleidomastoid muscles span both cervical regions.

# Control of cervical spine posture and motion

The role of individual cervical muscles in control of cervical spine posture and motion will be discussed according to the region of the spine about which they act (craniocervical/typical cervical regions) and their relative depth in relation to the vertebral column. There is a focus in discussion towards the interaction of the deep and superficial muscle groups. In general the superficial muscles have a greater capacity to exert torque than their deeper counterparts due to their larger lever arms and cross-sectional areas.[2, 18, 19] In contrast, the deeper muscles are more localized to either the craniocervical or typical cervical regions. They have segmental attachments, larger spindle densities, and muscle fiber compositions that enable them to guide and support vertebral motion segments.[20–22]

The following review is a guide only, based largely on gross anatomical observations, some of which are still poorly defined within the anatomical literature. Additionally, the redundancy of the cervical muscle system is well documented. It has been observed that mid-range head orientations common in daily function can be achieved with multiple combinations of movement strategies[23, 24] with motion characteristics of some cervical joints differing substantially depending on starting position and movement pattern.[13, 23, 24]

## Upright sustained postural tasks

An objective of rehabilitation is often to teach patients to achieve an upright "neutral" cervical spine posture, although the position of "neutral" is as yet undefined. The position of a patient's head relative to the thorax and the angulations of cervical lordosis at any moment in time are largely dependent on the orientation of the cervicothoracic junction and the orientation of the head as dictated by the requirements of vision. The integrity of the upright cervical spine is also dependent on the muscle system. It is estimated that, when devoid of muscles, the mobile cervical spine may buckle under a mass of less than one-fifth of the mass of the head.[25] A deep sleeve of muscles envelops both the craniocervical and typical cervical regions (Figure 3.3). These muscles have appropriate morphology and composition for segmental motion control.[21, 22, 26]

Posteriorly, the deep cervical extensor muscles of the typical cervical region (semispinalis cervicis and multifidus) have an anatomical arrangement well suited for support of the lordosis.[27, 28] The semispinalis cervicis forms a strong attachment to the spinous process of the axis with longitudinal bands forming extensor moments to the cervical spine. Its detachment during surgical procedures from the spinous process of C2 has been implicated in the loss of the cervical lordosis in patients postsurgery.[29-31] The distal attachments of the semispinalis cervicis to the thorax may also permit it a role in the maintenance of an upright orientation of the typical cervical spine over the thorax. In this manner these extensor muscles may function as postural synergists with the craniocervical flexor muscles in the prevention of forward head postures. The underlying cervical multifidus muscles have limited torque capacity; however, their attachments and proximity to the cervical motion segments and zygapophyseal joint capsules are appropriate for a segmental stability role.[32] From a gross anatomical perspective it appears that the deep extensor muscles of the typical cervical region provide a stable anchor for suboccipital muscle function (Figure 3.3). These suboccipital muscles are appropriately positioned to support and control the lordosis of the craniocervical region and perform the small head-on-neck movements required for daily function.

Anteriorly the cervical lordosis is supported by the deep cervical flexor muscles (longus capitis, longus colli, rectus capitis anterior). These muscles counter the accentuation of the lordotic angle induced by the extensor muscles and other external forces.[33, 34] The three divisions of the longus colli muscle intersect in the vicinity of the apex of the lordosis, and as such, a negative correlation has been found between the acuteness of the cervical lordosis and the cross-sectional area of the longus colli muscle.[26] The longus capitis muscle overlaps the superior portion of longus colli and extends on to the cranium. An increase in electromyographic (EMG) activity is evident in these deep cervical flexor muscles either when load is applied to the top of the head, that would tend to accentuate the lordosis, or when the lordosis is actively straightened during postural realignment tasks.[35, 36]

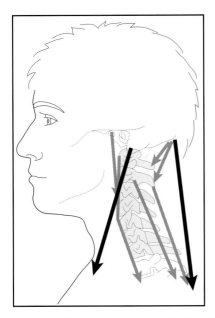

**Figure 3.3** The mass of the head and the integrity of the cervical lordosis are supported by the deep sleeve of cervical muscles (gray arrows) and torque produced on the head by the large superficial muscles (black arrows).

Neck pain is often associated with specific postures which are thought to expose the cervical spine to excessive mechanical load. Loading of cervical structures has been investigated with particular regard to the orientation and acuteness of the cervical lordosis.[37] Weight is borne anteriorly by the vertebral bodies and intervertebral disks and posteriorly by the articular processes and facets.[38-40] The shape of the ideal lordosis permits optimal sharing of loads between the anterior and posterior vertebral elements. A flattening of the cervical lordosis increases compressive forces on anterior vertebral elements and increases tensile forces at posterior vertebral elements. The reverse occurs in postures with an accentuated cervical lordosis.[41] Theoretically, an altered load distribution may irritate pain-sensitive structures. Certain sitting postures have been shown to position motion segments at the limit of their orientation with the potential for adverse load.[42]

There has been a long-standing interest in the relationship between the static cervical posture in the upright position and neck pain. A more forward posture of the cervical spine has been related to a reduced cervical lordosis.[43] Some clinical studies of external measurement of upright posture have drawn associations between changes in static postural angles and neck pain, while other have not.[44-46] Despite much clinical anecdotal evidence, direct scientific evidence linking static postural angles to painful cervical disorders remains inconclusive. Little association has been found between radiological measures of anatomical alignment and surface measurements of the head and neck posture.[47, 48] There are large interindividual variations in the angle of the lordotic curvature, which challenge interpretation of its clinical significance.[26] Furthermore there is disparity in results of radiological studies investigating any association between the angle of lordosis and neck pain.[49-52]

It is possible that external measurements of posture or the radiological measure of lordosis in the static upright posture might not be the critical point. Persons with neck pain have been shown to drift into a more forward head posture during computer work.[53, 54] Changes in cervical flexor and extensor muscle activity have been measured during such tasks in neck pain patients.[55-57] The posture adopted by the patient in function and the strategy by which it is maintained by the cervical muscles may be of greater importance.

## Motion in the sagittal plane

### Motion segment kinematics

Attempts have been made to analyze the dynamics (movement amplitude and timing) of individual cervical motion segments during active movements in the anatomical planes using radiographic techniques.[1, 58] Flexion and extension of the head and neck en masse have demonstrated some consistency of movement. During flexion, movement is initiated and terminated predominantly in the lower cervical spine (C4–7). The craniocervical (C0–2) and middle cervical (C2–4) regions contribute mostly during the middle phase of motion, but during the final phase, C0–2 motion segments usually move towards extension. A similar pattern of motion is observed during cervical extension, with the exception that C0–2 reaches its maximum extension during the final phase of the extension movement.[1, 58] The timing sequence of sagittal plane motion may be expected to change if the individual is asked to perform a different movement task such as a nodding action of the head. One may expect earlier motion of craniocervical motion segments following these commands, as opposed to sagittal plane motion of the head and neck en masse. Findings of nonuniform motion of the craniocervical and typical cervical regions when the cervical spine is moved en masse in the sagittal plane have underpinned the clinical practice of examining motion of the typical and craniocervical regions separately.

The sagittal movements of head protraction/retraction result in opposing motion at opposite ends of the cervical spine. Protraction places the lower motion segments near their end-range of flexion and the upper levels in progressively greater extension, with end-range extension achieved at C0–1 and C1–2. In contrast, cervical retraction positions the lower motion segments towards a mid-extension range with each superior level demonstrating more flexion, with C0–1 and C1–2 achieving full end-range of flexion.[59]

## Muscle function

*Extension* of the cervical spine to and from an upright position requires eccentric followed by concentric control of the cervical flexor muscles. Initially there is a slight burst of extensor muscle activity to initiate the motion. This is followed by extensor silence as the center of gravity of the head/neck moves posterior to the axis of motion to reach the end of available motion. The extensor muscles are then active in an effort to reach extreme cervical extension.[33] Eccentric control of the typical cervical spine upon the thorax is via the longus colli, sternocleidomastoid, anterior scalene, and hyoid muscles. It is estimated that as extension progresses, the flexor moment arms of sternocleidomastoid and the anterior scalene muscles reduce and in extreme extension are less than 25% of their value in neutral upright.[2] Consequently, as extension progresses, the deeper muscles play a larger role in the control of gravitational torque

(Figure 3.4). Gravitational torque imposed on the craniocervical motion segments by the mass of the head is restrained by the longus capitis and rectus capitis anterior muscles with assistance from the hyoid muscles. The sternocleidomastoid muscle does not contribute to flexor moments at the craniocervical region despite its large flexor moments at the typical cervical region.[2] The cleido-occipital portion of sternocleidomastoid has an extension moment arm at the craniocervical region that increases in extended postures and the portions that attach to the mastoid process have moment arms close to nil.[2] The role of the hyoid muscles in the production of cervical flexor torque is unknown. The suprahyoid muscles connect the mandible to the hyoid bone which in turn is connected to the thorax via the infrahyoid muscles. Their collective action when the mouth is closed will pull the mandible towards the sternum, inducing flexor moments to both the craniocervical and typical cervical regions. EMG activity of these muscles has been shown during both craniocervical and cervical flexion tasks.[60, 61] The infrahyoid muscles have large moment arms for neck flexion[2] but their total contribution to cervical flexion is unknown.

*Flexion* of the cervical spine and a return to an upright position require eccentric followed by concentric control of the cervical extensor muscles. The semispinalis capitis, splenius capitis, and the semispinalis cervicis and multifidus muscles have all been shown to be active through the eccentric and concentric stages of motion.[33] Only at the extreme of the cervical flexion range is there a cessation of EMG activity from the cervical extensor muscles,[33, 62] suggesting that load moments in this position are balanced by passive restraints, including the nuchal ligament.[42, 63]

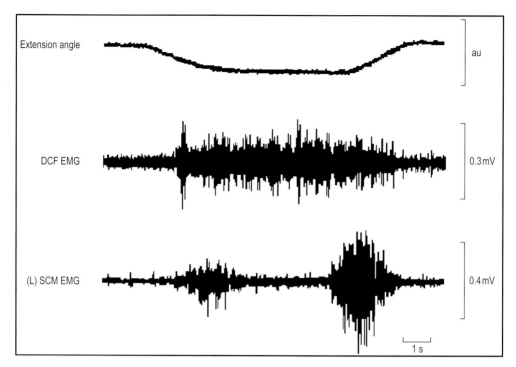

**Figure 3.4** Extension angle (au, arbitrary units) and electromyographic (EMG) data from the deep cervical flexors (DCF: longus colli, longus capitis) and left (L) sternocleidomastoid (SCM) muscles during cervical extension performed in standing. The EMG traces depict continuous activation of the DCF muscles during the eccentric phase of the motion compared to the more phasic activity of the SCM predominantly at the commencement of extension and at return from extension (Falla, O'Leary, Jull, unpublished data).

## Motion in the transverse and frontal planes

### Motion segment kinematics

Cervical motions in the horizontal and frontal planes are coupled. Axial rotation and lateral flexion of the typical cervical motion segments exhibit strong ipsilateral coupling, with the exception of the C2–3 motion segment that varies in coupling direction. This is in contrast to the craniocervical region that exhibits contralateral coupling.[1, 14] Therefore during cervical axial rotation the typical cervical spine flexes laterally to the side of rotation while the upper vertebrae tilt in the opposite direction.[14, 64] This mechanism permits the C1–2 complex and head to maintain vertical alignment during axial rotation, counterbalancing the lateral translation effect of the coupled lateral flexion of the typical cervical region.[65]

### Muscle function

The oblique orientation of most cervical spine muscles permits their contribution to axial rotation and lateral flexion motion. Studies investigating these movements have shown complex muscle patterns with many muscles contributing depending on the intensity of the contraction.[18, 24, 33] The sternocleidomastoid and splenius capitis muscles are strongly active during contralateral and ipsilateral axial rotation, respectively.[66, 67] Deeper cervical muscles (multifidus, the suboccipital muscles, and longus capitis and colli) have oblique orientations suited to contribute to motion in the transverse and frontal planes but, due to small moment arms, they have modest torque-producing capacity. These muscles may be more suited for segmental rotary stability rather than prime mover roles.[32] EMG activity recorded from the longus capitis and longus colli (superior portion) muscles during both ipsilateral and contralateral isometric cervical rotation and lateral flexion supports suggestions that these deeper muscles have a segmental stability role during these motions rather than a prime mover role (Figure 3.5).[36, 68] Biomechanical models suggest that tight rotary control of the deep craniocervical muscles is necessary to control unwanted rotary moments at C1–2 imposed by asymmetric contraction of larger

multisegmental muscles during motion in other anatomical planes.[23] This may explain the observations of bilateral EMG activity of the obliquus capitis inferior muscles recorded during unilateral axial rotation tasks.[69] Additionally, as the head is axially rotated to one side, activity of the contralateral cervical muscles would be expected to facilitate the contralateral side bending response of the craniocervical region observed in kinematic studies. In this manner sternocleidomastoid is ideally suited for its role in axial rotation as it produces both contralateral axial rotation and unilateral lateral flexion moments to the head.

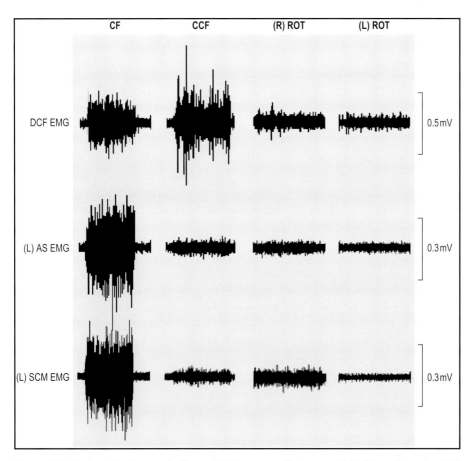

**Figure 3.5** Activation of the deep cervical flexors (DCF: longus capitis, longus colli), left (L) anterior scalene (AS), and sternocleidomastoid (SCM) muscles during typical cervical flexion (CF), craniocervical flexion only (CCF) and both ipsilateral and contralateral axial rotation (ROT). The DCF muscles are active during flexion of both regions of the neck and during both contralateral and ipsilateral rotation. In contrast SCM and AS are predominantly active during typical cervical flexion and contralateral axial rotation. EMG, electromyogram. (Adapted from Falla et al.[68] with permission.)

## Motion and neck pain

Alterations in movement accompany cervical disorders at the regional and segmental levels in the craniocervical and typical cervical spines. Reductions in regional motion have been shown to distinguish between healthy subjects and those with cervical disorders.[70, 71] In tandem with regional movement, motion at the segmental level may be reduced.[72] Conversely it may be excessive in either or both physiological and intervertebral translation and "neutral zone" motions.[72–74] Both the craniocervical and typical cervical regions have osteoligamentous structural characteristics that lend themselves to stability issues.

With injury to the craniocervical spine, a loss of integrity of the alar ligaments influences stability of both the C0–1 and C1–2 motion segments in multiple motion planes, but especially rotary stability.[75, 76] Transverse ligament injury permits anterior migration of the atlas from the dens during motion in the sagittal plane.[77] In the typical cervical region, fissuring of the intervertebral disk permits greater intervertebral translation during physiological motion that may place greater demands on other passive and active cervical restraints for stability. Degenerative change may also further perpetuate excessive intervertebral translation and "neutral zone" motion.[73] An anterolisthesis or retrolisthesis may develop with a loss of disk height and degenerative change.[78] There are difficulties in diagnosing motion segmental instability. Radiographic measurements may be used to detect excessive motion segment mobility[72, 75] but there is poor correlation between the magnitude of hypermobility/subluxation and presenting clinical signs and symptoms.[79] There are also challenges in detecting minor instabilities in the clinical setting (Chapter 12).[80, 81]

Degenerative changes are commonly noted in the lower cervical motion segments which also appear to be a common site of disk disorders,[82–85] but caution should be taken in assuming an association between degenerative changes and pain. Degenerative changes in the cervical spine are commonly found in asymptomatic individuals,[86] and the presence or severity of pain may not be related to the presence or degree of structural change.[87]

# Neurovascular structures of the cervical spine

A complex system of neurovascular structures is present in the neck. A basic description of the neurovascular structures is presented here but more detailed descriptions of these extensive systems are available in the literature.[3, 88–90]

The spinal cord in the cervical region is the thickest portion of the spinal cord and in accordance the cervical spinal canal is large. The canal is widest superiorly and narrows inferiorly. All cervical spinal nerves exit from the spinal canal through the intervertebral foramen except for the uppermost two cervical spinal nerves. Instead, the C1 spinal nerve exits the spinal canal through the posterior atlanto-occipital membrane, and the C2 spinal nerve through the foramen formed by the arch of the atlas and the lamina of the axis. Cervical intervertebral foramen are bordered superiorly and inferiorly by pedicles, dorsally by the facet joint and capsule, and ventrally by the posterolateral disk, uncovertebral joint, and vertebral artery. The foramina are largest at the C2–3 level, progressively reducing in size to the C6–7 level. In contrast, the cross-sectional area of the cervical spinal nerves increases in size towards the lower cervical levels, reducing available space through which the nerve travels. Cervical nerve roots are vulnerable to encroachment at their exit from the intervertebral foramen due to processes such as spondylosis, degenerative zygapophyseal or uncovertebral joints, herniated disks, or nerve root sleeve fibrosis, potentially causing radicular symptoms.[83, 91] It would appear the lower cervical nerve roots (C6, C7) are the most vulnerable due to the prevalent degenerative changes at the C5-6 and C6-7 motion segments, respectively.[82-84]

The brachial plexus is intimately related to the scalene muscles. The anterior and middle scalene muscles together with the first rib comprise the scalene triangle through which the brachial plexus and subclavian artery pass. Commonly the C5 and/or C6 ventral rami may penetrate the anterior scalene muscle[92] but mostly they penetrate the middle scalene along with the dorsal scapular nerve.[93] It is thought that atrophy, spasm, or the common presence of the additional scalenus minimus may compromise travel of neurovascular structures through the scalene triangle.[92, 94, 95]

The vertebral artery is the major source of blood supply to musculoskeletal structures of the cervical spine and the cervical spinal cord.[3] The bilateral vertebral arteries rise from the subclavian arteries before they enter and run through the foramen transversarium of C6 to C1. The vertebral arteries then wind posteriorly around the lateral masses of the atlas, pass over the posterior arch of C1 just behind its lateral mass, and join together after passing through the foramen magnum. The vertebral arteries are vulnerable to mechanical load due to their torturous course through the cervical spine and are therefore an important consideration during manual therapy techniques.[90]

## Relationship between the cervical spine and thorax

The cervical spine has a strong biomechanical relationship to the thorax, particularly with respect to the angulations of the cervical lordosis and the capacity to achieve full excursion of neck motion. The sagittal orientation of the cervicothoracic junction will largely dictate the resulting angle of the cervical lordosis.[96, 97] There is some evidence to suggest that as the angle of the thoracic kyphosis changes with age, there is an associated superior migration of the inflection point of the cervical lordosis.[98] Consequently the thoracic spine potentially dictates the loading mechanisms of the cervical spine.

Full excursion of cervical spine and shoulder girdle motion requires thoracic mobility, particularly at the cervicothoracic junction and upper thoracic motion segments.[99, 100] The transition of the mobile cervical spine to the more rigid thoracic spine occurs at the cervicothoracic junction. Mobility is required at both the upper thoracic motion segments and their corresponding articulations with the ribs.[101] Abnormal limitation in mobility of the upper thorax has consequently been implicated in conditions of abnormal loading and restricted motion of the cervical spine.[100]

## Relationship between the cervical spine and shoulder girdle

The shoulder girdle has muscular attachments to the cervical spine in the form of the axioscapular muscles and carries the trunks of the brachial plexus to the upper limb after their exit from the intervertebral foramen. Thus the dynamics of the shoulder girdle, and in particular the scapula, is of interest as it relates to the length–tension relationship of axioscapular muscles, their subsequent mechanical forces on the cervical spine, as well as their capacity to protect neurovascular structures. A comprehensive analysis of the shoulder girdle also includes the axiohumeral and scapulohumeral muscles; however, their inclusion is beyond the scope of this text.

## Kinematics of the scapula

There is consistency of "normal" scapular motion patterns recorded using electromagnetic devices during functional tasks of the upper limb, but variability in the amplitude of these movements between individuals is common. As the upper limb is elevated from its resting position there is initially minimal scapular motion (first 30–40° of upper-limb elevation), followed by progressive upward rotation, posterior tilt, and external rotation of the scapula on the thorax (Figure 3.6).[102-104] Posterior scapular tilt and rotation increase significantly once the upper limb is past 90° elevation.[103] These scapular rotations are associated with scapular elevation and retraction as well as elevation, posterior rotation, and retraction of the clavicle.[103, 105]

Of interest is the small change in scapular orientation in the initial phases of upper-limb elevation which would replicate scapular function demanded by many daily tasks of the upper limb in the neck pain patient, some of which would be prolonged and potentially fatiguing, for example during computer use. Interestingly, Tsai et al.[106] found that fatigue of shoulder girdle muscles had the most profound influence on scapular kinematics during the initial phase of arm elevation. Scapular stability is the primary task of the axioscapular muscles.

## Role of the axioscapular muscles

Interpreting the function of the individual axioscapular muscles in control of the scapula at rest and during elevation is challenging. Moments exerted to the scapula from the various muscles alter as the axis of scapular rotation migrates through range. The level of shoulder girdle muscle activity also appears to be dependent on factors such as the precision of the upper-limb task.[107]

The contribution of the trapezius muscle to scapular orientation at rest is evident in the presence of trapezius paralysis (post accessory nerve injury) that results in a downwardly rotated, protracted, and laterally displaced scapula at rest.[108-110] The patient is often unable to shrug and elevation motion is limited. EMG activity of all three portions of the trapezius has been demonstrated during elevation of the upper limb[111-114] with the three portions acting as a unit during arm elevation tasks.[115, 116] Timing of the three portions may differ depending on the task.[117] The upper trapezius elevates and retracts the outer end of the

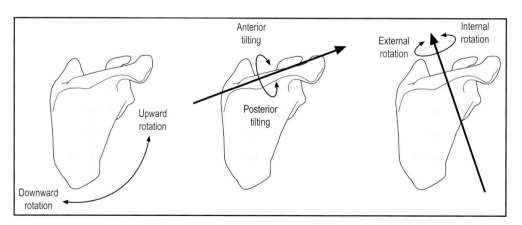

**Figure 3.6** During elevation of the upper limb the scapula rotates upwardly, tilts posteriorly, and externally rotates. These actions are controlled by the axioscapular muscles. (Adapted from Tsai et al.[106] with permission.)

clavicle about a pivot at the sternoclavicular joint,[118] thereby assisting in upward rotation of the scapula by elevating the acromion through the acromioclavicular joint. The orientation of the nuchal fibers, the middle fibers, and the lower fibers of trapezius dictates that they assist in drawing the clavicle and scapula backwards and medially.[118] This would assist in retraction and external rotation of the scapula. Lower trapezius may also contribute to posterior tipping and external rotation of the scapula.[111] The thoracic fibers of trapezius counteract lateral displacement of serratus anterior and upward motion of levator scapulae muscle, maintaining horizontal and vertical equilibrium rather than generating net torque.[118]

The role of the serratus anterior muscle during arm elevation is evident following its paralysis due to long thoracic nerve palsy. During elevation (especially flexion) there is inadequate fixation of the scapula against the ribcage (particularly the inferior angle of the scapula during flexion due to the strong anterior scapular tilt torque imposed by the weight of the upper limb) and a substantial loss of elevation range.[93, 119] These deformities reflect the major contribution of the serratus anterior muscle to upward rotation and posterior tilt of the scapula due to its high concentration of fibers on to the inferior scapular angle.[120, 121] The medial border also becomes prominent[93] due to inefficient external rotation of the scapula and there is a loss of scapular protraction during shoulder elevation.[122] Serratus anterior muscle activity gradually increases through elevation range of the upper limb.[113] Its fibers, particularly the lower ones, are oriented to exert moments about both the spine of the scapula and the acromio-clavicular joint during both the initial and later phases of elevation.[123] The clavicle offers a point of support for serratus anterior which can use the scapula as a lever to exert moments around the sternoclavicular and acromioclavicular joints.

Intramuscular fine-wire EMG techniques have been used to investigate the function of the levator scapulae muscle. Levator scapulae has been shown to be strongly active in upper-limb elevation,[33, 111, 124, 125] particularly in abduction. It contracts concentrically during the first half of abduction assisting scapular elevation, and eccentrically during the second half of abduction, allowing the scapular to rotate upwardly.[124]

There has been speculation as to the mechanical impact that the axioscapular muscles have on the cervical spine. The upper trapezius and levator scapulae muscles may have direct compressive effects on cervical motion segments due to their superior attachments. The mechanical effects of upper trapezius may be negligible due to its lack of cross-sectional area and its attachments primarily to the ligamentum nuchae.[24, 33, 114, 118] However, the vertical orientation of the levator scapulae fibers and its attachment to the upper four cervical vertebrae (Figure 3.7) may impose compressive forces to the cervical spine.[124] These vertical forces occur posterior to the axis of sagittal cervical spine motion, producing cervical spine extension when contracting bilaterally,[18] and assisting in ipsilateral cervical rotation when contracting unilaterally.[124]

In states of impaired shoulder girdle function or muscle fatigue, forces imposed to the cervical spine from the axioscapular muscle attachments may be potentially injurious[124] and contribute to the development of neck and shoulder pain during static work postures and repetitive arm movements.[126, 127] Additionally, shoulder girdle impairment may place detrimental loads on cervical neurovascular structures. Altered muscular control of the scapula resulting in positions of scapular depression and downward rotation is thought to contribute to adverse mechanical load to both nerve and vascular structures, potentially contributing to conditions such as thoracic outlet syndrome.[108, 109]

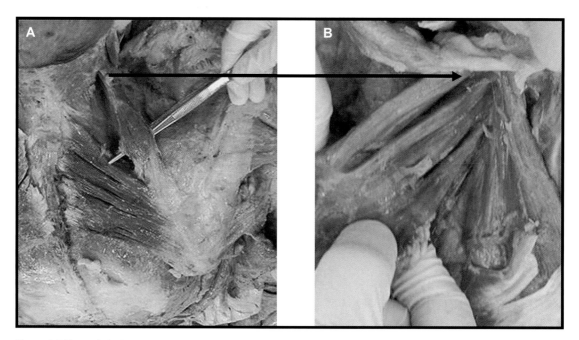

**Figure 3.7** The vertical orientation of the levator scapulae muscles (A) and their proximal attachments to the upper four cervical vertebrae (B) permits this muscle to exert vertical compressive forces to the cervical spine.

# Relationship between the cervical spine and temporomandibular region

There is a relationship between posture and motion of the cervical and temporomandibular regions. The orientation of the mandible is influenced by the posture adopted at the craniocervical region.[128–131] The mandible has been shown to pursue a more posterior path of opening when the head is positioned forward of its resting upright posture such that the craniocervical region is in extension.[130] This is most probably due to the change in resting length of the hyoid muscles. In reverse, alterations have been shown in craniovertebral angle following alterations in interocclusal relationships.[132] The head and the mandible also exhibit concomitant and well-coordinated movement when opening and closing the mouth, such that jaw opening and closing coincided with craniocervical extension and flexion respectively.[131, 133–135] These coordinated movement patterns may be disrupted by neck pain or injury, as has been demonstrated in cases of whiplash-associated disorders.[136, 137] Thus alterations may occur in the coordinated action of the muscles controlling the mandible and the head in disorders potentially involving either the cervical spine or temporomandibular regions. This may be one explanation for why disorders of the cervical spine and temporomandibular regions commonly coexist.[138–141]

# Conclusion

The structure of the cervical spine affords it sophisticated mobility and function. The cervical muscle system comprises numerous muscles, all with multiple functions and a high redundancy that makes description of their function difficult. Some simplification can be made by dividing the function of the muscles into deep and superficial muscle groups, and by describing the action of muscles into their action about the craniocervical and typical cervical regions. This chapter used these gross anatomical observations together with evidence from EMG studies to infer the function of the cervical muscle system. The description of the function of these muscles is made more complex by the integrated function of the craniomandibular and scapulothoracic regions. The juxtaposition of these regions to the cervical spine and their obvious mechanical and neurophysiological relationship to the cervical region indicates the necessity to assess their function within the scope of the cervical spine examination.

# References

1. *Bogduk N, Mercer S*. Biomechanics of the cervical spine. I: Normal kinematics. Clin Biomech 2000;15:633–648.

2. *Vasavada AN, Li S, Delp SL*. Influence of muscle morphometry and moment arms on the moment-generating capacity of human neck muscles. Spine 1998;23:412–422.

3. *Moore KL, Dalley AF*. Clinically Orientated Anatomy, 4th edn. Philadelphia: Lippincott/Williams and Wilkins, 1999.

4. *Dvorak J, Panjabi MM*. Functional anatomy of the alar ligaments. Spine 1987;12:183–189.

5. *Penning L*. Differences in anatomy, motion, development and aging of the upper and lower cervical disk segments. Clin Biomech 1988;3:37–47.

6. *Mestdagh H*. Morphological aspects and biomechanical properties of the vertebro-axial joint (C2–3). Acta Morphol Neerl-Scand 1976;14:19–30.

7. *Mercer S*. Comparative anatomy of the spinal disc. In: Boyling JD, Jull G (eds). Grieve's Modern Manual Therapy. The Vertebral Column, 3rd edn. Edinburgh: Elsevier, Churchill Livingstone, 2004:9–16.

8. *Mercer S, Bogduk N*. The ligaments and annulus fibrosus of human adult cervical intervertebral discs. Spine 1999;24:619–626.

9. *Tondury G*. The behaviour of the cervical discs during life. In: Hirsch C, Zotterman Y (eds) Cervical Pain. Oxford: Pergamon Press, 1972:59–66.

10. *Pooni J, Hukins D, Harris P, et al*. Comparison of the structure of human intervertebral discs in the cervical, thoracic, and lumbar regions of the spine. Surg Radiol Anat 1986;8:175–182.

11. *Scott JE, Bosworth TR, Cribb AM, et al*. The chemical morphology of age-related changes in human intervertebral disc glycosaminoglycans from cervical, thoracic and lumbar nucleus pulposus and annulus fibrosus. J Anat 1994;184:73–82.

12. *Nowitzke A, Westaway M, Bogduk N*. Cervical zygapophyseal joints: geometrical parameters and relationship to cervical kinematics. Clin Biomech 1994;9:342–348.

13. *Mercer SR, Bogduk N*. Joints of the cervical vertebral column. J Orthop Sports Phys Ther 2001;31:174–182.

14. *Mimura M, Moriya H, Watanabe T, et al*. Three-dimensional motion analysis of the cervical spine with special reference to the axial rotation. Spine 1989;14:1135–1139.

15. *Dutia MB*. The muscles and joints of the neck: their specialisation and role in head movement. Prog Neurobiol 1991;37:165–178.

16. *Richmond FJR, Bakker DA, Stacey MJ*. The sensorium: receptors of neck muscles and joints. In: Peterson BW, Richmond FJ (eds) Control of Head Movement. Oxford: Oxford University Press, 1988:49–62.

17. *Kamibayashi LK, Richmond FJR*. Morphometry of human neck muscles. Spine 1998;23:1314–1323.

18. *Conley MS, Meyer RA, Bloomberg JJ, et al*. Noninvasive analysis of human neck muscle function. Spine 1995;20:2505–2512.

19. *Roy RR, Ishihara A*. Overview: functional implications of the design of skeletal muscles. Acta Anat 1997;159:75–77.

20. *Peck D, Buxton DF, Nitz A*. A comparison of spindle concentrations in large and small muscles acting in parallel combinations. J Morphol 1984;180:243–252.

21. *Boyd-Clark LC, Briggs CA, Galea MP*. Comparative histochemical composition of muscle fibers in a pre- and a postvertebral muscle of the cervical spine. J Anat 2001;199:709–716.

22. *Boyd-Clark LC, Briggs CA, Galea MP*. Muscle spindle distribution, morphology, and density in longus colli and multifidus muscles of the cervical spine. Spine 2002;27:694–701.

23. *Winters JM, Peles JD*. Neck muscle activity and 3-D head kinematics during quasi-static and dynamic tracking movements. In: Winters JM, Woo SLY (eds) Multiple Muscle Systems: Biomechanics and Movement Organisation. New York: Springer-Verlag, 1990:461–480.

24. *Vasavada AN, Peterson BW, Delp SL*. Three-dimensional spatial tuning of neck muscle activation in humans. Exp Brain Res 2002;147:437–448.

25. *Panjabi MM, Cholewicki J, Nibu K, et al*. Critical load of the human cervical spine: an in vitro experimental study. Clin Biomech 1998;13:11–17.

26. *Mayoux Benhamou M, Revel M, Vallee C, et al*. Longus colli has a postural function on cervical curvature. Surg Radiol Anat 1994;16:367–371.

27. *Nolan JP, Sherk HH*. Biomechanical evaluation of the extensor musculature of the cervical spine. Spine 1988;13:9–11.

28. *Sherk HH*. Stability of the lower cervical spine. In: Kehr P, Weidner A (eds) Cervical Spine. New York: Springer Verlag, 1987:59–64.

29. *Sasai K, Saito T, Akagi S, et al*. Cervical curvature after laminoplasty for spondylotic myelopathy – involvement of yellow ligament, semispinalis cervicis muscle, and nuchal ligament. J Spinal Disord 2000;13:26–30.

30. *Takeuchi K, Yokoyama T, Aburakawa S, et al*. Anatomic study of the semispinalis cervicis for reattachment during laminoplasty. Clin Orthop Rel Res 2005;436:126–131.

31. *Iizuka H, Shimizu T, Tateno K, et al*. Extensor musculature of the cervical spine after laminoplasty: morphologic evaluation by coronal view of the magnetic resonance image. Spine 2001;26:2220–2226.

32. *Anderson JS, Hsu AW, Vasavada AN*. Morphology, architecture, and biomechanics of human cervical multifidus. Spine 2005;30:E86–E91.

33. *Mayoux Benhamou MA, Revel M, Vallee C*. Selective electromyography of dorsal neck muscles in humans. Exp Brain Res 1997;113:353–360.

34. *Oatis CA*. Kinesiology: The Mechanics and Pathomechanics of Human Movement. Philadelphia: Lippincott, Williams and Wilkins, 2004.

35. *Falla D, O'Leary S, Fagan A, et al*. Recruitment of the deep cervical flexor muscles during a postural-correction exercise performed in sitting. Man Ther 2007;12:139–143.

36. *Vitti M, Fujiwara M, Basmanjian JM, et al*. The integrated roles of longus colli and sternocleidomastoid muscles: an electromyographic study. Anat Rec 1973;177:471–484.

37. *Keller TS, Colloca CJ, Harrison DE, et al*. Influence of spine morphology on intervertebral disc loads and stresses in asymptomatic adults: implications for the ideal spine. Spine J 2005;5:297–309.

38. *Kumaresan S, Yoganandan N, Pintar FA*. Posterior complex contribution to the axial compressive and distractive behaviour of the cervical spine. J Musculoskel Res 1998;2:257–265.

39. *Pal GP, Routal RV*. A study of weight transmission through the cervical and upper thoracic regions of the vertebral column in man. J Anat 1986;148:245–261.

40. *Pal GP, Sherk HH*. The vertical stability of the cervical spine. Spine 1988;13:447–449.

41. *Harrison DE, Harrison DD, Janik TJ, et al*. Comparison of axial and flexural stresses in lordosis and three buckled configurations of the cervical spine. Clin Biomech 2001;16:276–284.

42. *Harms-Ringdahl K, Ekholm J, Schuldt K, et al*. Load moments and myoelectric activity when the cervical spine is held in full flexion and extension. Ergonomics 1986;29:1539–1552.

43. *Visscher CM, de Boer W, Naeije M*. The relationship between posture and curvature of the cervical spine. J Manipul Physiol Ther 1998;21:388–391.

44. *Zito G, Jull G, Story I*. Clinical tests of musculoskeletal dysfunction in the diagnosis of cervicogenic headache. Man Ther 2006;11:118–129.

45. *Griegel-Morris P, Larson K, Mueller-Klaus K, et al*. Incidence of common postural abnormalities in the cervical, shoulder, and thoracic regions and their association with pain in two age groups of healthy subjects. Phys Ther 1992;72:425–431.

46. *Watson DH, Trott PH*. Cervical headache: an investigation of natural head posture and upper cervical flexor muscle performance. Cephalalgia 1993;13:272–284.

47. *Refshauge KM, Goodsell M, Lee M*. The relationship between surface contour and vertebral body measures of upper spine curvature. Spine 1994;19:2180–2185.

48. *Johnson GM*. The correlation between surface measurement of head and neck posture and the anatomic position of the upper cervical vertebrae. Spine 1998;23:921–927.

49. *Harrison DD, Harrison DE, Janik TJ, et al*. Modeling of the sagittal cervical spine as a method to discriminate hypolordosis: results of elliptical and circular modeling in 72 asymptomatic subjects, 52 acute neck pain subjects, and 70 chronic neck pain subjects. Spine 2004; 29:2485–2492.

50. *Kristjansson E, Jonsson H, Jr*. Is the sagittal configuration of the cervical spine changed in women with chronic whiplash syndrome? A comparative computer-assisted radiographic assessment. J Manipul Physiol Ther 2002;25:550–555.

51. *Matsumoto M, Fujimura Y, Suzuki N, et al*. Cervical curvature in acute whiplash injuries: prospective comparative study with asymptomatic subjects. Injury 1998;29:775–778.

52. *Grob D*. The association between cervical spine curvature and neck pain. Eur Spine J 2007; 16:669–678.

53. *Szeto G, Straker L, Raine A*. A field comparison of neck and shoulder postures in symptomatic and asymptomatic office workers. Appl Ergon 2002;33:75–84.

54. *Falla D, Jull G, Russell T, et al*. Effect of neck exercise on sitting posture in patients with chronic neck pain. Phys Ther 2007;87:408–417.

55. *Szeto G, Straker L, O'Sullivan P*. A comparison of symptomatic and asymptomatic office workers performing monotonous keyboard work 1: Neck and shoulder muscle recruitment patterns. Man Ther 2005;10:270–280.

56. *Johnston V, Jull G, Souvlis T*. Alterations in cervical muscle activity in functional and stressful tasks in female office workers with neck pain. 2007; submitted for publication.

57. *Falla D, Bilenkij G, Jull G*. Patients with chronic neck pain demonstrate altered patterns of muscle activation during performance of a functional upper limb task. Spine 2004;29:1436–1440.

58. *van Mameren H*. Motion patterns in the cervical spine. Thesis. University of Limburg, 1988.

59. *Ordway NR, Seymour RJ, Donelson RG, et al*. Cervical flexion, extension, protrusion, and retraction: a radiographic segmental analysis. Spine 1999;24:240–247.

60. *Ferdjallah M, Wertsch JJ, Shaker R*. Spectral analysis of surface electromyography (EMG) of upper esophageal sphincter-opening muscles during head lift exercise. J Rehabil Res Dev 2000;37:335–340.

61. *O'Leary S, Falla D, Jull G, et al*. Muscle specificity in tests of cervical flexor muscle performance. J Electromyogr Kinesiol 2007;17:35–40.

62. *Meyer JJ, Berk RJ, Anderson AV*. Recruitment patterns in the cervical paraspinal muscles during cervical forward flexion: evidence of cervical flexion–relaxation. Electromyogr Clin Neurophysiol 1993;33:217–223.

63. *Takeshita K, Peterson ET, Bylski-Austrow D, et al*. The nuchal ligament restrains cervical spine flexion. Spine 2004;29:E388–E393.

64. *Winters JM, Peles JD, Osterbauer PJ, et al*. Three-dimensional head axis of rotation during tracking movements. A tool for assessing neck neuromechanical function. Spine 1993;18:1178–1185.

65. *White AA, Panjabi MM*. Clinical Biomechanics of the Spine, 2nd edn. Philadelphia: J.B. Lippincott, 1990.

66. *Takebe K, Vitti M, Basmajian J*. The functions of semispinalis capitis and splenius capitis muscles: an electromyographic study. Anat Rec 1974;179:477–480.

67. *Mayoux Benhamou MA, Revel M, Vallee C*. Surface electrodes are not appropriate to record selective myoelectric activity of splenius capitis muscle in humans. Exp Brain Res 1995;105:432–438.

68. *Falla D, Dall'Alba P, O'Leary S, et al*. Further evaluation of an EMG technique for assessment of the deep cervical flexor muscles. J Electromyogr Kinesiol 2006;16:621–628.

69. *Bexander CS, Mellor R, Hodges PW*. Effect of gaze direction on neck muscle activity during cervical rotation. Exp Brain Res 2005;167:422–432.

70. *Dall'Alba P, Sterling M, Treleavan J, et al*. Cervical range of motion discriminates between asymptomatic and whiplash subjects. Spine 2001;26:2090–2094.

71. *Zwart JA*. Neck mobility in different headache disorders. Headache 1997;37:6–11.

72. *Dvorak J, Froehlich D, Penning L, et al*. Functional radiographic diagnosis of the cervical spine: flexion/extension. Spine 1988;13:748–755.

73. *Panjabi MM*. The stabilizing system of the spine. Part II. Neutral zone and instability hypothesis. J Spinal Disord 1992;5:390–396.

74. *Panjabi MM, Lydon C, Vasavada A, et al*. On the understanding of clinical instability. Spine 1994;19:2642–2650.

75. *Dvorak J, Panjabi M, Gerber M, et al*. CT-functional diagnostics of the rotatory instability of upper cervical spine. 1. An experimental study on cadavers. Spine 1987;12:197–205.

76. *Panjabi M, Dvorak J, Crisco JJ, et al*. Effects of alar ligament transection on upper cervical spine rotation. J Orthop Res 1991;9:584–593.

77. *Fielding J, Cochran G, Lawsing J, et al*. Tears of the transverse ligament of the axis. J Bone Joint Surg Am 1974;56A:1683–1691.

78. *Pellengahr C, Pfahler M, Kuhr M, et al*. Influence of facet joint angles and asymmetric disk collapse on degenerative olisthesis of the cervical spine. Orthopedics 2000;23:697–701.

79. *Swinkels RA, Oostendorp RA*. Upper cervical instability: fact or fiction? J Manipul Physiol Ther 1996;19:185–194.

80. *Niere KR, Torney SK*. Clinicians' perceptions of minor cervical instability. Manual Ther 2004;9:144–150.

81. *Swinkels R, Beeton K, Alltree J*. Pathogenesis of upper cervical instability. Manual Ther 1996;1:127–132.

82. *Osborn A*. Diagnostic Neuroradiology. St. Louis: CV Mosby, 1994.

83. *Shedid D, Benzel EC*. Cervical spondylosis anatomy: pathophysiology and biomechanics. Neurosurgery 2007;60:S7–S13.

84. *Harrop JS, Hanna A, Silva MT, et al*. Neurological manifestations of cervical spondylosis: an overview of signs, symptoms, and pathophysiology. Neurosurgery 2007;60:S14–S20.

85. *Scoville WB*. Types of cervical disc lesions and their surgical approaches. JAMA 1966;196:479–481.

86. *Gore DR, Sepic SB, Gardner GM*. Roentgenographic findings of the cervical spine in asymptomatic people. Spine 1986;11:521–524.

87. *Gore DR, Sepic SB, Gardner GM, et al*. Neck pain: a long-term follow-up of 205 patients. Spine 1987;12:1–5.

88. *Bogduk N*. Anatomy and physiology of headache. Biomed Pharmacother 1995;49:435–445.

89. *Bogduk N*. The anatomy and pathophysiology of neck pain. Phys Med Rehabil Clin North Am 2003;14:455–472.

90. *Rivett DA*. The vertebral artery and vertebrobasilar insufficiency. In: Boyling JD, Jull G (eds) Grieve's Modern Manual Therapy. The Vertebral Column, 3rd edn. Edinburgh: Elsevier Churchill Livingstone, 2004:257–273.

91. *Epstein J, Epstein B, Lavine L, et al*. Cervical myelo-radiculopathy caused by arthrotic hypertrophy of the posterior facets and laminae. J Neurosurg 1978;49:387–392.

92. *Harry WG, Bennett JD, Guha SC*. Scalene muscles and the brachial plexus: anatomical variations and their clinical significance. Clin Anat 1997;10: 250–252.

93. *Wiater JM, Flatow EL*. Long thoracic nerve injury. Clin Orthop 1999;368:17–27.

94. *Rusnak-Smith S, Moffat M, Rosen E*. Anatomical variations of the scalene triangle: dissection of 10 cadavers. J Orthop Sports Phys Ther 2001;31:70–80.

95. *Makhoul RG, Machleder HI*. Developmental anomalies at the thoracic outlet: an analysis of 200 consecutive cases. J Vasc Surg 1992;16:534–542.

96. *Loder RT*. The sagittal profile of the cervical and lumbosacral spine in Scheuermann thoracic kyphosis. J Spinal Disord 2001;14:226–231.

97. *Hardacker JW, Shuford RF, Capicotto PN, et al*. Radiographic standing cervical segmental alignment in adult volunteers without neck symptoms. Spine 1997;22:1472–1480.

98. *Boyle JJ, Milne N, Singer KP*. Influence of age on cervicothoracic spinal curvature: an ex vivo radiographic survey. Clin Biomech 2002;17:361–367.

99. *Sobel JS, Kremer I, Winters JC, et al*. The influence of the mobility in the cervicothoracic spine and the upper ribs (shoulder girdle) on the mobility of the scapulohumeral joint. J Manipul Physiol Ther 1996;19:469–474.

100. *Edmondston S*. Clinical biomechanics of the thoracic spine including the ribcage. In: Boyling JD, Jull G (eds) Grieve's Modern Manual Therapy. The Vertebral Column, 3rd edn. Edinburgh: Elsevier, Churchill Livingstone, 2004:55–65.

101. *Lee D*. The Thorax: An Integrated Approach. White Rock, British Columbia: Distributed by OPTP, 2003.

102. *Ludewig PM, Cook TM*. Alterations in shoulder kinematics and associated muscle activity in people with symptoms of shoulder impingement. Phys Ther 2000;80:276–291.

103. *McClure PW, Michener LA, Sennett BJ, et al*. Direct 3-dimensional measurement of scapular kinematics during dynamic movements in vivo. J Shoulder Elbow Surg 2001;10:269–277.

104. *Lukasiewicz AC, McClure P, Michener L, et al*. Comparison of 3-dimensional scapular position and orientation between subjects with and without shoulder impingement. J Orthop Sports Phys Ther 1999;29:574–583.

105. *Ludewig PM, Behrens SA, Meyer SM, et al*. Three-dimensional clavicular motion during arm elevation: reliability and descriptive data. J Orthop Sports Phys Ther 2004;34:140–149.

106. *Tsai NT, McClure PW, Karduna AR*. Effects of muscle fatigue on 3-dimensional scapular kinematics. Arch Phys Med Rehabil 2003;84:1000–1005.

107. *Sporrong H, Palmerud G, Kadefors R, et al*. The effect of light manual precision work on shoulder muscles – an EMG analysis. J Electromyogr Kinesiol 1998;8:177–184.

108. *Al-Shekhlee A, Katirji B*. Spinal accessory neuropathy, droopy shoulder, and thoracic outlet syndrome. Muscle Nerve 2003;28:383–385.

109. *Novak CB, Mackinnon SE*. Patient outcome after surgical management of an accessory nerve injury. Otolaryngol Head Neck Surg 2002;127:221–224.

110. *Nori S, Soo KC, Green RF, et al*. Utilization of intraoperative electroneurography to understand the innervation of the trapezius muscle. Muscle Nerve 1997;20:279–285.

111. *Ludewig PM, Cook TM, Nawoczenski DA*. Three-dimensional scapular orientation and muscle activity at selected positions of humeral elevation. J Orthop Sports Phys Ther 1996;24:57–65.

112. *Filho JG, Furlani J, de Freitas V*. Electromyographic study of the trapezius muscle in free movements of the arm. Electromyogr Clin Neurophysiol 1991;31:93–98.

113. *Bagg SD, Forrest WJ*. Electromyographic study of the scapular rotators during arm abduction in the scapular plane. Am J Phys Med 1986;65:111–124.

114. *Bull ML, Vitti M, De Freitas V*. Electromyographic study of the trapezius (pars superior) and serratus anterior (pars inferior) muscles in free movements of the shoulder. Electromyogr Clin Neurophysiol 1989;29:119–125.

115. *Cools AM, Witvrouw EE, De Clercq GA, et al*. Scapular muscle recruitment pattern: electromyographic response of the trapezius muscle to sudden shoulder movement before and after a fatiguing exercise. J Orthop Sports Phys Ther 2002;32:221–229.

116. *Piacentini SC, Berzin F*. Electromyographic study of the upper, middle and lower portion of the trapezius muscle in the circumduction movement of the arm on a shoulder wheel apparatus. Electromyogr Clin Neurophysiol 1989;29:315–319.

117. *Wadsworth DJ, Bullock-Saxton JE*. Recruitment patterns of the scapular rotator muscles in freestyle swimmers with subacromial impingement. Int J Sports Med 1997;18:618–624.

118. *Johnson G, Bogduk N, Nowitzke A, et al*. Anatomy and actions of the trapezius muscle. Clin Biomech 1994;9:44–50.

119. *Truong XT, Rippel DV*. Orthotic devices for serratus anterior palsy: some biomechanical considerations. Arch Phys Med Rehabil 1979;60:66–69.

120. *Perry J*. Muscle control of the shoulder. In: Rowe CR (ed) The Shoulder. New York: Churchill Livingstone, 1988:1–17.

121. *Williams GR Jr, Shakil M, Klimkiewicz J, et al*. Anatomy of the scapulothoracic articulation. Clin Orthop 1999;359:237–246.

122. *Warner JJ, Navarro RA*. Serratus anterior dysfunction. Recognition and treatment. Clin Orthop Rel Res 1998;349:139–148.

123. *Dvir Z, Berme N*. The shoulder complex in elevation of the arm: a mechanism approach. J Biomech 1978;11:219–225.

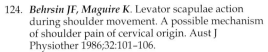
124. *Behrsin JF, Maguire K*. Levator scapulae action during shoulder movement. A possible mechanism of shoulder pain of cervical origin. Aust J Physiother 1986;32:101–106.

125. *de Freitas V, Vitti M, Furlani J*. Electromyographic study of levator scapulae and rhomboideous: major muscles in movements of the shoulder and arm. Electromyogr Clin Neurophysiol 1980;20:205–216.

126. *Sundelin G, Hagberg M*. Electromyographic signs of shoulder muscle fatigue in repetitive arm work paced by the methods–time measurement system. Scand J Work Environ Health 1992;18: 262–268.

127. *Sundelin G*. Patterns of electromyographic shoulder muscle fatigue during MTM-paced repetitive arm work with and without pauses. Int Arch Occup Environ Health 1993;64:485–493.

128. *Goldstein DF, Kraus SL, Williams WB, et al*. Influence of cervical posture on mandibular movement. J Prosthet Dent 1984;52:421.

129. *Makofsky HW, Sexton TR*. The effect of craniovertebral fusion on occlusion. Cranio 1994;12:38–46.

130. *Visscher CM, Huddleston Slater JJ, Lobbezoo F, et al*. Kinematics of the human mandible for different head postures. J Oral Rehabil 2000;27: 299–305.

131. *Zafar H*. Integrated jaw and neck function in man. Studies of mandibular and head–neck movements during jaw opening–closing tasks. Swed Dent J Suppl 2000;143:1–41.

132. *Moya H, Miralles R, Zuniga C, et al*. Influence of stabilization occlusal splint on craniocervical relationships. Part I; Cephalometric analysis. J Craniomandibular Pract 1994;12:47.

133. *Eriksson PO, Haggman-Henrikson B, Nordh E, et al*. Co-ordinated mandibular and head-neck movements during rhythmic jaw activities in man. J Dent Res 2000;79:1378–1384.

134. *Eriksson PO, Zafar H, Nordh E*. Concomitant mandibular and head–neck movements during jaw opening–closing in man. J Oral Rehabil 1998;25:859–870.

135. *Zafar H, Nordh E, Eriksson PO*. Temporal coordination between mandibular and head–neck movements during jaw opening–closing tasks in man. Arch Oral Biol 2000;45:675–682.

136. *Eriksson PO, Zafar H, Haggman-Henrikson B*. Deranged jaw–neck motor control in whiplash-associated disorders. Eur J Oral Sci 2004;112:25–32.

137. *Haggman-Henrikson B, Zafar H, Eriksson PO*. Disturbed jaw behavior in whiplash-associated disorders during rhythmic jaw movements. J Dent Res 2002;81:747–751.

138. *Stiesch-Scholz M, Fink M, Tschernitschek H*. Comorbidity of internal derangement of the temporomandibular joint and silent dysfunction of the cervical spine. J Oral Rehabil 2003;30:386–391.

139. *De Laat A, Meuleman H, Stevens A, et al*. Correlation between cervical spine and temporomandibular disorders. Clin Oral Invest 1998;2:54–57.

140. *Fink M, Tschernitschek H, Stiesch-Scholz M*. Asymptomatic cervical spine dysfunction (CSD) in patients with internal derangement of the temporomandibular joint. Cranio 2002;20:192–197.

141. *de Wijer A, Steenks MH, de Leeuw JR, et al*. Symptoms of the cervical spine in temporomandibular and cervical spine disorders. J Oral Rehabil 1996;23:742–750.

# 4

# Alterations in Cervical Muscle Function in Neck Pain

## Introduction

The combination of the number of muscles acting on the cervical spine together with its capacity for multiple degrees of freedom[1] makes the cervical muscle system highly redundant (Chapter 3). That is, specific forces may be produced by several combinations of muscle actions.[2] Given the complexity of the cervical spine, it is not surprising that neck pain induces a major reorganization of motor control strategies.

Many techniques, such as electromyography (EMG), magnetic resonance imaging, ultrasonography, muscle biopsy, laser Doppler flowmetry, and cervical dynamometry, have been used to expose a diverse range of neuromuscular adaptations in people with neck pain.[3-9] Studies utilizing experimental neck pain models have also shed light on the mechanisms underlying these changes.[10] Knowledge gained from cervical spine muscle research has underpinned our specific approach to the assessment and rehabilitation of cervical muscle function. This research has extended to the development of therapeutic exercise regimes (Chapter 14) that have shown positive therapeutic benefits when tested in clinical trials.[11-15]

This chapter reviews evidence which describes alterations cervical and axioscapular muscle function associated with neck pain, explores the physiological mechanisms underlying these observations, and provides the foundation for the therapeutic exercise approach described in Chapter 14.

# Changes in muscle strength and endurance

Traditionally, clinical studies have focused on mechanical measures of muscle function such as a change in cervical muscle strength and endurance in people with neck pain using dynamometry devices. Deficits in isometric strength and endurance have been consistently and variously documented in the cervical flexors,[16, 17] craniocervical flexors,[9, 18] and cervical extensor muscles,[19, 20] in association with neck disorders, inclusive of cervicogenic headache and neck pain of both an insidious and traumatic onset. Furthermore deficits in craniocervical flexor endurance have been observed over a range of contraction intensities (maximal voluntary contraction (MVC), 50% and 20% MVC).[9, 18] This is consistent with the finding that the neck flexors have reduced neuromuscular efficiency, particularly at lower contraction levels (25% MVC).[21] Interestingly, neck pain sufferers also exhibit a poorer steadiness of contraction at low load (20% MVC)[9] compared to controls and this may reflect other muscle fatigue manifestations such as muscle tremor.[22] These low-intensity contractile deficits of the cervical flexors observed in neck pain sufferers may be detrimental to the stability of the cervical spine, particularly during prolonged relatively static tasks commonly required in many occupations.

While mechanical measures may indicate changes in muscle performance which need to be addressed in the rehabilitation process, there are limitations. The immediate relevance of reductions in strength may not always be readily obvious in a person with neck pain as maximum strength of the neck muscles is infrequently utilized in everyday function of the cervical spine. In addition, while mechanical measures may provide a good general overview of the function of uniplanar muscle groups, they are less able to provide indications of how individual muscles may be affected by pain. This has prompted research in recent years to focus on the identification of more specific neuromuscular changes in people with neck pain. As a result, there has been an explosive growth in our knowledge of motor control changes in the presence of neck pain.

# Alterations in cervical motor control

There is an emerging body of research demonstrating changes in the amplitude and timing of cervical muscle activation associated with neck disorders.

## Spatial characteristics of muscle activation

EMG studies have demonstrated that neck pain is associated with an inhibition of the deep cervical flexor muscles,[7] longus colli and longus capitis, key postural muscles which support the cervical joints and lordosis.[23–28] Reduced activation of the deep cervical flexors muscles has been observed directly[7] and indirectly[5, 15, 29-34] when patients with neck pain perform a clinical test of craniocervical flexion (for further description of this test, see Chapter 12). The observed reduction in deep cervical flexor muscle activation is concomitant with increased activation of the superficial muscles – the sternocleidomastoid and anterior scalenes, indicating a reorganization of the motor strategy to perform the task[7] (Figure 4.1). Consistent with this observation, additional studies have demonstrated increased activity of superficial cervical flexor muscles in people with neck pain during isometric cervical flexion contractions[21] and during tasks involving dynamic movement of the upper limb.[35, 36] Similarly, greater co-activation of the superficial cervical flexor and extensor muscles has been observed in people with chronic headache during isometric contractions[37] and in office workers

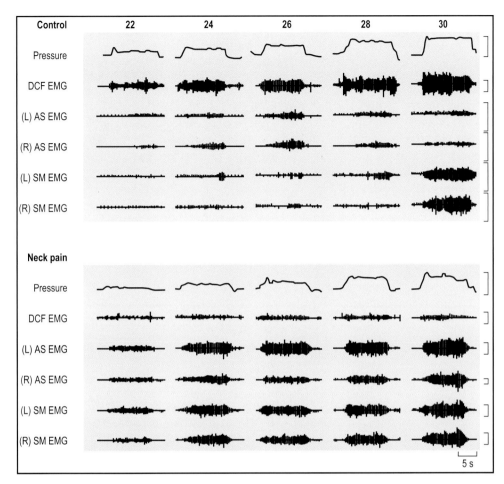

**Figure 4.1** Reorganization of cervical flexor muscle activity during craniocervical flexion: representative raw electromyogram (EMG) data are shown for a control subject and person with neck pain during a task of staged craniocervical flexion. Data are shown for the deep cervical flexors (DCF) and left (L) and right (R) anterior scalene (AS) and sternocleidomastoid (SM) muscles. Note the incremental increase in EMG activity for all muscles with increasing craniocervical flexion (recorded as an increase in pressure in a pressure sensor under the cervical spine) but with lesser activity in the deep cervical flexors and greater activity in the superficial muscles for the neck pain patient. EMG calibration, 0.5 mV. (Reprinted from Falla et al.[7] with permission.)

with neck pain during a typing task[38] which may also increase compressive loading on the spine. This may indicate a measurable compensation for poor passive or active segmental support.[39]

A reorganization of cervical extensor and axioscapular muscle activity has also been observed in persons with neck pain. Increased activity was found in the cervical extensors of office workers with neck pain in a 5-minute typing task.[38] However, reduced activation of the cervical extensor muscles concomitant with increased upper trapezius muscle activity was observed during a prolonged computer task.[40] Moreover, significantly higher amplitude ratios of upper trapezius/cervical extensor activity was identified for the patients complaining of the most discomfort throughout the task.

Altered axioscapular muscle function is a common clinical observation in people with cervical spine pain; however, its prevalence and role in the etiology of cervical spine disorders are not yet clearly understood. Alterations in scapular kinematics and axioscapular muscle activity have certainly been demonstrated in individuals with primary shoulder girdle disorders such as impingement syndromes.[41-44] However, axioscapular muscle function is yet to receive the same scientific attention in cervical spine disorders as it has for specific shoulder girdle conditions. Notwithstanding, observations of altered scapular orientation and motion, apparent impairment of axioscapular muscle function, and axioscapular muscle tenderness are common clinical findings. Changes in upper trapezius muscle activity have also been observed in patients with neck pain of both traumatic[45] and non-traumatic origin[35, 46] during repetitive movement of the upper limb. It is feasible that altered axioscapular muscle function and consequential alterations in the length–tension relationships within the axioscapular muscle group may jeopardize cervical spine stability. This is particularly so for muscles with attachments to the cervical spine such as the levator scapulae and trapezius muscles that induce motion[47] and mechanically load[48] cervical motion segments, potentially demanding greater amplitude of synergistic neck muscle activity to stabilize the head and neck.[49] It is likely that changes in axioscapular muscle coordination will abnormally load cervical spine structures as well as create fatigue within the axioscapular muscles, thus perpetuating the painful condition.

In addition to changes in muscle activation, people with neck pain demonstrate reduced ability to relax the anterior scalene and sternocleidomastoid muscles following activation,[17, 35] and this may indicate a deficit in the sensory system or a change in the descending drive to the motor neuron pool.[50] Upper trapezius also shows decreased ability to relax between[51] and following[35, 46] repetitive arm movements, has reduced muscle rest periods during repetitive tasks,[52, 53] and is generally susceptible to increased activity during tasks involving mental demand.[54-56]

## Temporal characteristics of muscle activation

A change in the timing of the cervical muscles has also been observed in people with neck pain, providing further evidence for a change in motor control of the cervical spine. For example, when a perturbation to the spine occurs, such as during a rapid arm movement, the cervical muscles are co-activated in a feedforward manner in painfree individuals.[6, 57-59] That is, onset of the neck muscles occur within 50 ms of the deltoid, indicating that the response is too fast to be mediated by a reflex. Instead these responses are preplanned by the nervous system prior to the onset of movement. In contrast, when people with neck pain perform a rapid arm movement, onset of both the deep and superficial cervical muscles is delayed.[6] The delay in onset of the neck muscles exceeds the criteria for feedforward contraction during movements, which indicates a significant deficit in the automatic feedforward control of the cervical spine (Figure 4.2). In view of the function of the deep cervical muscles (Chapter 3), this is consistent with a compromise in the control of the cervical spine which may leave the cervical spine vulnerable to further strain.[6] Accordingly, a cervical spine model has shown regions of local segmental instability when large superficial muscles of the neck are simulated to produce movement in the absence of deep muscle activation.[28] A further observation in people with neck pain is that activation of the deep cervical flexor muscles adopts a direction-specific response which is in contrast to that observed in healthy individuals.[6] This indicates that the change is not simply a delay that could be explained by factors such as decreased motor neuron excitability, but instead is consistent with the change in the strategy used by the central nervous system to control the cervical spine.

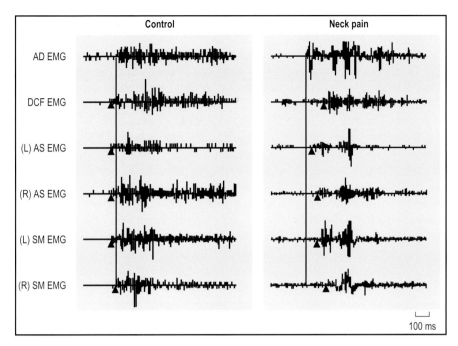

**Figure 4.2** Delayed activation of the cervical flexor muscles during a perturbation: representative raw electromyogram (EMG) data are shown for the anterior deltoid (AD), deep cervical flexors (DCF), left (L) and right (R) sternocleidomastoid (SM) and the anterior scalene (AS) muscles for a control subject and person with neck pain during rapid upper-limb flexion. Line indicates onset of the anterior deltoid; filled triangle denotes onset of neck muscle activation. Note the delayed activation of the neck muscles for the neck pain patient. (Reprinted from Falla et al.[6] with permission.)

In summary, a consistent finding in people with neck pain is impaired activation (both temporal and spatial domains) of the deep cervical muscles, concomitant with augmented superficial muscle activity, which often persists even following completion of a movement or muscle contraction. This has been predominantly observed during tasks of low biomechanical load.[7, 31, 35, 40] However, it must also be noted that there is considerable variability in the change of muscle activity between individuals, as demonstrated by the large standard deviation of EMG data often reported for people with neck pain.[35] There is some evidence that this may be related to the magnitude of pain and disability[35, 36, 38] and thus the individual variability of presentation. It is also in accordance with the notion of redundancy in the cervical muscle system.

## Peripheral adaptations of the cervical muscles

In addition to the concept that pain has a differential effect on motor control of the deep and superficial muscles of the cervical spine, there is complementary evidence from the investigation of the peripheral properties of the cervical muscles in people with neck pain which supports this hypothesis.

Muscle biopsies on ventral (sternocleidomastoid, omohyoid, and longus colli) and dorsal neck muscles (rectus capitis posterior major, obliquus capitis inferior, splenius capitis) in individuals with neck pain have demonstrated a significant increase in the proportion of type IIC fibers with respect to control subjects; this increase is unrelated to the patient diagnosis or presence of neurological symptoms.[60] The

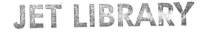

observation of increased type IIC transitional fibers is consistent with a transformation of slow-twitch oxidative type I fibers to fast-twitch glycolytic type IIB fibers. This would suggest a diminution of the tonic contractile capacity of the cervical muscles and is consistent with reduced endurance of the cervical muscles in patients with neck pain,[18,20,61] particularly the reduced endurance determined for low force contractions, as demonstrated in the craniocervical flexors.[9]

Atrophy and connective tissue infiltration of the deep suboccipital muscles have also been documented in people with chronic neck pain.[8, 62-64] In a recent study, fatty infiltrate of both deep and superficial cervical extensor muscles was identified in people with whiplash-associated disorders.[8] Although fatty infiltrate was generally higher in all muscles investigated for the patient group, it was highest in the deeper muscles – the rectus capitis minor/major and multifidi and in particular at the level of the third cervical vertebrae (Figure 4.3). Consistent with this observation, reduced cross-sectional area (CSA) has also been demonstrated in the deep multifidus in chronic whiplash[65] and in the intermediate semispinalis capitis measured at the C2 level in people with chronic cervicogenic headache.[32] However, a recent magnetic resonance imaging study of persons with chronic whiplash showed larger CSAs of multifidus and variable reductions in the CSAs in semispinalis cervicis and capitis. The CSAs mirrored the degree of fatty infiltrate, indicating that both measures need to be considered in defining muscle changes in neck pain.[66]

Muscle biopsies and laser Doppler flowmetry have also shown specific morphological and histological changes in the upper trapezius muscle in people with trapezius myalgia, including morphological signs of disturbed mitochondrial function (ragged red and cytochrome-$c$ oxidase negative fibers),[67, 68] reduced adenosine triphosphate content,[3, 69] and increased CSA of type I muscle fibers despite a lower capillary-to-fiber-area ratio.[3, 67, 68] Such changes may be associated with overload of low-threshold motor units[70] that may explain pain development in individuals performing repetitive tasks at low forces.[71, 72]

The observed greater proportion of type IIC fibers and lower capillary-to-fiber area in the muscles of people with neck pain is also indirectly in agreement with the finding of greater myoelectric manifestations of cervical muscle fatigue during sustained contraction.[73, 74] People with chronic neck pain were shown to have a greater decrease of the mean frequency of EMG signal detected from the sternocleidomastoid and

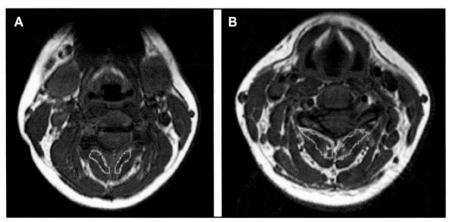

**Figure 4.3** Fatty tissue infiltration of the cervical multifidus: bilateral axial magnetic resonance images of the segmental cervical multifidus muscle at the level of the third cervical vertebra in (A) a healthy control and (B) a person with whiplash-associated disorder. (Reprinted from Elliott et al.[8] with permission.)

anterior scalene muscles during sustained isometric contractions.[74] Moreover people with chronic neck pain demonstrate a greater decrease of upper trapezius muscle fiber conduction velocity during repetitive shoulder elevation[75] (Figure 4.4).

In view of the observation that pain may result in motor control and peripheral modifications of the cervical muscles, it is necessary to consider the possible mechanisms for this effect.

## Mechanisms underlying neuromuscular adaptations in neck pain

Despite our expanding knowledge of changes in muscle function in people with neck pain, interpretations of the mechanisms underlying these observations have been limited and to some degree speculative. That is, it is often difficult to differentiate the potential physiological mechanisms which may contribute to a specific change in cervical neuromuscular function. Furthermore, given the spectrum of neck pain disorders it would be naive to consider that stimulation of peripheral nociceptors is solely responsible for all the neuromuscular changes that have been observed in patients. Rather, it is necessary to consider the interaction between biological, psychological, and social elements of the pain experience and the effect that each factor may have on neuromuscular function of the cervical spine. It is beyond the scope of this chapter to address all aspects and therefore readers are referred to Chapter 7 for a discussion of the psychosocial aspects of neck pain disorders. Rather, this section will consider the direct effects that pain has on muscle function.

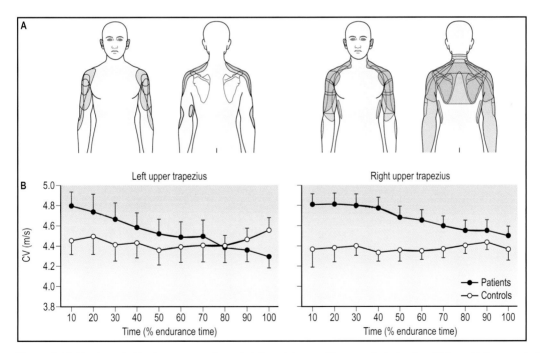

**Figure 4.4** Subjective and objective measures of muscle fatigue during repetitive upper-limb elevation. (A) Area of fatigue reported by control subjects (left) and neck pain patients (right) following performance of a repetitive upper-limb task performed for up to 5 minutes. Note the more widespread area of fatigue for the neck pain patient group. (B) Mean and standard error of the upper trapezius muscle fiber conduction velocity (CV) calculated across the duration of the repetitive upper-limb task. Note the higher initial values and greater decrease of CV estimates across the duration of the task for the patient group. (Reprinted from Falla and Farina[75] with permission.)

## Possible mechanisms underlying changes in cervical motor control

There is continuous debate in the literature as to whether pain changes motor control or whether motor control changes lead to pain. For instance, it has been proposed that deficits in motor control lead to poor control of joint movement, repeated microtrauma, and thus, eventually, to pain.[76] Whilst this hypothesis cannot be ruled out entirely, some of the changes in motor control which have been identified in people with neck pain are also observed following experimental induction of pain in healthy subjects, suggesting that pain may provide the initial trigger for changes in motor control.

The most frequently utilized method of experimentally exciting cervical nociceptors is intramuscular injection of hypertonic saline.[77–79] Hypertonic saline induces a central inhibition within the muscle without modification of the muscle fiber membrane properties.[80] Thus, experimental muscle pain provides a method to assess the effect of pain on cervical motor control in the absence of altered muscle properties, such as those documented in clinical neck pain conditions.[60]

From experimental pain studies it is known that neck muscle pain induces an immediate inhibition of the cervical muscles when acting as agonists.[78, 81–83] For example, during cervical flexion contractions of linearly increasing force, sternocleidomastoid muscle pain results in a force-dependent reduction of sternocleidomastoid EMG amplitude ipsilateral to the side of pain[78] (Figure 4.5). Similarly, splenius capitis muscle pain results in a reduction in splenius capitis EMG amplitude during isometric cervical extension[78] and upper trapezius muscle pain reduces upper trapezius muscle activity in both isometric[81, 82] and dynamic upper-limb tasks.[83, 84]

In addition to a change in the activation of the painful muscle, experimental neck muscle pain induces a dynamic reorganization of the coordination among synergist and/or antagonist muscles. For example, during cervical flexion isometric contractions, pain-induced decreased sternocleidomastoid EMG activity is associated with concomitant bilateral reduction of splenius capitis (Figure 4.5) and trapezius muscle activity.[78] Reduced sternocleidomastoid muscle activity has also been reported during cervical rotation following hypertonic saline-evoked splenius capitis muscle pain[85] and, during dynamic contraction of the upper limb, hypertonic saline-evoked unilateral upper trapezius muscle pain induces a bilateral reorganization in the coordinated activity of the three subdivisions of the trapezius.[83]

In summary, experimental pain studies demonstrate that muscle nociception induces an immediate reorganization of the motor strategy which appears to be adaptive in order to minimize the use of the painful muscle and minimize disruption to the task. Reorganization of cervical motor strategies has also been identified in people with clinical neck pain disorders.[7, 40] Thus, there is convincing evidence that pain leads to changes in motor control of the cervical spine, even though in some cases pain may come secondary to poor motor control. Although it has not been established, it is likely that altered motor control would also be evident following experimental induced pain in deeper structures such as the zygapophyseal joints.

If pain induces a change in cervical motor control, then what are the mechanisms for this effect? Nociceptors project into spinal motor neurons and into the sensorimotor cortex. Thus, it is evident that pain will have a direct impact on motor neuron output through altered synaptic input and on motor planning and muscle control at the cortical level.

The task-dependent nature of pain-induced reorganization of cervical muscle coordination observed in experimental pain studies supports the notion of a change in central

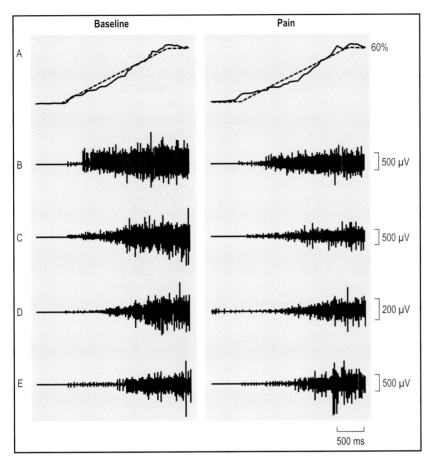

**Figure 4.5** Pain-induced reorganization of cervical muscle activity during isometric contraction: representative force and electromyogram (EMG) data are presented from one subject performing a linearly increasing cervical flexion force contraction from 0 to 60% of the maximum voluntary contraction. Data are presented before (baseline) and during (pain) hypertonic saline-induced sternocleidomastoid muscle pain. A, force; B, sternocleidomastoid EMG ipsilateral to the injection; C, sternocleidomastoid EMG contralateral to the injection; D, splenius capitis EMG ipsilateral to the injection; E, splenius capitis contralateral to the injection. Note the reduction in both sternocleidomastoid and splenius capitis EMG amplitude following sternocleidomastoid muscle pain. (Reprinted from Falla et al.[78] with permission.)

strategies[78] rather than simply a change in motor neuron excitability. Moreover, it has been observed that experimental excitation of cervical nociceptors results in bilateral inhibition of the sternocleidomastoid muscle during cervical flexion, whereas during cervical extension, the agonist (splenius capitis) demonstrated a unilateral inhibition.[78] This finding further supports inhibitory effects at the cortical level in response to nociceptive input.[86]

In clinical neck pain conditions, there are also findings which suggest that alterations in muscle activity are not just simply a change in excitability or delayed transmission of the motor command. As described previously, when people move an arm rapidly, the onset of activation of the deep cervical flexor muscles is independent of the direction of the arm movement.[6] If the delayed response observed during neck pain was a result of a change in excitability, it may be predicted that the response would remain consistent between movement directions, although delayed when people have pain. However, this is not the case and rather the direction-specific response observed in neck pain suggests that there is a change in motor planning. Consistent with this hypothesis, studies have reported that experimental pain changes the activity of regions of the brain involved in movement planning and performance.[87]

Modified cervical afferent input may also affect control of movement. Several studies have reported decreased proprioceptive acuity,[88–90] disturbances of eye movement control[91, 92] and balance[93–95] in people with neck pain disorders which may reflect abnormal input from cervical afferents (Chapter 5). It has also been proposed that neck muscle fatigue may affect mechanisms of postural control by producing abnormal sensory input to the central nervous system and a lasting sense of instability.[96] More-over, psychological stress and anxiety with consequent enhancement in sympathetic drive have the potential to affect the contractility of muscle fibers and to modulate the proprioceptive information arising from the muscle spindle receptors, thus affecting motor control of the cervical muscles.[97] This leads us to explore the mechanisms underlying changes in the peripheral properties of the cervical muscles and the link between muscular and neural changes in people with neck pain.

## Possible mechanisms underlying changes in the peripheral properties of cervical muscles

In addition to the controversial cause–effect relationship between pain and neuromuscular changes, the association between motor control changes and modification of the peripheral properties of the cervical muscles is also not fully understood. Some data suggest that pain by itself does not explain all electrophysiological observations in patients with neck pain. For

example, larger changes in upper trapezius muscle fiber conduction velocity observed in neck pain patients during repetitive shoulder elevation[75] cannot be reproduced in healthy subjects by experimental stimulation of the nociceptors.[83] Similarly, larger myoelectric manifestations of fatigue observed in neck pain patients during sustained cervical contractions[74] cannot be reproduced in healthy subjects by experimental neck pain.[98] Thus, greater fatigue of the cervical muscles, which has been observed in people with neck pain,[74] is more likely to reflect a chronic adaptation to pain, i.e., changes in muscle composition.[60, 67, 68] It has also been proposed that vasoconstriction due to increased sympathetic outflow may explain the observed changes in muscle microcirculation in people with trapezius myalgia.[97] In turn, an altered metabolite concentration in the intercellular muscle interstitium may activate chemosensitive group III and IV muscle afferents that are known to exert complex reflex actions on spinal neurons, thus leading to altered motor control strategies.[97]

Although fatty infiltration of the neck muscles may be the consequence of either a minor nerve injury or irritated and subsequently demyelinated nerve tissue resulting from an acute inflammatory process,[99] it may also be perpetuated by a change in motor strategy. The observation that connective tissue infiltration of the cervical extensor muscles is widespread and not isolated suggests that the degeneration may be a consequence of generalized disuse.[8] It has been argued that atrophic changes in muscle are not uniform and are more likely to affect slow-twitch muscle fibers.[100, 101] For example, rapid atrophy of type I fibers has been observed following injury to the knee[100] and painful stimulation of the sural nerve results in selective inhibition of type I muscle fibers.[102] Consistent with this hypothesis, greatest changes in people with neck pain were identified for the deeper multifidus and suboccipital muscles.[8] Likewise, the smaller amounts of fatty infiltrate in the more superficial muscles may reflect the larger proportion of type II fibers,[69] which have been shown to be more resistant to fiber transformation in patients with cervical spine dysfunction.[60]

In summary, our current evidence suggests that perpetuation of an altered control strategy induced by pain may contribute to muscle overload or disuse and this induces additional adaptations at the muscle level. Thus, although pain-induced reorganization of motor control strategies may be effective in the short term to minimize use of the painful muscle and/or maintain motor output, in the long term this may lead to additional adaptations at the muscle level (Figure 4.6).[103] Likewise, modification of muscle properties may further perpetuate altered motor control. This has implications for selection of therapeutic exercise for the rehabilitation of patients with neck pain.

# Implications for rehabilitation of people with neck pain

People with neck pain demonstrate an array of complex changes in cervical neuromuscular function. These include changes in the deep cervical muscles which are vital for cervical segment support,[6-8, 31, 63, 64] changed motor control strategies, which may result in poor support and potential overload on cervical structures,[31, 35, 45] insufficiency in the preprogrammed activation of cervical muscles,[6] greater fatigability,[73-75] decreased strength and endurance,[9, 17, 18, 20, 32, 61] and morphological and histological changes within the cervical muscles.[60, 68] This section will outline some of the key principles for therapeutic exercise selection for the rehabilitation of muscle function in people with neck pain. The practical aspects of this rehabilitation program are detailed in Chapter 14.

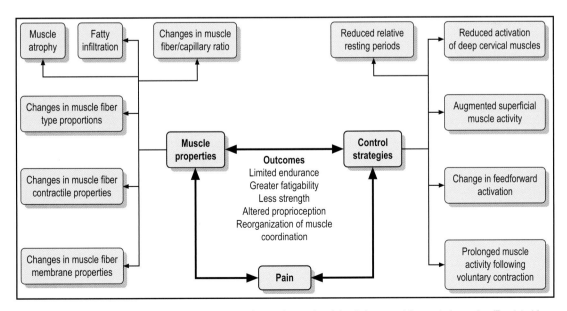

**Figure 4.6** Interrelationships between pain, altered control strategies, and peripheral changes of the cervical muscles. (Reprinted from Falla and Farina[103] with permission.)

## Selectivity and specificity of exercise

Modifications of muscle activity in people with chronic neck pain are likely to be the result of a combination of altered neural input to muscles and changed muscle properties.[10] Consequently, therapeutic exercise approaches for the rehabilitation of people with neck pain should address both peripheral and central neuromuscular adaptations which have been identified in these patients. This approach has been supported in a series of clinical trials which investigated the efficacy of specific therapeutic exercise interventions for the rehabilitation of cervical muscle function.[12-14] For example, a low-load exercise regime which trains the deep craniocervical flexors, longus colli and longus capitis,[104] is effective at increasing the activation of the deep cervical flexor muscles, enhancing the speed of their activation when challenged by a postural perturbation,[12] and improving the ability to maintain an upright posture of the cervical spine during prolonged sitting.[14] Similar benefits were not achieved following 6 weeks of higher-load strength and endurance training for the cervical muscles.[12, 14] However, provision of load to challenge the neck flexor muscles is required to reduce the fatigability of the sternocleidomastoid and anterior scalene muscles in people with neck pain (Figure 4.7).[13] Likewise, higher-load strength training is required to improve the strength of the cervical muscles,[13] an outcome which may not occur following lower-load muscle retraining. This observation is consistent with low-back pain literature, which indicates that low-level activation of the multifidus is not sufficient to reverse multifidus atrophy in people with chronic low-back pain.[105]

The need for specificity in therapeutic exercise selection is also highlighted by studies demonstrating selective changes within muscle groups and/or regions in response to pain. For example, experimentally induced knee joint effusions result in a preferential inhibition of the vastus medialis muscle of the quadriceps group.[106, 107] In the cervical spine, fatty infiltration of the rectus capitis posterior minor and major muscles and the multifidi were most obvious at particular segmental levels.[8] Side specificity of neuromuscular changes has also been demonstrated in patients with unilateral pain. For example, atrophy of the semispinalis cervicis occurs ipsilateral to the side of headache in cervicogenic headache sufferers[32] and sternocleidomastoid muscle fatigue is greater on the side of pain in people with unilateral neck pain.[108] An experimental pain study has also shown that there may be reorganization of activity within the same muscle in response to painful stimulation.[81] These studies demonstrate that exercise should be selected based on careful and precise assessment of neuromuscular changes and thus be specific to the impairments of the presenting patient.

## Early rehabilitation

Changes in cervical motor control have been documented soon after the onset of neck pain.[109] Experimental pain studies also indicate that pain induces an immediate yet complex reorganization of muscle activity.[78, 83] Failure to rehabilitate altered motor control may result in further long-term changes in cervical muscle properties, such as selective muscle fiber atrophy,[60] which have been documented in people with chronic neck pain. This knowledge suggests the need for early management of altered cervical neuromotor control.

## Painfree rehabilitation

Since pain induces a change in muscle activity,[78, 83] performing exercises which provoke neck pain is unlikely to be beneficial for encouraging normal motor control of the cervical spine. Therefore, the type, load, and frequency of exercise should be tailored

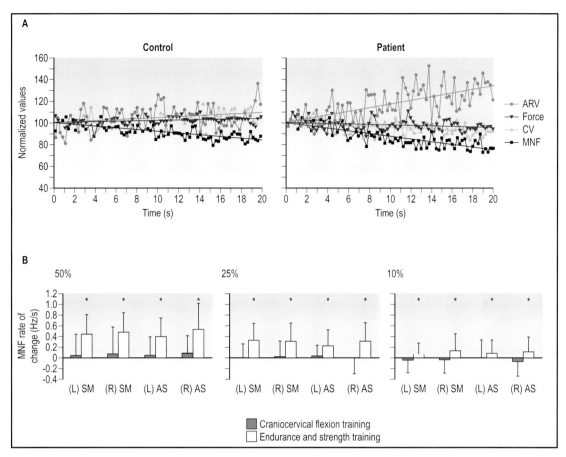

**Figure 4.7** Greater cervical muscle fatigability is reduced following specific exercise intervention. (A) Example of fatigue plots obtained from the sternocleidomastoid muscle of a control subject and a neck pain patient contracting at 50% of maximum force. The data represent the electromyogram (EMG) average rectified value (ARV), conduction velocity (CV), and mean frequency (MNF) normalized with respect to the intercept of the regression line. Greater fatigue of the sternocleidomastoid muscle is evident for the neck pain patient, as characterized by the faster rate of change of the MNF over time. (Reprinted from Falla et al.[13] with permission) (B) Change in muscle fatigue following exercise intervention: data (mean and sd) are shown for the change (pre- to postintervention) in MNF rate of change for the left (L) and right (R) sternocleidomastoid (SM) and anterior scalene (AS) muscles contracting at 50%, 25%, and 10% of the maximum voluntary contraction. Patients with chronic neck pain were randomized into two groups: endurance and strength training of the cervical flexors or low-load craniocervical flexion retraining. Following 6 weeks of exercise intervention, a reduction in cervical muscle fatigue was identified only for the patients who participated in the strength and endurance training program. *$P < 0.05$ between groups. (Reprinted from Falla et al.[74] with permission.)

towards the patient to ensure that this criterion can be met. Other therapeutics which assist in resolving pain will also play an important role in the management of motor control dysfunction.

## Rehabilitation for prevention of recurrence

The observed changes in motor control of the cervical spine in people with neck pain have often been detected in patients who are currently in remission of symptoms at the time of testing.[74] Furthermore, changes in cervical muscle activation have been shown to persist in people who have had a whiplash injury, even if full recovery of symptoms is reported.[109, 110] Similar findings of continuous muscle inhibition have been reported for the multifidus muscle in low-back pain patients[111] and the quadriceps muscle following knee surgery[112] despite recovery of symptoms and return to normal activity. Although not confirmed, ongoing changes in muscle function may explain the high recurrence rate of neck pain symptoms.[113] Moreover, actual pain may not necessarily have to be present for motor control changes to be existent. Factors such as fear of pain may have similar effects and may explain motor control changes in patients with musculoskeletal pain when they are in remission.[50] Taken together, these observations further emphasize the need for early and effective rehabilitation of altered cervical muscle function.

# Conclusion

Pain induces an immediate change in cervical muscle function. Accordingly, a complex array of cervical neuromuscular adaptations has been documented in people with neck pain. These include both modification of cervical motor control as well as peripheral modifications, including atrophy of specific muscle fibers and changes in muscle microcirculation. Our progressive understanding of changes in cervical muscle function in the presence of neck pain has directed rehabilitation programs to include more specific therapeutic exercise regimes as a component of a multimodal intervention. Moreover, clinical trials have demonstrated that exercise programs should be tailored towards the impairments and thus based on a detailed and specific assessment to detect these changes. An evidence-based detailed clinical assessment and rehabilitation approach are provided in Chapters 12 and 14.

# References

1. *Keshner EA*. Motor control of the cervical spine. In: Boyling JD, Jull G (eds) Grieve's Modern Manual Therapy: The Vertebral Column, 3rd ed. Edinburgh: Elsevier, 2004:105-117.

2. *Peterson BW, Pellionisz AJ, Baker JF, et al.* Functional morphology and neural control of neck muscles in mammals. Am Zool 1989;29:139–149.

3. *Larsson R, Cai H, Zhang Q, et al.* Visualization of chronic neck-shoulder pain: impaired microcirculation in the upper trapezius muscle in chronic cervico-brachial pain. Occup Med 1998;48:189–194.

4. *Larsson B, Bjork J, Elert J, et al.* Fibre type proportion and fibre size in trapezius muscle biopsies from cleaners with and without myalgia and its correlation with ragged red fibres, cytochrome-c-oxidase-negative fibres, biomechanical output, perception of fatigue, and surface electromyography during repetitive forward flexions. Eur J Appl Physiol 2001;84:492–502.

5. *Jull G, Kristjansson E, Dall'Alba P.* Impairment in the cervical flexors: a comparison of whiplash and insidious onset neck pain patients. Man Ther 2004;9:89–94.

6. *Falla D, Jull G, Hodges PW.* Feedforward activity of the cervical flexor muscles during voluntary arm movements is delayed in chronic neck pain. Exp Brain Res 2004;157:43–48.

7. *Falla D, Jull G, Hodges PW.* Patients with neck pain demonstrate reduced electromyographic activity of the deep cervical flexor muscles during performance of the craniocervical flexion test. Spine 2004;29:2108–2114.

8. *Elliott J, Jull G, Noteboom JT, et al.* Fatty infiltration in the cervical extensor muscles in persistent whiplash-associated disorders: a magnetic resonance imaging analysis. Spine 2006;31:847–855.

9. *O'Leary S, Jull G, Kim M, et al.* Craniocervical flexor muscle impairment at maximal, moderate, and low loads is a feature of neck pain. Man Ther 2007;12:34–39.

10. *Falla D, Farina D.* Neuromuscular adaptation in experimental and clinical neck pain. J Electromyogr Kinesiol 2006:In Press.

11. *Jull G, Trott P, Potter H, et al.* A randomized controlled trial of exercise and manipulative therapy for cervicogenic headache. Spine 2002;27:1835–1843.

12. *Jull G.* Cervical flexor muscle retraining: physiological mechanisms of efficacy. 2nd International Conference on Movement Dysfunction. Cairns M, Comerford M, Gibbons S et al (eds). Kinetic Control and Manipulation Association of Chartered Physiotherapists (UK). Edinburgh, Scotland: 2005:L01.

13. *Falla D, Jull G, Hodges P, et al.* An endurance-strength training regime is effective in reducing myoelectric manifestations of cervical flexor muscle fatigue in females with chronic neck pain. Clin Neurophysiol 2006;117:828–837.

14. *Falla D, Jull G, Russell T, et al.* Effect of neck exercise on sitting posture in patients with chronic neck pain. Phys Ther 2007;87:408-417.

15. *Jull G, Sterling M, Kenardy J, et al*. Does the presence of sensory hypersensitivity influence outcomes of physical rehabilitation for chronic whiplash? A preliminary RCT. Pain 2007;129:28-34.

16. *Silverman JL, Rodriquez AA, Agre JC*. Quantitative cervical flexor strength in healthy subjects and in subjects with mechanical neck pain. Arch Phys Med Rehabil 1991;72:679-681.

17. *Barton PM, Hayes KC*. Neck flexor muscle strength, efficiency, and relaxation times in normal subjects and subjects with unilateral neck pain and headache. Arch Phys Med Rehabil 1996;77:680-687.

18. *Watson DH, Trott PH*. Cervical headache: an investigation of natural head posture and upper cervical flexor muscle performance. Cephalalgia 1993;13:272-284.

19. *Vernon HT, Aker P, Aramenko M, et al*. Evaluation of neck muscle strength with a modified sphygmomanometer dynamometer: reliability and validity. J Manipul Physiol Ther 1992;15:343-349.

20. *Placzek JD, Pagett BT, Roubal PJ, et al*. The influence of the cervical spine on chronic headache in women: a pilot study. J Manual Manipul Ther 1999;7:33-39.

21. *Falla D, Jull G, Edwards S, et al*. Neuromuscular efficiency of the sternocleidomastoid and anterior scalene muscles in patients with chronic neck pain. Disabil Rehabil 2004;26:712-717.

22. *Gandevia SC*. Spinal and supraspinal factors in human muscle fatigue. Physiol Rev 2001;81:1725-1789.

23. *Boyd Clark LC, Briggs CA, Galea MP*. Comparative histochemical composition of muscle fibres in a pre- and a postvertebral muscle of the cervical spine. J Anat 2001;199:709-716.

24. *Boyd Clark LC, Briggs CA, Galea MP*. Muscle spindle distribution, morphology, and density in longus colli and multifidus muscles of the cervical spine. Spine 2002;27:694-701.

25. *Conley MS, Meyer RA, Bloomberg JJ, et al*. Noninvasive analysis of human neck muscle function. Spine 1995;20:2505-2512.

26. *Mayoux-Benhamou MA, Revel M, Vallee C, et al*. Longus colli has a postural function on cervical curvature. Surg Radiol Anat 1994;16:367-371.

27. *Vasavada AN, Li S, Delp SL*. Influence of muscle morphometry and moment arms on the moment-generating capacity of human neck muscles. Spine 1998;23:412-422.

28. *Winters JM, Peles JD*. Neck muscle activity and 3D head kinematics during quasistatic and dynamic tracking movements. In: Winters JM, Woo SL-Y (eds) Multiple Muscle Systems: Biomechanics and Movement Organisation. New York: Springer-Verlag, 1990:461-480.

29. *Sterling M, Jull G, Wright A*. The effect of musculoskeletal pain on motor activity and control. J Pain 2001;2:135-145.

30. *Jull G, Barrett C, Magee R, et al*. Further clinical clarification of the muscle dysfunction in cervical headache. Cephalalgia 1999;19:179-185.

31. *Jull GA*. Deep cervical flexor muscle dysfunction in whiplash. J Musculoskel Pain 2000;8:143-154.

32. *Jull G, Amiri M, Bullock-Saxton J, et al*. Cervical musculoskeletal impairment in frequent intermittent headache. Part 1: subjects with single headaches. Cephalalgia 2007;27:793-802.

33. *Chiu TT, Law E, Chiu TH*. Performance of the craniocervical flexion test in subjects with and without chronic neck pain. J Orthop Sports Phys Ther 2005;35:567-571.

34. *Amiri M, Jull G, Bullock-Saxton J, et al*. Cervical musculoskeletal impairment in frequent intermittent headache. Part 2: subjects with multiple headaches. Cephalalgia 2007;27:891-898.

35. *Falla D, Bilenkij G, Jull G*. Patients with chronic neck pain demonstrate altered patterns of muscle activation during performance of a functional upper limb task. Spine 2004;29:1436-1440.

36. *Johnston V, Jull G, Souvlis T, et al*. Neck movement and muscle activity characteristics in office workers with neck pain. Spine 2008:In Press.

37. *Fernandez-de-las-Penas C, Falla D, Arendt-Nielsen L, et al*. Cervical muscle co-contraction in isometric contraction is enhanced in chronic tension type headache patients. Cephalalgia 2008:In Press.

38. *Johnston V, Jull G, Souvlis T, et al*. Alterations in cervical muscle activity in functional and stressful tasks in female office workers with neck pain. 2007: Submitted for publication.

39. *Cholewicki J, Panjabi MM, Khachatryan A*. Stabilizing function of trunk flexor-extensor muscles around a neutral spine posture. Spine 1997;22:2207-2212.

40. *Szeto GP, Straker LM, O'Sullivan PB*. A comparison of symptomatic and asymptomatic office workers performing monotonous keyboard work 1: Neck and shoulder muscle recruitment patterns. Man Ther 2005;10:270-280.

41. *Ludewig PM, Cook TM*. Alterations in shoulder kinematics and associated muscle activity in people with symptoms of shoulder impingement. Phys Ther 2000;80:276-291.

42. *Lukasiewicz A, McClure P, Michener L, et al*. Comparison of 3-dimensional scapular position and orientation between subjects with and without shoulder impingement. J Orthop Sports Phys Ther 1999;29:574-586.

43. *Endo K, Ikata T, Katoh S, et al*. Radiographic assessment of scapular rotational tilt in chronic shoulder impingement syndrome. J Orthop Sci 2001;6:3-10.

44. *Cools AM, Witvrouw EE, Declercq GA, et al*. Scapular muscle recruitment patterns: trapezius muscle latency with and without impingement syndrome. Am J Sports Med 2003;31:542-549.

45. *Nederhand MJ, Ijzerman MJ, Hermens HJ, et al*. Cervical muscle dysfunction in the chronic whiplash associated disorder grade II (WAD-II). Spine 2000;25:1938-1943.

46. *Nederhand MJ, Hermens H, Ijzerman MJ, et al*. Cervical muscle dysfunction in the chronic whiplash associated disorder grade 2: the relevance of the trauma. Spine 2002;27:1056–1061.

47. *Moore KL, Dalley AF*. Clinically Orientated Anatomy, 4th ed. Philadelphia: Lippincott Williams and Wilkins, 1999.

48. *Behrsin JF, Maguire K*. Levator scapulae action during shoulder movement. A possible mechanism of shoulder pain of cervical origin. Aust J Physiother 1986;32:101–106.

49. *Eliot DJ*. Electromyography of levator scapulae: new findings allow tests of a head stabilization model. J Manipul Physiol Ther 1996;19:19–25.

50. *Hodges P*. Pain Models. In: Richardson C, Hodges P, Hides J (eds) Therapeutic Exercise for Lumbopelvic Stabilization: A Motor Control Approach for the Treatment and Prevention of Low Back Pain. Edinburgh: Churchill Livingstone, 2004:129–137.

51. *Fredin Y, Elert J, Britschgi N, et al*. A decreased ability to relax between repetitive muscle contractions in patients with chronic symptoms after whiplash trauma of the neck. J Musculoskel Pain 1997;5:55–70.

52. *Hägg GM, Anstrom A*. Load pattern and pressure pain threshold in the upper trapezius muscle and psychosocial factors in medical secretaries with and without shoulder/neck disorders. Int Arch Occup Environ Health 1997;69:423–432.

53. *Veiersted KB, Westgaard RH, Andersen P*. Pattern of muscle activity during stereotyped work and its relation to muscle pain. Int Arch Occup Environ Health 1990;62:31–41.

54. *Bansevicius D, Sjaastad O*. Cervicogenic headache: the influence of mental load on pain level and EMG of shoulder–neck and facial muscles. Headache 1996;36:372–378.

55. *Laursen B, Jensen BR, Garde AH, et al*. Effect of mental and physical demands on muscular activity during the use of a computer mouse and a keyboard. Scand J Work Environ Health 2002;28:215–221.

56. *Westgaard RH*. Muscle activity as a releasing factor for pain in the shoulder and neck. Cephalalgia 1999;19:251–258.

57. *Falla D, Rainoldi A, Merletti R, et al*. Spatio-temporal evaluation of neck muscle activation during postural perturbations in healthy subjects. J Electromyogr Kinesiol 2004;14:463–474.

58. *Gurfinkel VS, Lipshits MI, Lestienne FG*. Anticipatory neck muscle activity associated with rapid arm movements. Neurosci Lett 1988;94:104–108.

59. *van der Fits IBM, Kilp AWJ, van Eykern LA, et al*. Postural adjustments accompanying fast pointing movements in standing, sitting and lying adults. Exp Brain Res 1998;120:202–216.

60. *Uhlig Y, Weber BR, Grob D, et al*. Fiber composition and fiber transformations in neck muscles of patients with dysfunction of the cervical spine. J Orthop Res 1995;13:240–249.

61. *Treleaven J, Jull G, Atkinson L*. Cervical musculoskeletal dysfunction in post-concussional headache. Cephalalgia 1994;14:273–279.

62. *Andary MT, Hallgren RC, Greenman PE, et al*. Neurogenic atrophy of suboccipital muscles after a cervical injury: a case study. Am J Phys Med Rehabil 1998;77:545–549.

63. *Hallgren RC, Greenman PE, Rechtien JJ*. Atrophy of suboccipital muscles in patients with chronic pain: a pilot study. J Am Osteopath Assoc 1994;94:1032–1038.

64. *McPartland JM, Brodeur RR, Hallgren RC*. Chronic neck pain, standing balance, and suboccipital muscle atrophy – a pilot study. J Manipul Physiol Ther 1997;20:24–29.

65. *Kristjansson E*. Reliability of ultrasonography for the cervical multifidus muscle in asymptomatic and symptomatic subjects. Man Ther 2004;9:83–88.

66. *Elliott J, Jull G, Noteboom T, et al*. MRI study of the cross sectional area for the cervical extensor musculature in patients with persistent whiplash associated disorders (WAD). Man Ther 2007:In Press.

67. *Kadi F, Waling K, Ahlgren C, et al*. Pathological mechanisms implicated in localized female trapezius myalgia. Pain 1998;78:191–196.

68. *Lindman R, Hagberg M, Angqvist K, et al*. Changes in muscle morphology in chronic trapezius myalgia. Scand J Work Environ Health 1991;17:347–355.

69. *Lindman R, Eriksson A, Thornell LE*. Fiber type composition of the human female trapezius muscle: enzyme-histochemical characteristics. Am J Anat 1991;190:385–392.

70. *Hägg GM*. Static work loads and occupational myalgia – a new explanation model. In: Anderson PA, Hobart DJ, Danoff JV (eds) Electromyographical Kinesiology. Amsterdam: Elsevier, 1991:141–143.

71. *Sjøgaard G, Lundberg U, Kadefors R*. The role of muscle activity and mental load in the development of pain and degenerative processes at the muscle cell level during computer work. Eur J Appl Physiol 2000;83:99–105.

72. *Mork PJ, Westgaard RH*. Low-amplitude trapezius activity in work and leisure and the relation to shoulder and neck pain. J Appl Physiol 2006;100:1142–1149.

73. *Gogia PP, Sabbahi MA*. Electromyographic analysis of neck muscle fatigue in patients with osteoarthritis of the cervical spine. Spine 1994;19:502–506.

74. *Falla D, Rainoldi A, Merletti R, et al*. Myoelectric manifestations of sternocleidomastoid and anterior scalene muscle fatigue in chronic neck pain patients. Clin Neurophysiol 2003;114:488–495.

75. *Falla D, Farina D*. Muscle fiber conduction velocity of the upper trapezius muscle during dynamic contraction of the upper limb in patients with chronic neck pain. Pain 2005;116:138–145.

76. *Panjabi MM*. The stabilizing system of the spine. Part II. Neutral zone and instability hypothesis. J Spinal Disord 1992;5:390–396.

77. *Birch L, Arendt-Nielsen L, Graven-Nielsen T, et al*. An investigation of how acute muscle pain modulates performance during computer work with digitizer and puck. Appl Ergon 2001;32:281–286.

78. *Falla D, Farina D, Kanstrup Dahl M, et al*. Muscle pain induces task-dependent changes in cervical agonist/antagonist activity. J Appl Physiol 2007;102:601–609.

79. *Schmidt-Hansen PT, Svensson P, Jensen TS, et al*. Patterns of experimentally induced pain in pericranial muscles. Cephalalgia 2006;26:568–577.

80. *Farina D, Arendt-Nielsen L, Merletti R, et al*. Effect of experimental muscle pain on motor unit firing rate and conduction velocity. J Neurophysiol 2004;91:1250–1259.

81. *Madeleine P, Leclerc F, Arendt-Nielsen L, et al*. Experimental muscle pain changes the spatial distribution of upper trapezius muscle activity during sustained contraction. Clin Neurophysiol 2006;117:2436–2445.

82. *Ge HY, Arendt-Nielsen L, Farina D, et al*. Gender-specific differences in electromyographic changes and perceived pain induced by experimental muscle pain during sustained contractions of the upper trapezius muscle. Muscle Nerve 2005;32:726–733.

83. *Falla D, Farina D, Graven-Nielsen T*. Experimental muscle pain results in reorganization of coordination among trapezius muscle subdivisions during repetitive shoulder flexion. Exp Brain Res 2007;178:385-393.

84. *Madeleine P, Lundager B, Voigt M, et al*. Shoulder muscle co-ordination during chronic and acute experimental neck-shoulder pain. An occupational pain study. Eur J App Physiol Occup Physiol 1999;79:127–140.

85. *Svensson P, Wang K, Sessle BJ, et al*. Associations between pain and neuromuscular activity in the human jaw and neck muscles. Pain 2004;109:225–232.

86. *Le Peru D, Graven-Nielsen T, Valeriani M, et al*. Inhibition of motor system excitability at cortical and spinal level by tonic muscle pain. Clin Neurophysiol 2001;112:1633–1641.

87. *Derbyshire SW, Jones AK, Gyulai F, et al*. Pain processing during three levels of noxious stimulation produces differential patterns of central activity. Pain 1997;73:431–445.

88. *Revel M, Andre Deshays C, Minguet M*. Cervicocephalic kinesthetic sensibility in patients with cervical pain. Arch Phys Med Rehabil 1991;72:288–291.

89. *Heikkila H, Astrom P*. Cervicocephlic kinesthetic sensibility in patients with whiplash injury. J Rehabil Med 1996;28:133–138.

90. *Treleaven J, Jull G, Sterling M*. Dizziness and unsteadiness following whiplash injury: characteristic features and relationship with cervical joint position error. J Rehabil Med 2003;35:36–43.

91. *Tjell C, Rosenhall U*. Smooth pursuit neck torsion test: a specific test for cervical dizziness. Am J Otol 1998;19:76–81.

92. *Treleaven J, Jull G, LowChoy N*. Smooth pursuit neck torsion test in whiplash-associated disorders: relationship to self-reports of neck pain and disability, dizziness and anxiety. J Rehabil Med 2005;37:219–223.

93. *Kogler A, Lindfors J, Odkvist LM, et al*. Postural stability using different neck positions in normal subjects and patients with neck trauma. Acta Otolaryngol 2000;120:151–155.

94. *Michaelson P, Michaelson M, Jaric S, et al*. Vertical posture and head stability in patients with chronic neck pain. J Rehabil Med 2003;35:229–235.

95. *Treleaven J, Jull G, LowChoy N*. Standing balance in persistent whiplash: a comparison between subjects with and without dizziness. J Rehabil Med 2005;37:224–229.

96. *Schieppati M, Nardone A, Schmid M*. Neck muscle fatigue affects postural control in man. Neuroscience 2003;121:277–285.

97. *Passatore M, Roatta S*. Influence of sympathetic nervous system on sensorimotor function: whiplash associated disorders (WAD) as a model. Eur J Appl Physiol 2006;98:423–449.

98. *Falla D, Farina D, Kanstrup Dahl M, et al*. Pain induced changes in cervical muscle activation do not affect muscle fatigability during sustained isometric contraction. J Electromyogr Kinesiol 2007:In Press.

99. *Nukuda H, McMorran D, Shimizu J*. Acute inflammatory demyelination in reperfusion nerve injury. Ann Neurol 2000;47:71–79.

100. *Haggmark T, Jansson E, Eriksson E*. Fiber type area and metabolic potential of the thigh muscle in man after knee surgery and immobilization. Int J Sports Med 1981;2:12–17.

101. *Meyer DC, Pirkl C, Pfirrmann CW, et al*. Asymmetric atrophy of the supraspinatus muscle following tendon tear. J Orthop Res 2005;23:254–258.

102. *Gydikov AA*. Pattern of discharge of different types of alpha motor units during voluntary and reflex activities under normal physiological conditions. In: Komi PV (ed) Biomechanics. Baltimore, MD: University Park Press, 1976:45–57.

103. *Falla D, Farina D*. Altered muscle activity during clinical and experimental neck pain. Curr Rheumatol Rep 2007:In Press.

104. *Jull G, Falla D, Treleaven J, et al*. A therapeutic exercise approach for cervical disorders. In: Boyling JD, Jull G (eds) Grieve's Modern Manual Therapy: The Vertebral Column, 3rd edn. Edinburgh: Elsevier, 2004:451-470.

105. *Danneels LA, Vanderstraeten GG, Cambier DC, et al*. Effects of three different training modalities on the cross sectional area of the lumbar multifidus muscle in patients with chronic low back pain. Br J Sports Med 2001;35:186–191.

106. *Kennedy JC, Alexander IJ, Hayes KC*. Nerve supply of the human knee and its functional importance. Am J Sports Med 1982;10:329–335.

107. *Spencer JD, Hayes KC, Alexander IJ*. Knee joint effusion and quadriceps reflex inhibition in man. Arch Phys Med Rehabil 1984;65:171–177.

108. *Falla D, Jull G, Rainoldi A, et al*. Neck flexor muscle fatigue is side specific in patients with unilateral neck pain. Eur J Pain 2004;8:71–77.

109. *Sterling M, Jull G, Vicenzino B, et al*. Development of motor dysfunction following whiplash injury. Pain 2003;103:65–73.

110. *Sterling M, Jull G, Vicenzino B, et al*. Physical and psychological factors predict outcome following whiplash injury. Pain 2005;114: 141–148.

111. *Hides JA, Richardson CA, Jull GA*. Multifidus muscle recovery is not automatic after resolution of acute, first-episode low back pain. Spine 1996;21:2763–2769.

112. *Stokes M, Young A*. Investigations of quadriceps inhibition: implications for clinical practice. Physiother 1984;70:425–428.

113. *Gore DR, Sepic SB, Gardner GM, et al*. Neck pain: a long term follow-up of 205 patients. Spine 1987;12:1–5.

# 5

# The Cervical Spine and Sensorimotor Control

## Introduction

People with neck pain may demonstrate other alterations in sensorimotor function in addition to changes in muscle activation (Chapter 4). These alterations include changes in eye movement control, reduced proprioceptive acuity, and disturbed balance. Understanding how and why cervical spine disorders can influence such sensorimotor control, as well as being able to quantify impairments, provides direction for precise assessment and interventions for people with neck pain. Thus the mechanisms associated with disturbed cervical somatosensory input to the sensorimotor control system will first be reviewed. The impairments in sensorimotor control that may present in patients with neck pain will then be discussed (Chapter 6).

Afferent information from the vestibular, visual, and somatosensory systems converges in multiple areas within the central nervous system and is important for general equilibrium, body orientation, and oculomotor control. The abundance of mechanoreceptors in the muscles and joints of the cervical spine and the central and reflex connections from cervical afferents to the vestibular, visual, and postural control systems suggests that cervical proprioceptive information provides important somatosensory information, influencing postural stability, head orientation, and eye movement control.[1] Abnormal afferent input from the vestibular, visual, or somatosensory systems can result in abnormal sensorimotor control. The resulting mismatch, which may occur in the presence of conflicting afferent information, is thought to underlie symptoms of dizziness or unsteadiness, problems in maintaining a stable upright posture, and measurable deficits in head and eye movement control in people with neck pain.[2–6]

There are many possible mechanisms that may disturb cervical somatosensory input in those with neck pain or neck pain and headache, especially following neck injury. Firstly, afferent information from the cervical receptors (mechanoreceptors and nociceptors) can be altered either by direct trauma or as a consequence of impaired muscle function.[3] Secondly, inflammatory mediators may activate chemosensitive nerve endings in joints and muscles, leading to altered muscle spindle activity.[7, 8] Thirdly, the direct effect of nociception on mechanoreceptors can influence the central modulation of cervical somatosensory input, thus affecting sensorimotor control.[9, 10] Fourthly, the sympathetic nervous system may exert effects on muscle spindle activity,[11] thus affecting cervical somatosensory input.

The purpose of this chapter is to review the potential effects of disturbed cervical somatosensory input on sensorimotor control. The morphology of cervical mechanoreceptors and their central and reflex connections will be reviewed, followed by discussion of the signs and symptoms that present following artificial disturbance to the cervical mechanoreceptors. The discussion will then review how disturbed somatosensory input from the cervical spine influences sensorimotor control and conclude with possible mechanisms and etiology of disturbed somatosensory cervical input in people with neck pain.

# Morphology of cervical mechanoreceptors

Sensory information provided by receptors in the cervical structures conveys information for sensorimotor control. Muscle receptors, particularly muscle spindles, are probably the most significant receptors and are found in high densities in the cervical region. There is a higher density of mechanoreceptors in the upper cervical joints compared to the lower cervical joints; however, mechanoreceptors are present in greater proportions in muscle compared to joints.[12, 13] This suggests that mechanoreceptors in articular structures only supplement information from the abundant muscle spindles.[14–16] Nevertheless, joint and ligament receptors, via their influence on muscle spindles and the gamma motor neurons, are considered to be important for the initiation of protective muscle activation to prevent joint degeneration and instability.[9, 17]

The segmental and multisegmental muscles of the neck contain relatively high densities of mechanoreceptors. Muscle spindles, Golgi tendon organs, and paciniform corpuscles have been identified in the human cervical spine. The density of muscle spindles is highest in the suboccipital muscles and, even more specifically, in the deeper sections of these muscles.[12, 13] The average number of muscle spindles found per gram of muscle is: 242 in the obliquus capitis inferior; 190 in obliquus capitis superior; 98 in the rectus capitis posterior minor; 48.6 in the longus colli at the C5-6 level (concentrated away from the vertebral body); and 24.3 in the multifidus at the C5-6 segmental level.[13] For comparison, the first lumbrical in the hand has 16 and the superficial trapezius muscle has 2 muscle spindles per gram of muscle.

In addition to the high density of muscle spindles, the cervical region appears to be quite unique with respect to the arrangements of muscle spindles.[18] Spindles exist as single muscle spindles or are linked in pairs, parallel or tandem, with up to 35–50% of the total spindles being in tandem. In contrast, a tandem arrangement is less common in leg muscles (10–25%).[19, 20] Neck muscle spindles are also compartmentalized in series within the muscle, allowing a response to both stretch and contraction, leading to effective tension generation in the muscle.[21] The density and distinct morphological features of muscle spindles in the deep neck muscles demonstrate their importance for movement precision, proprioception, control of head position, and eye–head coordination.[18] The muscle fiber composition of the deep suboccipital muscles also supports their key role in proprioception of the cervical spine,[12, 22, 23] with particularly high numbers of slow-twitch muscle fibers and muscle spindles found in the deepest portion of the obliquus capitis inferior[20] and rectus capitis posterior minor muscles.[24]

# Central connections

Cervical afferents provide input to the ventral and dorsal horn in the spinal cord. They can directly excite the spinothalamic, spinocerebellar, and long propriospinal neurons in the upper cervical cord. This relay to the thalamus, cerebellum, and somatosensory cortex serves to integrate and formulate appropriate efferent neuromuscular responses.[25] Cervical afferents also provide input to the dorsal column nuclei and the central cervical nucleus[26] (Figure 5.1). Cervical afferents play an important role in the mediation of reflex responses and subsequent connections between the visual and vestibular apparatus. Neck afferents project to the medial and lateral vestibular nuclei as well as the superior colliculus, a reflex center for coordination between vision and neck movement.[27, 28] Cervical afferents may also influence the sympathetic nervous system via beta receptors within muscle tissue.[29-31] Conversely, sympathetic nerve stimulation may have direct effects on the dorsal muscle spindles.[32]

It appears that the deep suboccipital muscles, in tandem with their important proprioceptive role, are particularly important for relaying and receiving information for sensorimotor control to and from the central nervous system.[18] There is evidence from feline studies that the central cervical nucleus, which projects to the cerebellum, is powerfully influenced by

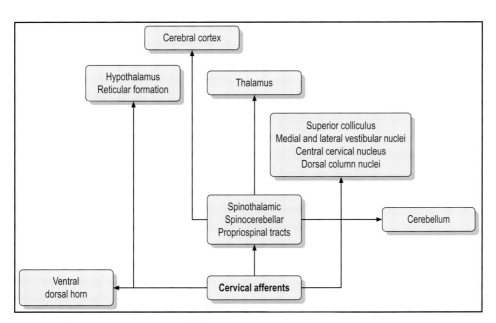

**Figure 5.1** Central connections from cervical afferents.

mechanoreceptors in the deep neck muscles.[30] In addition, many descending systems, which have been implicated in the control of head movement, have dense projections into the C1 and C2 segments, which contain the motor neurons for the deep suboccipital muscles. It has also been shown in the cat that motor neurons of neck muscles have their own characteristic patterns of input from the six semicircular canals of the vestibular apparatus. Interestingly, the obliquus capitis inferior muscle has a different pattern to the rectus capitis major and minor and mutifidus muscles.[33] This may translate to functional differences between these muscles in humans where different morphological characteristics have been shown to exist.

## Reflex-mediated activity

Synaptic connections from the cervical receptors to other areas of the central nervous system play an important role in neck reflex activity. Neck afferents are involved in reflexes which influence head orientation, eye movement control, and postural stability, namely, the cervicocollic reflex (CCR), the cervico-ocular reflex (COR), and the tonic neck reflex (TNR). These reflexes work in conjunction with other cervical, vestibular, and visual reflexes acting on the neck musculature, for coordinated stability of posture as well as head and eye control (Figure 5.2).

### Head position

The CCR causes activation of neck muscles when they are stretched with movement of the head in relation to the body. The CCR is integrated with the vestibulocollic reflex (VCR) to activate neck muscles to assist in the maintenance of head position and limit unintentional displacements of the head.[1, 5] The CCR has a high sensitivity to small stimuli and a lower sensitivity for larger neck rotations, which suggests that muscle spindles rather than joint receptors provide the major input to the CCR. More specifically, responses have been demonstrated in the obliquus capitis inferior, the rectus capitis posterior major, and splenius muscles when the CCR has been elicited during rotation of the body with the head held fixed. Chan et al.[34] in their feline study confirmed the role of the perivertebral muscles in evoking the CCR. The VCR, which is evoked by vestibular stimuli acting on the neck muscles, is also related to the movement of the head in space together with the CCR. The behavior of the VCR is similar to that of the CCR, but it occurs in response to faster neck movements.[1, 5]

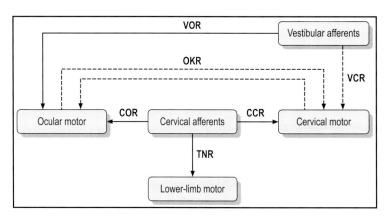

**Figure 5.2** Sensorimotor control reflex activity relating to the cervical spine. VOR, vestibulo-ocular reflex; VCR, vestibulocollic reflex; COR, cervico-ocular reflex; CCR, cervicocollic reflex; OKR, optokinetic reflex; TNR, tonic neck reflex. The bold lines indicate the cervical afferent effects. Dashed lines indicate reflex activity relating to cervical motor afferents.

## Visual control

The COR works together with the vestibulo-ocular reflex (VOR) and optokinetic reflex to control the extraocular muscles. The COR serves to assist in maintaining eye position such that head movement results in equal but opposite movement of the eyes, creating clear vision with low-frequency movement. The COR is evoked by stretch of the neck muscles. The importance of the COR in humans has been debated[35, 36] and speculation continues about its precise role.[37, 38] It has been suggested that, although the slow phase of the COR has no functional significance in humans, the quick phase of the COR may be important for both stabilization and reorientation of gaze.[39, 40] The VOR provides for eye movement control at high-frequency movements.

The optokinetic reflex activates neck muscles in response to movement of the visual field over the retina. Cervical input has been shown to affect "optokinetic afternystagmus," that is, the nystagmus produced after an optokinetic stimulus has been presented.[41] Ocular influences on cervical muscles in humans have been demonstrated by the presence of neck muscle activity in association with eye movements while the head is still. Specifically, a close relationship has been observed between activity in the deep cervical extensors and horizontal eye movement.[42] It is thought that this synergy is mediated by tectoreticulospinal nuclei at the brainstem.[43]

## Balance

The TNR is responsible for alteration in limb muscle activity when the body moves with respect to the head. It acts to maintain a stable posture. The TNR is integrated with the vestibulospinal reflex to achieve postural stability.[44] Again, it is thought that neck muscle spindles play a key role in this reflex.[34]

When the cervical muscle spindle characteristics, central connections, and their role in reflex pathways are considered, it is apparent that the sensory properties of the cervical region are important for somatosensory information and for their influence on postural stability and eye–head coordination. The importance of the cervical sensory system can also be demonstrated by reviewing the signs and symptoms to artificial disturbances of this system.

# Artificial disturbance of cervical somatosensory input

The association between disturbances to cervical afferent input and disturbances in sensorimotor control has been demonstrated in several ways. DeJong and DeJong[45] injected lidocaine in the area around the C2–3 level unilaterally in human subjects. Symptoms of disequilibrium began immediately and were more pronounced on the side of the injection. Symptoms of ataxia, hypotonia of the ipsilateral arm and leg muscles, and a strong sensation of ipsilateral falling or tilting were also reported. These symptoms were suggested to be due to a disturbance in the flow of afferent information from neck joint and muscle receptors. In support of this finding, Ishikawa et al.[46] showed that sectioning the cervical dorsal root ganglions or injecting anesthetic into deep neck structures caused nystagmus and severe ataxia in guinea pigs.

Less invasive techniques in humans include vibrating the neck muscles, which stimulates the muscle spindle afferents, induces eye position changes, visual illusory movements and, to a lesser extent, head movement illusions.[47-49] Vibration of neck muscles has similar effects on postural sway in standing to that seen with vibration of the calf[50] and has a greater influence on postural sway in standing than vibration of other areas, such as the gluteal, hamstrings, tibialis anterior, abdominal, or lumbar muscles.[50, 51] Neck muscle vibration also influences the velocity and direction of gait.[52, 53] Similarly, Karlberg et al.[54] showed that restraining cervical mobility (wearing a restrictive brace for 5 days) resulted in altered eye movement control and increased postural sway, reflecting a consequence of decreased cervical somatosensory input. Sustained isometric contractions to neck muscle fatigue were shown to affect postural sway, gait, and head position awareness in healthy persons.[55–60]

There is some evidence to suggest that the deeper structures of the cervical spine have a greater role in reflex connections with the visual and vestibular systems. TNRs in the cat were abolished by cutting the nerve supply to deep intervertebral tissues but were not abolished with removal of the large dorsal muscles.[61] Similarly, sensory input to the deeper region of the vertebrae changed the VOR in cats whereas input to the large dorsal muscles had no effect.[62]

# Mechanisms underlying disturbances in sensorimotor control

The likely mechanism for disturbances in postural control and eye movement control in people with neck pain is a conflict between converging inputs from the different sensory systems due to alterations in cervical somatosensory afferent activity.[2] Information from the muscle spindles is of primary importance for cervical proprioceptive acuity and this information is combined with input from the vestibular and visual systems. A changed or disturbed sensitivity of the muscle spindles may result in one or more complaints of dizziness, disturbance of sense of head movement, eye–head coordination, or postural stability. There is

also some evidence that the neck may directly influence vestibular function. For example, stimulation of the deep neck mechanoreceptors has a measurable impact on the VOR in cats.[62] Altered cervical proprioceptive input may give rise to a mismatch of sensory input or an asymmetry to the VOR.[63] In people with neck pain, altered cervical proprioceptive input may cause an asymmetry of the VOR,[29, 64] which may explain some of the reported symptoms such as dizziness and unsteadiness. Thus management may need to address both the cervical spine's primary and secondary influences on the postural control system.

Either a decrease or increase of cervical somatosensory input may result in altered sensorimotor control. Anesthetizing cervical structures reduces somatosensory input yet produces symptoms of ataxia, visual disturbances, and disequilibrium.[45] Likewise, increasing the activity of cervical mechanoreceptors by applying low-frequency pulse stimulation has been shown to increase disequilibrium of the eyes and body. Hinoki and Niki[65] also found that, when a procaine solution, known to interrupt gamma fibers, was injected into deep muscles of the upper neck in people with whiplash-associated disorders, it often led to an improvement in their disequilibrium and pain, which suggests that an overactivity of the muscle spindles was contributing to their symptoms.

Overactivity of cervical sympathetic nerves may cause an abnormal increase in neck muscle spindle activity.[29] However, it has also been found that activation of the sympathetic nervous system leads to a profound inhibition of muscle spindle afferents.[11, 32]

It has been postulated that, in trauma-induced neck pain, the injury may initiate a perpetual cycle of incorrect somatosensory afferent information.[66, 67] The proposed mechanism is that a sudden barrage of abnormal input from cervical proprioceptors and nociceptors, particularly following the deceleration phase of a whiplash injury, results in incorrect somatosensory information. This is followed by compensatory muscle tension to prevent the person from falling. In turn this leads to further altered cervical somatosensory information, which perpetuates the cycle. The cycle may be augmented from the effects of pain and inflammation from damaged neck structures.

In summary, there is evidence to suggest that disturbances in sensorimotor control may result from either a decrease or increase in cervical somatosensory afferent activity.

## Possible causes of altered cervical somatosensory input

There are several possible causes of altered cervical somatosensory input that could lead to disturbances in postural stability and eye movement control (Table 5.1 and Figure 5.3). These include direct damage to the mechanoreceptors from trauma, which could affect proprioceptive functioning and motor control, leading to a functional impairment of the cervical mechanoreceptors.[3] Morphological changes of the neck muscles have been documented in persons with neck pain,[23, 68, 69] which could affect their proprioceptive capability. In addition, pain and inflammation may alter cervical mechanoreceptor function at the spinal level as well as influence the central nervous system's modulation of cervical somatosensory information. There are also suggestions that stress and subsequent sympathetic nervous system activation may be a factor in the modulation of cervical somatosensory information.

## Effects of trauma and changes in muscle function

Trauma to cervical structures at the time of injury, inflammation, ischemia, excessive joint loading, or stretching can either directly injure nerve terminals or cause abnormal

**Table 5.1** Processes other than pain which may have deleterious effects on muscle spindle function

| Cause | Mechanism |
| --- | --- |
| Mechanical disruption[71, 95] | Direct damage |
| Excessive joint loading[70, 96] | Direct damage/functional impairment |
| Facet joint stretch[74, 75] | Direct damage |
| Muscle damage[97] | Direct damage/functional impairment |
| Local ischemia[73] | Direct damage |
| Joint inflammation [72 98] | Direct damage/functional impairment |
| Altered protective muscle responses[83] | Functional impairment |
| Inhibition of deep musculature[99] | Functional impairment |
| Altered feedforward neuromuscular control[100] | Functional impairment |
| Increased superficial muscle activity[101, 102] | Functional impairment |
| Altered neuromuscular efficiency[103] | Functional impairment |
| Muscle fatigue[104] | Functional impairment |
| Muscle fiber transformations[78] | Morphological change |
| Fatty infiltration into muscle[68, 105] | Morphological change |
| Muscle atrophy (reduced cross-sectional area) | Morphological change |
| Enhanced sympathetic nervous system activation[11, 32] | Functional impairment |

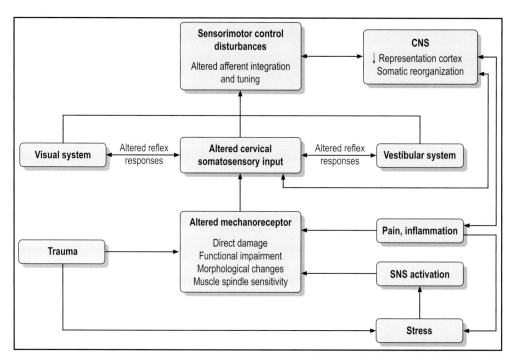

**Figure 5.3** Impact of somatosensory dysfunction in the cervical spine on sensorimotor control. Several peripheral mechanisms can alter mechanoreceptor function and cervical somatosensory input to the sensorimotor control system. Such changes can also alter the central nervous system (CNS) processing and subsequent descending information to the periphery. This can further contribute to altered somatosensory input. Visual and vestibular input to the sensorimotor control system can also be affected indirectly by altered cervical mechanoreceptor function. SNS, sympathetic nervous system.

afferent impulses from the cervical mechanoreceptors.[70–75] Mechanoreceptor input influences motor control primarily via the muscle spindles.[25] Conversely, altered motor control may desensitize mechanoreceptors and further perpetuate cervical somatosensory dysfunction. Motor control is affected by neck pain (Chapter 4). Changes in muscle function occur in the acute state[76, 77] and may persist despite the patient reporting recovery.[76, 77] Recent studies have demonstrated the deleterious effects of neck muscle extensor fatigue on standing balance in humans.[56–58] Likewise, standing balance has been shown to be adversely affected by scapular muscle fatigue and sustained isometric contractions.[55, 60] Thus persistent long-term alterations in cervical mechanoreceptors due to disturbed motor control may lead to additional changes in sensorimotor control such as balance disturbances.

Morphological changes have been observed in neck muscles, which may alter their proprioceptive capabilities (Chapter 4). These changes are often most prominent in the deep suboccipital muscles.[23, 68, 69, 78, 79] Furthermore, in a preliminary study, McPartland et al.[69] found a relationship between poor control of standing balance and fatty infiltration of the rectus capitis posterior major, suggesting that the sensory properties of the muscle had been altered. These changes may suggest changes in the proprioceptive capabilities of the muscles and thus adversely influence the input for sensorimotor control.

## Effects of pain

Pain may modulate proprioceptive input at many levels, including the information locally from the mechanoreceptors in the spinal cord and during the supraspinal control and evaluation of cervical somatosensory information (Figure 5.4). At the local level, an increase in nociceptor input occurs as a result of chemical mediators released in response to injury. This may cause temporary peripheral sensitization, in which normally high thresholds of receptors are lowered and spontaneous receptor activity is increased. Painful responses can occur to nonnoxious stimuli such as light touch.[80, 81] It has also been speculated that generation of pain from mechanoreceptors that normally only generate innocuous responses may result in an increase in nociceptive input and also a decrease in nonnociceptive input, which might also disturb somatosensory input for sensorimotor control.[81]

In chronic pain, mechanoreceptors may continue to be sensitive to noxious stimuli, due to changes in the central nervous system and decreased central inhibition.[80] Sensitivity following a neck injury often occurs at regions both local and remote to the original injury[82] and is a feature in many patients with chronic whiplash disorders (Chapter 2).[76, 80, 82] Chronic sensitivity may further prolong disruption of somatosensory input from the cervical region.

Experimentally induced pain has been shown to change muscle activity,[10, 83, 84] including reflex activity[85, 86] and muscle spindle sensitivity. In the cervical region several studies in cats have demonstrated experimentally induced, long-lasting increased activity in the gamma muscle spindle system following excitation of chemosensitive afferents in and around the cervical joint complex.[7, 8, 87, 88] Interestingly, lower doses of bradykinin were needed to evoke responses from the fusimotor neurons in neck muscles compared to hind-limb muscles, suggesting that the neck muscles may be more sensitive to pain.[8, 87, 88] These long-lasting and extensive changes in muscle spindle activation in superficial muscles of the cervical region in response to pain would certainly lead to altered cervical somatosensory input.[89, 90]

Pain has also been shown to alter spinal inhibition via effects on the somatosensory cortex and subcortical levels in humans. Tonic muscle pain caused a long-lasting depression of the primary motor area in the contralateral cerebral cortex in humans.[10] The effects lasted several hours, even after the pain had ceased. Further, Rossi et al.[91] demonstrated that tonic muscle pain discharge strongly interacted with nonnociceptive input arising from the same site and it altered proprioception. It was suggested that this was due to a gating of input at the cortical or precortical level. There is also evidence to suggest a possible role of pain in subcortical and cortical reorganization at many levels of the somatosensory system in humans. The

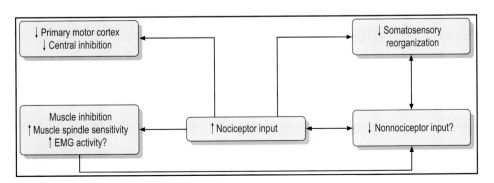

**Figure 5.4** Direct effects of pain on afferent function. EMG, electromyogram.

removal of mechanoreceptive inputs and enhancement of nociceptive inputs could contribute to this neural reorganization.[92-94]

## Sympathetic nervous system

Sympathetic nervous system activation has been shown to influence muscle spindle activity directly.[32] Animal studies have shown that experimental activation of the cervical sympathetic nerve depresses the discharge rate of cervical muscle spindle afferents and affects the sensitivity of changes in muscle length. This was independent of changes in blood flow and inflammatory responses.[32] A recent review discussed possible links between pain, stress, and activation of the sympathetic nervous system and the effect that this may have on muscle spindle activation. This could be another factor to consider as a cause of altered modulation of cervical somatosensory information in those with neck pain.[11]

## Conclusion

The abundance of mechanoreceptors in the muscles and joints of the cervical spine, as well as their central and reflex connections to the vestibular and visual systems, indicates that they have an important role in postural stability, head orientation, and eye movement. The observed changes in balance and eye movement control in people with neck pain may reflect altered somatosensory input from a variety of structures in the cervical spine. Alterations in cervical somatosensory information in neck pain may be due to a number of mechanisms, including direct trauma, functional impairment, or morphological changes in the cervical muscles, as well as the direct effects of pain itself. Psychosocial and/or work-related stresses may also affect cervical somatosensory function via activation of the sympathetic nervous system. It is likely that a combination of features leads to an immediate, sustained alteration in cervical somatosensory input, which in turn influences sensorimotor control. The numerous reflex connections between cervical structures and the vestibular and visual systems imply that changes in somatosensory information could result in disturbances in reflex activity relating to postural stability and coordinated stability of the head and eyes in the presence of neck pain.

## References

1. *Peterson BW*. Current approaches and future directions to understanding control of head movement. Brain mechanisms for the integration of posture and movement. Prog Brain Res 2004;143:369–381.

2. *Baloh R, Halmagyi G*. Disorders of the Vestibular System. New York: Oxford University Press, 1996.

3. *Heikkila H, Astrom PG*. Cervicocephalic kinesthetic sensibility in patients with whiplash injury. Scand J Rehabil Med 1996;28:133–138.

4. *Karlberg M, Johansson R, Magnusson M, et al*. Dizziness of suspected cervical origin distinguished by posturographic assessment of human postural dynamics. J Vestibul Res Equil 1996;6:37–47.

5. *Peterson B, Goldberg J, Bilotto G, et al*. Cervicocollic reflex: its dynamic properties and interaction with vestibular reflexes. J Neurophysiol 1985;54:90–108.

6. *Revel M, Andre-Deshays C, Minguet M*. Cervicocephalic kinesthetic sensibility in patients with cervical pain. Arch Phys Med Rehabil 1991;72:288–291.

7. *Thunberg J, Hellstrom F, Solander P, et al*. Influences on the fusimotor-muscle spindle system from chemosensitive nerve endings in the cervical facet joints in the cat; possible implications for whiplash induced disorders. Pain 2001;91:15–22.

8. *Wenngren B, Pedersen J, Sjolander P, et al*. Bradykinin and muscle stretch alter contralateral cat neck muscle spindle output. Neurosci Res 1998;32:119–129.

9. *Ageborg E*. Consequences of a ligament injury on neuromuscular function and relevance to rehabilitation – using the anterior cruciate ligament-injured knee as a model. J Electromyogr Kinesiol 2002;12:205–212.

10. *Le Pera D, Graven-Nielsen T, Valeriani M, et al*. Inhibition of motor system excitability at cortical and spinal level by tonic muscle pain. Clin Neurophysiol 2001;112:1633–1641

11. *Passatore M, Roatta S*. Influence of sympathetic nervous system on sensorimotor function: whiplash associated disorders (WAD) as a model. Eur J Appl Physiol 2006;98:423–449.

12. *Kulkarni V, Chandy M, Babu K*. Quantitative study of muscle spindles in suboccipital muscles of human foetuses. Neurol India 2001;49:355–359.

13. *Boyd Clark L, Briggs C, Galea M*. Muscle spindle distribution, morphology and density in the longus colli and multifidus muscles of the cervical spine. Spine 2002;27:694–701.

14. *Strasmann T, Feilscher T, Baumann K, et al*. Distribution of sensory receptors in joints of the upper cervical column in the laboratory marsupial *Monodelphis domestica*. Ann Anat 1999;181:199–206.

15. *Mendel T, Wink CS, Zimny ML*. Neural elements in human cervical intervertebral disks. Spine 1992;17:132–135.

16. *McLain RF*. Mechanoreceptor endings in human cervical facet joints. Spine 1994;19:495–501.

17. *Krogsgaard M, Dyre-Poulsen P, Fischer-Rasmussen T*. Cruciate ligament reflexes. J Electromyogr Kinesiol 2002;12:177–182.

18. *Liu J, Thornell L, Pedrosa-Domellof F*. Muscle spindles in the deep muscles of the human neck: a morphological and immunocytochemical study. J Histochem Cytochem 2003;51:175–186.

19. *Bolton PS, Holland CT*. An in vivo method for studying afferent fibre activity from cervical paravertebral tissue during vertebral motion in anaesthetised cats. J Neurosci Meth 1998;85: 211–218.

20. *Richmond F, Singh K, Corneil B*. Marked non-uniformity of fiber-type composition in the primate suboccipital muscle obliquus capitis inferior. Exp Brain Res 1999;125:14–18.

21. *Dutia MB*. The muscles and joints of the neck: their specialisation and role in head movement. Prog Neurobiol 1991;37:165–178.

22. *Richmonds FJR, Bakker VC*. Anatomical organisation and sensory content of the soft tissues surrounding upper cervical vertebrae in the cat. J Neurophysiol 1982;48:49–61.

23. *Andary MT, Hallgren RC, Greenman PE, et al*. Neurogenic atrophy of suboccipital muscles after a cervical injury. Am J Phys Med Rehabil 1998;77:545–549.

24. *Selbie WS, Thomson DB, Richmond FJ*. Suboccipital muscles in the cat neck: morphometry and histochemistry of the rectus capitis muscle complex. J Morphol 1993;216:47–63.

25. *Swanik C, Lephart F, Giannantonio F, et al*. Re-establishing proprioception and muscle control in the ACL injured athlete. J Sport Rehabil 1997;6:182–206.

26. *Bolton PS, Tracey DJ*. Spinothalamic and propriospinal neurons in the upper cervical cord of the rat – terminations of primary afferent fibers on soma and primary dendrites. Exp Brain Res 1992;92:59–68.

27. *Werner J*. Neuroscience – A Clinical Perspective. Canada: W.B. Saunders, 1980.

28. *Corneil BD, Olivier E, Munoz DP*. Neck muscle responses to stimulation of monkey superior colliculus. I. Topography and manipulation of stimulation parameters. J Neurophysiol 2002;88:1980–1999.

29. *Hinoki M*. Vertigo due to whiplash injury: a neuro-otological approach. Acta Otolaryngol 1975;419: 9–329.

30. *Hirai N, Hongo T, Sasaki S et al*. Neck muscle afferent input to spinocerebellar tract cells of the central cervical nucleus in the cat. Exp Brain Res 1984;55:286–300.

31. *Bolton PS, Kerman IA, Woodring SF, et al*. Influences of neck afferents on sympathetic and respiratory nerve activity. Brain Res Bull 1998;47:413–419.

32. *Hellstrom F, Roatta S, Thunberg J, et al*. Responses of muscle spindles in feline dorsal neck muscles to electrical stimulation of the cervical sympathetic nerve. Exp Brain Res 2005;165:328–342.

33. *Shinoda Y, Sugiuchi Y, Futami T, et al*. Input patterns and pathways from the six semicircular canals to motoneurons of neck muscles. I. The multifidus muscle group. J Neurophysiol 1994;72:2691–2702.

34. *Chan YS, Kasper J, Wilson VJ*. Dynamics and directional sensitivity of neck muscle – spindle responses to head rotation. J Neurophysiol 1987;57:1716–1729.

35. *Bronstein AM, Morland AB, Ruddock KH, et al*. Recovery from bilateral vestibular failure: implications for visual and cervico-ocular function. Acta Otolaryngol 1995;520:405–407.

36. *Doerr M, Hong SH, Thoden U*. Eye movements during active head turning with different vestibular and cervical input. Acta Otolaryngol 1984;98:14–20.

37. *Barnes GR, Forbat LN*. Cervical and vestibular afferent control of oculomotor response in man. Acta Otolaryngol 1979;88:79–87.

38. *Barlow D, Freedman W*. Cervico-ocular reflex in the normal adult. Acta Otolaryngol 1980;89:487–496.

39. *Mergner T, Schweigart G, Botti F, et al*. Eye movements evoked by proprioceptive stimulation along the body axis in humans. Exp Brain Res 1998;120:450–460.

40. *Jurgens R, Mergner T*. Interaction between cervico-ocular and vestibulo-ocular reflexes in normal adults. Exp Brain Res 1989;77:381–390.

41. *Karlberg M, Magnusson M*. Asymmetric optokinetic after nystagmus-induced by active or passive sustained head rotations. Acta Otolaryngol 1996;116:647–651.

42. *Vidal PP, Roucoux A, Berthoz A*. Horizontal eye position-related activity in neck muscles of the alert cat. Exp Brain Res 1982;46:448–453.

43. *Berthoz A, Grantyn A*. Neuronal mechanisms underlying eye–head coordination. Prog Brain Res 1986;64:325–343.

44. *Yamagata Y, Yates BJ, Wilson VJ*. Participation of Ia reciprocal inhibitory neurons in the spinal circuitry of the tonic neck reflex. Exp Brain Res 1991;84:461–464.

45. *DeJong PI, DeJong JM*. Ataxia and nystagmus induced by injection of local anaesthetics in the neck. Ann Neurol 1977;1:240–246.

46. *Ishikawa K, Matsuzaki Z, Yokomizo M, et al*. Effect of unilateral section of cervical afferent nerve upon optokinetic response and vestibular nystagmus induced by sinusoidal rotation in guinea pigs. Acta Otolaryngol 1998;537:6–10.

47. *Lennerstrand G, Han Y, Velay JL*. Properties of eye movements induced by activation of neck muscle proprioceptors. Graefes Arch Clin Exp Ophthalmol 1996;234:703–709.

48. *Taylor JL, McCloskey DI*. Illusions of head and visual target displacement induced by vibration of neck muscles. Brain 1991;114:755–759.

49. *Karnath HO, Reich E, Rorden C, et al*. The perception of body orientation after neck-proprioceptive stimulation – effects of time and of visual cueing. Exp Brain Res 2002;143:350–358.

50. *Pyykko I, Aalto H, Seidel H et al*. Hierarchy of different muscles in postural control. Acta Otolaryngol 1989;468:175–180.

51. *Kavounoudias A, Gilhodes JC, Roll R, et al*. From balance regulation to body orientation: two goals for muscle proprioceptive information processing? Exp Brain Res 1999;124:80–88.

52. *Bove M, Courtine G, Schieppati M*. Neck muscle vibration and spatial orientation during stepping in place in humans. J Neurophysiol 2002;88:2232–2241.

53. *Courtine G, Papaxanthis C, Laroche D, et al*. Gait-dependent integration of neck muscle afferent input. Neuroreport 2003;14:2365–2368.

54. *Karlberg M, Magnusson M, Johansson R*. Effects of restrained cervical mobility on voluntary eye movements and postural control. Acta Otolaryngol 1991;111:664–670.

55. *Duclos C, Roll R, Kavounoudias A, et al*. Long-lasting body leanings following neck muscle isometric contractions. Exp Brain Res 2004;158:58–66.

56. *Schmid M, Schieppati M*. Neck muscle fatigue and spatial orientation during stepping in place in humans. J Appl Physiol 2005;99:141–153.

57. *Schieppati M, Nardone A, Schmid M*. Neck muscle fatigue affects postural control in man. Neuroscience 2003;121:277–285.

58. *Gosselin G, Rassoulian H, Brown I*. Effects of neck extensor muscles fatigue on balance. Clin Biomech 2004;19:473–479.

59. *Owens EF Jr, Henderson CN, Gudavalli MR, et al*. Head repositioning errors in normal student volunteers: a possible tool to assess the neck's neuromuscular system. Chiropr Osteopat 2006;14:1–5.

60. *Vuillerme N, Pinsault N, Vaillant J*. Postural control during quiet standing following cervical muscular fatigue: effects of changes in sensory inputs. Neurosci Lett 2005;378:135–139.

61. *McCouch G, Deering I, Ling T*. Location of receptors for tonic neck reflexes. J Neurophysiol 1951;14:191–195.

62. *Hikosaka O, Maeda M*. Cervical effects on abducens motoneurons and their interaction with vestibulo-ocular reflex. Exp Brain Res 1973;18:512–530.

63. *Fischer A, Verhagen WIM, Huygen PLM*. Whiplash injury. A clinical review with emphasis on neurootological aspects. Clin Otolaryngol 1997;22:192–201.

64. *Padoan S, Karlberg M, Fransson PA, et al*. Passive sustained turning of the head induces asymmetric gain of the vestibulo-ocular reflex in healthy subjects. Acta Otolaryngol 1998;118:778–782.

65. *Hinoki M, Niki H*. Neurotological studies on the role of the sympathetic nervous system in the formation of traumatic vertigo of cervical origin. Acta Otolaryngol 1975;330:185–196.

66. *Davis C*. Chronic pain dysfunction in whiplash-associated disorders. J Manipul Physiol Ther 2001;24:44–51.

67. *Tjell C*. Diagnostic considerations in whiplash associated disorders. Thesis. Department of Otorhinlaryngology, Central Hospital Skovde, Sweden, 1998.

68. *Elliott J, Jull G, Noteboom JT, et al*. Fatty infiltration in the cervical extensor muscles in persistent whiplash-associated disorders – a magnetic resonance imaging analysis. Spine 2006;31:E847–E855.

69. *McPartland JM, Brodeur RR, Hallgren RC*. Chronic neck pain, standing balance, and suboccipital muscle atrophy – a pilot study. J Manipul Physiol Ther 1997;20:24–29.

70. *Loescher AR, Holland GR, Robinson PP*. The distribution and morphological characteristics of axons innervating the periodontal ligament of reimplanted teeth in cats. Arch Oral Biol 1993;38:813–822.

71. *Quick D*. Acute lesion of the intrafusal muscle of muscle spindles. Ultrastructural and electrophysiological consequences. J Neurosci 1986;6:2097–2105.

72. *Gentle M, Thorp B*. Sensory properties of ankle joint capsulemechanoreceptors in acute monoarthritic chickens. Pain 1994;57:361–374.

73. *Diwan F, Milburn A*. The effects of temporary ischemia on rat muscle spindles. J Embryol Exp Morphol 1986;92:223–254.

74. *Lu Y, Chen C, Kallakuri S, et al*. Neural response of cervical facet joint capsule to stretch: a study of whiplash pain mechanism. Stapp Car Crash J 2005;49:49–65.

75. *Chen CY, Lu Y, Kallakuri S, et al*. Distribution of A-delta and C-fiber receptors in the cervical facet joint capsule and their response to stretch. J Bone Joint Surg 2006;88A:1807–1816.

76. *Sterling M, Jull G, Vicenzino B, et al*. Development of motor system dysfunction following whiplash injury. Pain 2003;103:65–73.

77. *Hides JA, Jull GA, Richardson CA*. Long-term effects of specific stabilizing exercises for first-episode low back pain. Spine 2001;26: E243–E248.

78. *Uhlig Y, Weber BR, Grob D, et al*. Fiber composition and fiber transformation in neck muscles of patients with dysfunction of the cervical spine. J Orthop Res 1995;13:240–249.

79. *Kristjansson E*. Reliability of ultrasonography for the cervical multifidus muscle in asymptomatic and symptomatic subjects. Man Ther 2004;9: 83–88.

80. *Curatolo M, Petersen-Felix S, Arendt-Nielsen L, et al*. Central hypersensitivity in chronic pain after whiplash injury. Clin J Pain 2001;17:306–315.

81. *Seaman D*. Dysafferentation: a novel term to describe the neuropathological effects of joint complex dysfunction – a look at likely mechanisms of symptom generation – in reply. J Manipul Physiol Ther 1999;22:493–494.

82. *Sterling M, Treleaven J, Edwards S, et al*. Pressure pain thresholds in chronic WAD. Further evidence of altered central pain processing. J Musculoskelet Pain 2002;10:69–81.

83. *Holm S, Aage I, Solomonow M*. Sensorimotor control of the spine. J Electromyogr Kinesiol 2002;12:219–234.

84. *Zedka M, Prochazka A, Knight B, et al*. Voluntary and reflex control of human back muscles during induced pain. J Physiol 1999;520:591–604.

85. *Matre D, Arendt-Nielsen L, Knardahl S*. Effects of localization and intensity of experimental muscle pain on ankle joint proprioception. Eur J Pain 2002;6:245–260.

86. *Wang K, Svensson P, Arendt-Nielsen L*. Effect of tonic muscle pain on short latency jaw-stretch reflexes in humans. Pain 2000;88:189–197.

87. *Pedersen J, Sjolander P, Wenngren B, et al*. Increased intramuscular concentration of bradykinin increases the static fusimotor drive to muscle spindles in neck muscles of the cat. Pain 1997;70:83–91.

88. *Hellstrom F, Thunberg J, Bergenheim M, et al*. Elevated intramuscular concentration of bradykinin in jaw muscle increases the fusimotor drive to neck muscles in the cat. J Dent Res 2000;79:1815–1822.

89. *Ro J, Capra N*. Modulation of jaw muscle spindle afferent activity following intramuscular injections with hypertonic saline. Pain 2001;92: 117–127.

90. *Proske U, Wise AK, Gregory JE*. The role of muscle receptors in the detection of movements. Prog Neurobiol 2000;60:85–96.

91. *Rossi S, Della Volpe R, Ginanneschi F, et al*. Early somatosensory processing during tonic muscle pain in humans: relation to loss of proprioception and motor 'defensive' strategies. Clin Neurophysiol 2003;114:1351–1358.

92. *Tinazzi M, Fiaschi A, Rosso T, et al*. Neuroplastic changes related to pain occur at multiple levels of the human somatosensory system: a somatosensory-evoked potentials study in patients with cervical radicular pain. J Neurosci 2000;20:9277–9283.

93. *Gandevia SC, Phegan CM*. Perceptual distortions of the human body image produced by local anaesthesia, pain and cutaneous stimulation. J Physiol 1999;514:609–616.

94. *Flor H*. Cortical reorganisation and chronic pain: implications for rehabilitation. J Rehabil Med 2003;35:66–72.

95. *Garret W, Nikolaou P, Ribbeck B, et al*. The effect of muscle architecture on the biomechanical failure properties of skeletal muscle under passive extension. Am J Sports Med 1988;16:7–12.

96. *Solomonow M, Zhou BH, Baratta RV, et al*. Biomechanics of increased exposure to lumbar injury caused by cyclic loading: part 1. Loss of reflexive muscular stabilization. Spine 1999;24:2426–2434.

97. *Bani D, Bergamini M*. Ultrastructural abnormalities of muscle spindles in the rat masseter muscle with malocclusion-induced damage. Histol Histopathol 2002;17:45–54.

98. *Gedalia U, Solomonow M, Zhou BH, et al*. Biomechanics of increased exposure to lumbar injury caused by cyclic loading – part 2. Recovery of reflexive muscular stability with rest. Spine 1999;24:2461–2467.

99. *Falla D, Jull G, Dall'Alba P, et al*. An electromyographic analysis of the deep cervical flexor muscles in performance of craniocervical flexion. Phys Ther 2003;83:899–906.

100. *Falla D, Jull G, Hodges PW*. Feedforward activity of the cervical flexor muscles during voluntary arm movements is delayed in chronic neck pain. Exp Brain Res 2004;157:43–48.

101. *Jull G*. Deep cervical flexor muscle dysfunction in whiplash. J Musculoskelet Pain 2000;8: 143–154.

102. *Falla D*. Unravelling the complexity of muscle impairment in chronic neck pain. Man Ther 2004;9:125–133.

103. *Falla D, Jull G, Edwards S et al*. Neuromuscular efficiency of the sternocleidomastoid and anterior scalene muscles in patients with chronic neck pain. Disabil Rehabil 2004;26:712–717.

104. *Falla D, Jull G, Rainoldi A, et al*. Neck flexor muscle fatigue is side specific in patients with unilateral neck pain. Eur J Pain 2004;8:71–77.

105. *Andary MT, Hallgren RC, Greenman PE, et al*. Neurogenic atrophy of suboccipital muscles after a cervical injury: a case study. Am J Phys Med Rehabil 1998;77:545–549.

# Disturbances in Postural Stability, Head and Eye Movement Control in Cervical Disorders

## Introduction

Cervical mechanoreceptors are vital for providing proprioceptive input. They have reflex connections to both the vestibular and visual systems and thus can influence the function of these systems and vice versa. Somatosensory information from the cervical spine can be altered through several mechanisms (Chapter 5). Cervical somatosensory disturbances can influence the control, interaction, and tuning of afferent input and thus sensorimotor control. Disturbances in cervical joint position sense, eye movement control, and postural stability have been identified in patients with idiopathic neck pain and neck pain following a whiplash injury. In addition, there may or may not be complaints of dizziness or unsteadiness. This chapter will explore the symptom of dizziness and impairments in cervical joint position sense, postural stability, and eye movement control which may present in the neck pain patient, as well as their measurement. Evidence for management will be presented.

## Dizziness

Cervical vertigo is not the unique cause of the symptom of dizziness or light-headedness in patients with a neck disorder. There are several other potential causes, including vertebral artery insufficiency, minor brain injury in cases of whiplash and, commonly, peripheral vestibular disorders. The clinician should be cognizant of all causes to allow differentiation of dizziness in the patient presenting with neck pain.

## Cervical vertigo

A cervical disorder can cause the symptom of dizziness, but there has been considerable controversy with respect to its frequency. The main limitation is that there are no reliable clinical tests that differentiate cervical vertigo from other causes of dizziness. Nevertheless, evidence is emerging to support cervical disorders as a genuine and frequent cause of dizziness when it is associated with neck pain and disability.[1-4] Humphreys et al.[2] found a 33% incidence of dizziness in 180 patients with neck pain. Dizziness correlated with duration of neck pain, higher neck pain and disability scores, and a history of neck trauma, all of which imply a cervical origin. Dizziness or light-headedness is not an uncommon complaint of those presenting with cervicogenic headache.[5] We determined a 74% incidence of dizziness and, more specifically, unsteadiness in a group with chronic whiplash-associated disorders.[3] It has also been established that people with neck pain complaining of dizziness have greater deficits in specific tests of sensorimotor control than those without dizziness, which is reasoned to reflect abnormal somatosensory input.[3, 6-8] A cervical cause of dizziness is also supported by evidence of improvement in these symptoms with treatments directed specifically towards the cervical spine.[1, 9-11]

A cervical disorder is more readily accepted as the cause of dizziness when neck pain is of an idiopathic origin. Other causes of dizziness need to be considered when it is associated with a trauma such as whiplash injury. Some believe that dizziness and unsteadiness following a whiplash injury are due to side-effects of medication and the anxiety caused by either the ongoing pain or financial gain.[12] Nevertheless we found no difference between chronic whiplash patients with and without dizziness with respect to medication intake, anxiety levels, or compensation status. Neither did these features influence our selected measures of sensorimotor control, that is, balance, eye movement control, and proprioceptive acuity.[3,6,7,13] However, damage to the vertebral artery, vestibular receptors, or neck receptors or a mild head injury are all possible causes of dizziness following a whiplash injury, making it difficult to determine the exact cause of the symptoms.[4, 14-17] It is considered that in the absence of traumatic brain injury following a whiplash injury, the symptom of dizziness is most frequently ascribed to disturbed sensory properties of cervical joint and muscle receptors resulting from the trauma or subsequent functional impairment.[3, 17-21] However other possible causes of dizziness must be considered.

## Vertebral artery insufficiency

Vertebral artery insufficiency can cause dizziness and is a primary concern of clinicians managing patients with neck pain, especially in the context of the use of manipulative therapy procedures. The reader is directed to a recent review of cervical arterial dysfunction to assist differential diagnosis of vertebral artery dysfunction.[22] Spontaneous dissections of either the vertebral or internal carotid arteries often present initially with severe neck pain and headache and often other neurological symptoms.[23, 24] The clinician must be alert to patients presenting with spontaneous onset, acute suboccipital pain, and headache with or without dizziness and arrange immediate medical attention. Equally, due care is needed in patients with peripheral vascular disease or gross degenerative change, even with the use of low-velocity manipulative therapy techniques in management.[25, 26]

Damage to the vertebral artery and abnormalities in blood flow can occur in a whiplash injury[27, 28] and the symptom of dizziness could result from disturbances in cerebral blood flow. However, damage to the vertebral artery is rare in a whiplash injury without a fracture or dislocation[29, 30] and, if it occurs, it may be either asymptomatic, because of compensation by collateral arteries,[22, 31, 32] or cause symptoms, indicating an ischemic event soon after the injury.[33] Further recent studies have also found the report of dizziness was uncommon even in the presence of vertebral artery blood flow abnormalities.[33–35] However caution is always warranted.

## Minor brain injury

In the whiplash patient, dizziness can result from a minor brain injury sustained in a motor vehicle crash. Brain injury should not be excluded automatically, especially when there has been a direct blow to the head or reports of amnesia or concussion.[36] This does not occur in the majority of people who sustain a whiplash injury and disturbance in afferent input from the cervical region is probably a more likely cause of dizziness.[37] Interestingly, a cervical cause of dizziness is still a relatively common cause of vertigo in those sustaining blunt head trauma.[4]

## Peripheral vestibular lesions

Vestibular disorders are a primary consideration in the differential diagnosis of dizziness, although conversely, a cervical source should be considered in the absence of any diagnosable vestibular disorder. Discussion here will center on vestibular disorders in relation to neck trauma. Forces generated during a whiplash injury can shear the delicate structures of the peripheral vestibular system, resulting in several possible peripheral vestibular causes of dizziness. These include benign paroxysmal positional vertigo (BPPV), damage to the endolymphatic sac which could cause hydrops (Ménière's disease), labyrinthine concussion, otolith disorders,[4] or rupture of the otic capsule window resulting in perilymph fistula.[38]

There is considerable controversy regarding the frequency of a vestibular versus a cervical cause of dizziness in the whiplash-injured patient who reports dizziness. At one extreme, many consider vestibular disorders are the primary cause of dizziness, although these reports are based largely on clinical patterns rather than tests of the vestibular system.[16, 17, 39] Other studies of whiplash patients, which have screened with vestibular tests, report variable proportions. Ernst et al.[4] reported a 73% incidence of vestibular disorders (mostly a diagnosis of BPPV) and a 23% incidence of cervical vertigo. Hinoki[40] found only a 5.6% incidence of a pure or near-pure peripheral labyrinthine dysfunction in a cohort of 136 whiplash patients. Fischer et al.[41] reported normal vestibular test results in most of their whiplash group, although half of them had some vestibular hyperactivity. Interestingly, these authors proposed a cervical basis for the vestibular hypersensitivity; a result of limited neck movement and pain, with subsequent vestibule-ocular reflex enhancement.

There is a greater likelihood of peripheral vestibular damage when there has been a mild head injury associated with the whiplash injury.[4, 38] In the absence of a mild head injury, most concur that brain damage and peripheral vestibular dysfunction are less likely causes of dizziness, which points to abnormal cervical somatosensory input from damaged neck joint and muscle receptors.[17–20, 37] Thus a cervical cause of dizziness is likely in cases of whiplash or other neck trauma, but other causes of dizziness in such patients are possible and should always be considered.

## Symptom differentiation

Table 6.1 presents a summary of the characteristic features of dizziness of various origins which need to be considered in making a differential diagnosis. Attention here will focus on cervical vertigo whose diagnosis is usually made on the description of symptoms, the association of dizziness with neck pain, and the exclusion of vestibular disorders.[42, 43] Cervical vertigo is usually described as a nonspecific sensation of altered orientation in space and disequilibrium,[44] rather than the true vertigo (environment and self-spinning) which is characteristic of vestibular pathology.[15] Perceptual symptoms of disorientation and vague unsteadiness are described, occurring in episodes lasting minutes to hours.[44, 45] Visual complaints such as blurred vision, words jumping on the page, unclear contours of objects, or difficulty focusing may be reported,[46] possibly reflecting disturbances in the cervico-ocular and cervicocollic reflexes.[20] There may also be complaints of difficulty with specific activities such as walking in the dark or on stairs or negotiating doorways. Cervical vertigo is exacerbated with neck movements and increased neck pain and has a close temporal relationship with pain, injury, or pathology. Accordingly, relief of dizziness often occurs with relief of neck pain.[42, 44] We found in our chronic whiplash cohort that the descriptions of dizziness were in accordance with these descriptions[3, 47] which in turn were different from those described by patients with vestibular pathology.[47] It was notable that there was no difference between the whiplash and vestibular groups in their scores for the handicap associated with dizziness (Dizziness Handicap Inventory[48]).

# Measures of proprioception, eye movement control, and postural stability

There are three groups of measures that are currently commonly used in the clinical setting to assess disturbances in sensorimotor control in those with neck pain: cervical joint position error (JPE), postural stability, and eye movement control.

## Cervical joint position error

The measure of cervical JPE tests a patient's ability to relocate the position of the head to a natural head posture or to a predetermined target whilst vision is occluded[49] (Figure 6.1). Deficits in relocation accuracy are considered to reflect abnormal afferent input from the neck joint and muscle receptors rather than vestibular input, especially if neck movements are performed slowly, that is, when the vestibular system is below threshold.[50, 51] Greater cervical JPEs have been shown in persons with both insidious and traumatic-onset neck pain.[3, 21, 49, 52-54] There is some evidence to suggest that greater JPEs are exhibited by patients with chronic whiplash compared to those with idiopathic neck pain,[54, 55] in those reporting higher levels of pain and disability,[53, 56] and in those who report dizziness.[3] This suggests that patients with greater pain, a traumatic onset of neck pain, and symptoms of dizziness may have more disturbed cervical somatosensory input.

Deficits in relocation accuracy may not be unique to cervical disorders as previously thought.[21, 50] We recently found no difference in JPE between persons with whiplash and vestibular disorders.[47] Nevertheless there were differences in the features of dizziness and other tests of the postural control system, implying that the causes of the disturbances differ between whiplash and discrete vestibular pathology. Both groups

**Table 6.1** Characteristic features of cervical vertigo and other causes of dizziness which may be present in the neck pain patient*

| | Cervical vertigo[12, 44, 92] | BPPV[93, 94] | Perilymph fistula[15, 93, 94] | Ménière's disease[15, 93, 94] | Vertebral artery[33, 34, 95] | Psychogenic[15, 96, 97] |
|---|---|---|---|---|---|---|
| Description | Vague unsteadiness<br>Light-headedness | Severe vertigo lasting several minutes | Vertigo<br>Disequilibrium<br>Motion intolerance | Whirling vertigo<br>Unsteadiness<br>Motion intolerance | Faintness<br>Blurred vision<br>Dizziness | Apart from self<br>Floating<br>Fullness in head |
| Frequency | Episodic | Discrete attacks related to specific head/body movements | Constant | Episodic severe vertigo<br>Constant unsteadiness | Episodic | Episodic |
| Duration | Minutes to hours | Seconds to minutes | Constant | Hours | Several seconds | Minutes/hours |
| Exacerbated by | Increased neck pain<br>Neck movement | Rolling in bed<br>Quick head movements<br>Changing body position | Visual challenges<br>↑Intracranial pressure<br>Loud noises | Nil | Neck extension and/or rotation | Hyperventilation<br>Panic, stress |
| Relieved by | Lessening neck pain<br>Local neck treatment | Subsides if stay in provoking position | | | Neck back to neutral | Relaxation |
| Associated symptoms | Blurred vision<br>Nausea<br>Neck pain | Nausea<br>Vomiting<br>Aging | Unilateral tinnitus<br>Aural pressure<br>Hearing loss | Nausea<br>Vomiting<br>Hearing loss<br>Tinnitus<br>Ear fullness | Dysarthria<br>Hemiparesis<br>Dysesthesia<br>Diplopia<br>Dysphagia<br>Drop attacks<br>Nystagmus<br>Nausea<br>Numbness | Perioral numbness<br>Paresthesia in extremities<br>Lump in throat<br>Tight chest<br>Fatigue<br>Tightness in head |
| Onset | Neck pain<br>Neck injury<br>Neck pathology | Spontaneous<br>Posttrauma | 24–72 hours posttrauma | Often several years after trauma | Immediate or few hours after trauma | |
| Suggested cause | Abnormal cervical afferent input | Debris in endolymph | Leak of perilymph fluid into middle ear | Endolymph hydrops | Vertebral artery dissection<br>Peripheral vascular disease | Anxiety<br>Panic<br>Psychosomatic |
| Other | | Often spontaneous improvement<br>Positive Hallpike Dix maneuver<br>Nystagmus often observed | | | VBI may be present without symptoms | |

*The superscript numbers in the headings refer to the reference source.
BPPV, benign paroxysmal positional vertigo; VBI, vertebrobasilar injury.

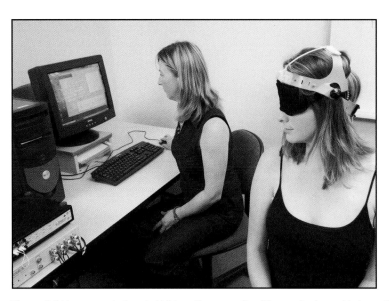

**Figure 6.1** Measurement of cervical joint position error – the difference (in degrees) between the starting and relocated position from rotation, measured using a Fastrak (Polhemus, Kaiser Aerospace, Vermont).

demonstrated greater cervical JPE than controls. Thus the test of JPE might be useful to determine changes in sensorimotor control due to mismatched afferent input from either abnormal vestibular or cervical origins, but not to differentiate between a vestibular and cervical cause. In circumstances that are not dissimilar, tests that use vision to determine the straight-ahead position in a darkened room have demonstrated that artificial disturbances to either cervical or vestibular input can alter the performance.[57–59]

In those with neck pain, measures of JPE are still relevant as deficits in relocation accuracy have been shown in people with either insidious-onset or trauma-induced neck pain. Moreover, reduced dizziness and improved relocation accuracy have been shown to occur following treatment directed specifically to the cervical spine.[1, 60, 61] Interestingly, evidence is emerging that JPE in the shoulder and elbow are also impaired following a whiplash injury[62, 63] which could affect the coordination and movement of the upper limb. Future research will undoubtedly reveal implications of such findings and any need for specific management.

## Postural stability

Disturbed postural stability has been found in patients with insidious-onset neck pain.[9, 45, 64–67] In relation to whiplash, some research has been inconclusive.[65, 68–70] In the case of a whiplash injury, patients may have vestibular disturbances or a mild head injury associated with the injury which can confuse interpretation of measures. In studies of whiplash which eliminated persons with a mild head injury or known vestibular disorder, balance disturbances were found to be present.[7, 71] Moreover, postural instability was greatest in those who reported the symptom of dizziness (Figure 6.2). Most whiplash patients were also unable to maintain postural stability in tandem stance. The level of anxiety, medication use, and compensation status did not influence the balance responses, which refutes the assertion that these factors primarily underlie postural stability deficits in this group.[12] Although a vestibular cause cannot

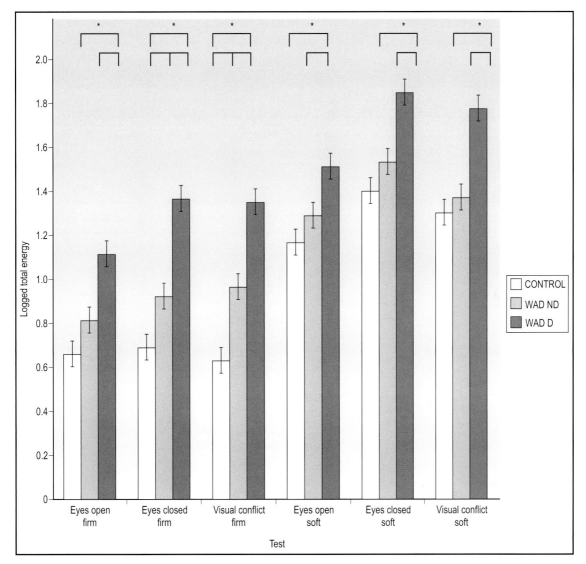

**Figure 6.2** Differences in balance measured in comfortable stance between whiplash patients with (WAD D) and without dizziness (WAD ND) and control subjects. The measures (mean and standard error) are of total energy of sway measured with eyes open, eyes closed, and visual conflict for both firm and soft surfaces. *$P < 0.05$. (Adapted from Treleaven et al.[7] with permission.)

be ruled out entirely, the results point to a cervical cause of balance disturbances in whiplash.[7] In support of a cervical cause, Stapley et al.[72] demonstrated that whiplash subjects with cervical muscle fatigue induced by sustained neck extension had increased postural sway.

Balance disturbances can be present in both insidious-onset and whiplash-induced neck pain; however, people with whiplash generally show greater disturbances.[66] Interestingly, Field et al.[66] showed that neither patient group can maintain tandem stance with their eyes closed for 30 seconds, which is in accordance with the findings of Michaelson et al.[65] We have also compared patients with chronic whiplash to patients with unilateral vestibular pathology.[47] Not unexpectedly, both groups had balance disturbances, but they had dissimilar characteristics, suggesting different underlying causes. In general, the whiplash group had greater deficits in comfortable stance (possibly reflecting somatosensory deficits) whereas the vestibular group had few deficits in comfortable stance, but greater deficits in the more challenging positions for the vestibular system, e.g., narrow stance on a foam surface.[73–76] Alpini et al.[77] also compared patients with whiplash injury and vestibular pathology during the Fuduka stepping test. This test assesses the distance and amount of angular turn of the person when stepping on the spot with the eyes closed for 30 seconds. In a subset of the whiplash group, a pattern of postural instability was observed that was comparable to neither the control group nor the subjects with vestibular pathology. Alpini et al.[77] considered this to be indicative of disturbed cervical somatosensory input in the neck pain patients. Future research into the discriminatory power of this and other tests may help to distinguish better patients with vestibular and cervical somatosensory dysfunction.

Age is another factor that affects balance. In a recent study we determined that elderly subjects with neck pain had greater balance disturbances when compared to elderly subjects without neck pain.[67] Older patients are likely to have more profound deficits in balance than younger patients with neck pain and this consideration should be given in assessment and management.

## Eye movement control

Control of vision can be divided into three types of eye movement control: the smooth-pursuit system, the saccadic system, and the optokinetic system. The smooth-pursuit system ensures stable images of a moving target with slow eye follow. The saccadic system allows rapid eye movements to change a point of fixation. The optokinetic system allows fixation of a target when a person is moving. To date deficits in oculomotor control have been demonstrated in subjects with both insidious-onset and traumatic neck pain, although the majority of research has been in subjects with whiplash.[6, 8, 20, 37, 78–83] In those with whiplash, Heikkila and Wenngren[78] demonstrated decreased smooth-pursuit velocity gain, i.e., decreased ability to follow the target smoothly with the eyes, altered peak velocity, and latency of saccadic eye movements. More recently an increased gain of the cervico-ocular reflex was demonstrated over a wide range of neck movement velocities, but especially with slower neck movements.[81, 82] This was reasoned to be related to either an increased proprioceptive sensitivity to neck movements, due to a decrease in range of motion, or altered cervical somatosensory input.[81, 82] Problems with convergence and diplopia have also been associated with whiplash disorders.[83] There is also some evidence that eye movement dysfunction may be prognostic.[79, 84] Hildingsson and Toolanen[84] found that those with eye movement dysfunction on smooth-pursuit and/or saccadic eye movement on initial assessment soon after the accident (20% of the cohort) continued to have persistent disabling symptoms at least 8 months postinjury. In contrast, the 80% with normal eye movement on initial assessment recovered fully or only had minor discomfort at this time point.

Tjell and Rosenhall[20] introduced the smooth-pursuit neck torsion test (SPNT), which is considered to be specific for detecting eye movement disturbances due to altered cervical afferent input. This test measures the difference in smooth-pursuit eye movement control with the head and trunk in a neutral position and when the neck is torsioned, i.e., the trunk and neck are rotated relative to the stationary head (Figure 6.3). Poor eye movement control in the torsioned position when compared to the neutral position is thought to reflect disturbances in the cervicocollic and cervico-ocular reflexes.[8] Tjell and Rosenhall[20]

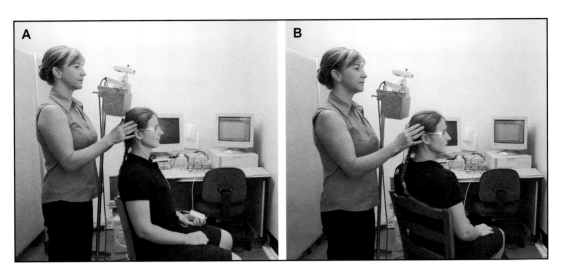

**Figure 6.3** The smooth-pursuit neck torsion test. The patient's eyes follow a laser beam moving horizontally at a speed of 20°/s through a total visual angle of 40°. Eye movement control is first tested (A) with the head and neck in neutral and (B) when the neck is torsioned or rotated relative to the stationary head. The measure is the difference in eye follow when the neck is in a torsioned position compared to the neutral position. Electrodes are placed laterally to the eyes and measure voltage change as the eye moves.

demonstrated that the altered smooth-pursuit eye movement control in torsion was evident in persons with whiplash but not in persons with vestibular disorders and central nervous system dysfunction. In addition, greater loss of eye movement control was identified for people with whiplash complaining of dizziness. Our research has confirmed these findings.[6, 47] The differences between people with whiplash and persons with vestibular or central nervous system dysfunction suggest that somatosensory input dysfunction from the cervical spine structures is the cause of loss of eye movement control in whiplash.

Disturbances of eye movement control have also been demonstrated in association with insidious-onset cervical vertigo and cervical spondylosis but not in fibromyalgia or control subjects.[8] However, greatest deficits have been observed in people with whiplash compared to idiopathic neck disorders. It is speculated that this is due to the sudden acceleration and deceleration forces imposed on the neck muscles and subsequent muscle tension.

It has also been suggested that cognitive disturbance, another common complaint after whiplash, may manifest from disturbances in sensorimotor control resulting from abnormal cervical somatosensory input. Gimse et al.[19] found a close correlation between technical reading ability, information uptake, and SPNT results. Similarly, driving skills were associated with altered eye movement control in the absence of other possible causes such as premorbid state and brain injury.[85]

## Relationship between measures of proprioception, eye movement control, and postural stability

Evidence has been presented that disturbed cervical somatosensory input associated with neck pain may affect postural stability, head orientation, and oculomotor control. Such changes in sensorimotor control have been shown to occur to a greater extent in those with traumatic-origin neck pain and in those complaining of dizziness. It could be postulated that there is a relationship between these three measures; however, we have shown no correlation between them.[13] Thus a patient with neck pain may present with disturbances to eye movement control but may not demonstrate any disturbance in cervical joint position sense or postural stability. Moreover, the degree of dizziness reported by the patient does not correlate with these measures. While subjects with whiplash complaining of dizziness demonstrated greater impairments in postural stability, cervical JPE and the SPNT, 50% of subjects with whiplash not complaining of dizziness had deficits in two or more of the objective tests of sensorimotor control.[13] At this time it is not known whether dizziness reflects an overall greater degree of cervical somatosensory dysfunction or relates to more specific areas of dysfunction.

## Onset of disturbances in sensorimotor control

The majority of studies investigating changes in sensorimotor control have been conducted in people with chronic neck disorders with little research to date into the acute state. Nevertheless, Karlberg et al.[86] demonstrated altered postural stability and eye movement control in healthy subjects within 5 days of wearing a restrictive neck brace. Hildingsson and Toolanen[84] noted disturbances in eye movement in 20% of their whiplash cohort within 1.7 months (0.5–3 months) postinjury. In addition, Sterling et al.[53] found increased JPE in whiplash patients with moderate to severe pain within 1 month of injury. Dizziness was reported in 20% of this group. Thus evidence is emerging to suggest that disturbances in sensorimotor control begin early in the history of the disorder.

## Management of disturbances in proprioception, eye movement control, and postural stability

Management of disturbances in proprioception, eye movement control, and postural stability has not been studied extensively in people with neck pain. However, there is some evidence for the efficacy of specific

rehabilitation strategies to change altered sensorimotor control.

Acupuncture has been shown to improve cervical joint position sense, vertigo,[1] and standing balance.[87] Improvements in dizziness, JPE, and range of motion have also been demonstrated with manipulative therapy.[1, 11, 60] Recently craniocervical flexion training was shown to have a demonstrable benefit on impaired cervical JPE in people with neck pain.[61] Stapley et al.[72] demonstrated a reduction in the deleterious effect of fatiguing contractions on postural stability in those with whiplash following physiotherapy, which included muscle endurance training. This suggests that improving muscle endurance may assist in the management of balance deficits in those with neck pain. Revel et al.[88] showed that 8 weeks of gaze stability, eye–head coordination and/or head-on-trunk relocation practice improved neck pain and disability and cervical JPE. Similar findings were described by Jull et al.[61] and Humphreys and Irgens.[54] Balance has also been shown to improve following a program of oculomotor rehabilitation.[83]

Other programs have been tested. Heikkila and Astrom[21] devised a multimodal approach which included body awareness retraining and demonstrated improvements in JPE as well as a tendency for improved range of motion following 5 weeks of training. Moreover, Hansson et al.[89] demonstrated that balance is improved and dizziness reduced in chronic whiplash with a vestibular rehabilitation program.

Based on the evidence to date, management of disturbances in proprioception, eye movement control, and postural stability should address not only impairments but also the source of altered cervical somatosensory input (e.g., impaired muscle function, painful and restricted joints). Thus we advocate a multimodal program, inclusive of manipulative therapy, specific muscle rehabilitation in conjunction with tailored programs including cervical joint

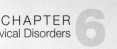

position retraining, gaze stability, and eye–head coordination exercises, as well as balance training. This program aims to address potential causes of altered cervical somatosensory input and to consider the important association between the cervical somatosensory, vestibular, and ocular systems. It is similar to vestibular rehabilitation programs designed to retrain the sensory and motor aspects of postural control and has proved to be successful for the management of postural control disturbances in patients with vestibular deficits.[90, 91]

## Conclusion

Deficits in cervical joint position sense, balance, and eye movement control have been demonstrated in both insidious-onset and traumatic neck pain and are likely reflecting disturbances in cervical somatosensory afferent information. It is recommended that cervical JPE, eye movement control, and postural stability are assessed routinely in the patient with neck pain. The lack of direct relationships between these measures and a lack of a direct relationship to patients' reported pain and disability indicates that each aspect should be assessed. The clinician should also be aware of other possible causes of dizziness and associated impairments, especially when neck pain is associated with trauma. Management tailored specifically to deficits in sensorimotor control in conjunction with treatment addressing the potential causes of abnormal cervical somatosensory input is advocated. Rehabilitation strategies to enhance cervical joint position sense, balance, and eye movement control are provided in Chapter 14.

## References

1. *Heikkila H, Johansson M, Wenngren BI*. Effects of acupuncture, cervical manipulation and NSAID therapy on dizziness and impaired head repositioning of suspected cervical origin: a pilot study. Man Ther 2000;5:151–157.

2. *Humphreys BK, Bolton J, Peterson C, et al*. A cross-sectional study of the association between pain and disability in neck pain patients with dizziness of suspected cervical origin. J Whiplash Relat Disord 2003;1:63–73.

3. *Treleaven J, Jull G, Sterling M*. Dizziness and unsteadiness following whiplash injury: characteristic features and relationship with cervical joint position error. J Rehabil Med 2003;35:36–43.

4. *Ernst A, Basta D, Seidl RO, et al*. Management of posttraumatic vertigo. Otolaryngol Head Neck Surg 2005;132:554–558.

5. *Jull G, Stanton W*. Predictors of responsiveness to physiotherapy treatment of cervicogenic headache. Cephalalgia 2005;25:101–108.

6. *Treleaven J, Jull G, Low Choy N*. Smooth pursuit neck torsion test in whiplash associated disorders – relationship to self reports of neck pain and disability, dizziness and anxiety. J Rehabil Med 2005;37:219–223.

7. *Treleaven J, Jull G, Low Choy N*. Standing balance in persistent WAD – comparison between subjects with and without dizziness. J Rehabil Med 2005;37:224–229.

8. *Tjell C, Tenenbaum A, Sandström S*. Smooth pursuit neck torsion test – a specific test for whiplash associated disorders? J Whiplash Relat Disord 2003;1:9–24.

9. *Karlberg M, Magnusson M, Malmstrom EM, et al*. Postural and symptomatic improvement after physiotherapy in patients with dizziness of suspected cervical origin. Arch Phys Med Rehabil 1996;77:874–882.

10. *Galm R, Rittmeister M, Schmitt E, et al*. Vertigo in patients with cervical spine dysfunction. Eur Spine J 1998;7:55–58.

11. *Reid S, Rivett D, Katekar M, et al*. Sustained natural apophyseal glides (SNAGs) are an effective treatment for cervicogenic dizziness. Man Ther 2008: In press.

12. *Ferrari R, Russell AS*. Development of persistent neurologic symptoms in patients with simple neck sprain. Arthritis Care Res 1999;12:70–76.

13. *Treleaven J, Jull G, LowChoy N*. The relationship of cervical joint position error to balance and eye movement disturbances in persistent whiplash. Man Ther 2006;11:99–106.

14. *Sturzenegger M, Stefano GD, Radanov B, et al*. Presenting symptoms and signs after whiplash

injury: the influence of accident mechanisms. Neurology 1994;44:688–693.

15. *Baloh R, Halmagyi G*. Disorders of the Vestibular System. New York: Oxford University Press, 1996.

16. *Chester JB*. Whiplash, postural control, and the inner ear. Spine 1991;16:716–720.

17. *Rubin AM, Woolley SM, Dailey VM, et al*. Postural stability following mild head or whiplash injuries. Am J Otol 1995;16:216–221.

18. *Hildingsson C, Wenngren BI, Toolanen G*. Eye motility dysfunction after soft-tissue injury of the cervical spine – a controlled, prospective study of 38 patients. Acta Orthop Scand 1993;64:129–132.

19. *Gimse R, Bjorgen IA, Tjell C, et al*. Reduced cognitive functions in a group of whiplash patients with demonstrated disturbances in the posture control system. J Clin Exp Neuropsychol 1997;19:838–849.

20. *Tjell C, Rosenhall U*. Smooth pursuit neck torsion test: a specific test for cervical dizziness. Am J Otol 1998;19:76–81.

21. *Heikkila H, Astrom PG*. Cervicocephalic kinesthetic sensibility in patients with whiplash injury. Scand J Rehabil Med 1996;28:133–138.

22. *Kerry R, Taylor AJ*. Cervical arterial dysfunction assessment and manual therapy. Man Ther 2006;11:243–253.

23. *Sturzenegger M*. Headache and neck pain: the warning symptoms of vertebral artery dissection. Headache 1994;34:187–193.

24. *Lee V, Brown RB Jr, Mandrekar J, et al*. Incidence and outcome of cervical artery dissection: a population-based study. Neurology 2006;67: 1809–1812.

25. *Cagnie B, Barbaix E, Vinck E, et al*. Atherosclerosis in the vertebral artery: an intrinsic risk factor in the use of spinal manipulation? Surg Radiol Anat 2006;28:129–134.

26. *Cagnie B, Barbaix E, Vinck E, et al*. Extrinsic risk factors for compromised blood flow in the vertebral artery: anatomical observations of the transverse foramina from C3 to C7. Surg Radiol Anat 2005;27:312–316.

27. *Panjabi MM, Cholewicki J, Nibu K, et al*. Mechanism of whiplash injury. Clin Biomech 1998;13:239–249.

28. *Endo K, Ichimaru K, Komagata M, et al*. Cervical vertigo and dizziness after whiplash injury. Eur Spine J 2006;15:886–890.

29. *Kloen P, Patterson JD, Wintman BI, et al*. Closed cervical spine trauma associated with bilateral vertebral artery injuries. Arch Orthop Trauma Surg 1999;119:478–481.

30. *Biffl WL, Moore EE, Elliott JP, et al*. The devastating potential of blunt vertebral arterial injuries. Ann Surg 2000;231:672–681.

31. *Taylor J, Taylor M*. Cervical spinal injuries: an autopsy study of 109 blunt injuries. J Musculoskel Pain 1996;4:61–79.

32. *Inamasu J, Guiot BH*. Vertebral artery injury after blunt cervical trauma: an update. Surg Neurol 2006;65:238–245.

33. *Michaud TC*. Uneventful upper cervical manipulation in the presence of a damaged vertebral artery. J Manipul Physiol Ther 2002;25:472–483.

34. *Arnold C, Bourassa R, Langer T, et al*. Doppler studies evaluating the effect of a physical therapy screening protocol on vertebral artery blood flow. Man Ther 2004;9:13–21.

35. *Thomas L, Rivett D, Bolton P*. Changes in vertebral artery blood flow during neck rotation. 13th Biennial conference Musculoskeletal Physiotherapy Australia. Sydney, Australia: 2003.

36. *Taylor AE, Cox CA, Mailis A*. Persistent neuropsychological deficits following whiplash: evidence for chronic mild traumatic brain injury? Arch Phys Med Rehabil 1996;77:529–535.

37. *Wenngren B, Pettersson K, Lowenhielm G, et al*. Eye motility and auditory brainstem response dysfunction after whiplash injury. Acta Orthop Scand 2002;122:276–283.

38. *Grimm RJ*. Inner ear injuries in whiplash. J Whiplash Relat Disord 2002;1:65–75.

39. *Toglia JU*. Acute flexion–extension injury of neck – electronystagmographic study of 309 patients. Neurology 1976;26:808–814.

40. *Hinoki M*. Vertigo due to whiplash injury: a neuro-otological approach. Acta Otolaryngol 1975;419: 9–29.

41. *Fischer A, Huygen PLM, Folgering HT, et al*. Vestibular hyperreactivity and hyperventilation after whiplash injury. J Neurol Sci 1995;132:35–43.

42. *Wrisley DM, Sparto PJ, Whitney SL, et al*. Cervicogenic dizziness: a review of diagnosis and treatment. J Orthop Sports Phys Ther 2000;30: 755–766.

43. *Reid SA, Rivett DA*. Manual therapy treatment of cervicogenic dizziness: a systematic review. Man Ther 2005;10:4–13.

44. *Bracher ES, Almeida CI, Almeida RR, et al*. A combined approach for the treatment of cervical vertigo. J Manipul Physiol Ther 2000;23:96–100.

45. *Karlberg M, Persson L, Magnusson M*. Impaired postural control in patients with cervico-brachial pain. Acta Oto-Laryngol 1995;520:440–442.

46. *Hulse M, Holzl M*. Vestibulospinal reflexes in patients with cervical disequilibrium ("the cervical staggering"). HNO 2000;48:295–301.

47. *Treleaven J, Low Choy N, Jull G, et al*. Comparison of postural control disturbance between subjects with persistent whiplash associated disorder and subjects with unilateral vestibular loss. Arch Phys Med Rehabil 2008; In press.

48. *Tesio L, Alpini D, Cesarani A, et al*. Short form of the Dizziness Handicap Inventory. Am J Phys Med Rehabil 1999;78:233–241.

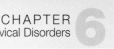
49. *Revel M, Andre-Deshays C, Minguet M*. Cervicocephalic kinesthetic sensibility in patients with cervical pain. Arch Phys Med Rehabil 1991;72:288–291.

50. *Mergner T, Schweigart G, Botti F, et al*. Eye movements evoked by proprioceptive stimulation along the body axis in humans. Exp Brain Res 1998;120:450–460.

51. *Blouin J, Okada T, Wolsley C, et al*. Encoding target-trunk relative position: cervical versus vestibular contribution. Exp Brain Res 1998;122:101–107.

52. *Kristjansson E, Dall'Alba P, Jull G*. New approaches to testing cervicocephalic kinaesthesia. Physiother Res Int 2002;6:224–235.

53. *Sterling M, Jull G, Vicenzino B, et al*. Development of motor system dysfunction following whiplash injury. Pain 2003;103:65–73.

54. *Humphreys B, Irgens P*. The effect of a rehabilitation exercise program on head repositioning accuracy and reported levels of pain in chronic neck pain subjects. J Whiplash Relat Disord 2002;1:99–112.

55. *Kristjansson E, Dall'Alba P, Jull G*. A study of five cervicocephalic relocation tests in three different subject groups. Clin Rehabil 2003;17:768–774.

56. *Feipel V, Salvia P, Klein H, et al*. Head repositioning accuracy in patients with whiplash-associated disorders. Spine 2006;31:E51–E58.

57. *Karnath HO, Reich E, Rorden C, et al*. The perception of body orientation after neck-proprioceptive stimulation – effects of time and of visual cueing. Exp Brain Res 2002;143:350–358.

58. *Strupp M, Arbusow V, Dieterich M, et al*. Perceptual and oculomotor effects of neck muscle vibration in vestibular neuritis – ipsilateral somatosensory substitution of vestibular function. Brain 1998;121:677–685.

59. *Karlberg M, Aw ST, Halmagyi GM, et al*. Vibration-induced shift of the subjective visual horizontal: a sign of unilateral vestibular deficit. Arch Otolaryngol Head Neck Surg 2002;128:21–27.

60. *Palmgren PJ, Sandstrom PJ, Lundqvist FJ, et al*. Improvement after chiropractic care in cervicocephalic kinesthetic sensibility and subjective pain intensity in patients with nontraumatic chronic neck pain. J Manipul Physiol Ther 2006;29:100–106.

61. *Jull G, Falla D, Treleaven J, et al*. Retraining cervical joint position sense: the effect of two exercise regimes. J Orthop Res 2007;5:404-412.

62. *Knox JJ, Beilstein DJ, Charles SD, et al*. Changes in head and neck position have a greater effect on elbow joint position sense in people with whiplash-associated disorders. Clin J Pain 2006;22:512–518.

63. *Sandlund J, Djupsjobacka M, Ryhed B, et al*. Predictive and discriminative value of shoulder proprioception tests for patients with whiplash-associated disorders. J Rehabil Med 2006;38:44–49.

64. *Alund M, Ledin T, Odkvist L, et al*. Dynamic posturography among patients with common neck disorders. A study of 15 cases with suspected cervical vertigo. J Vestib Res Equil Orient 1993;3:383–389.

65. *Michaelson P, Michaelson M, Jaric S, et al*. Vertical posture and head stability in patients with chronic neck. J Rehabil Med 2003;35:229–235.

66. *Field S, Treleaven J, Jull G*. Standing balance. A comparison between idiopathic and whiplash-induced neck pain. Man Ther 2008: In press.

67. *Poole E, Treleaven J, Jull G*. The influence of neck pain on balance and gait parameters in community dwelling elders. Man Ther 2008; In press.

68. *El-Kahky A, Kingma H, Dolmans M, et al*. Balance control near the limit of stability in various sensory conditions in healthy subjects and patients suffering from vertigo or balance disorders: impact of sensory input on balance control. Acta Otolaryngol 2000;120:508–516.

69. *Madeleine P, Prietzel H, Svarrer H, et al*. Quantitative posturography in altered sensory conditions: a way to assess balance instability in patients with chronic whiplash injury. Arch Phys Med Rehabil 2004;85:432–438.

70. *Sjostrom H, Allum JH, Carpenter MG, et al*. Trunk sway measures of postural stability during clinical balance tests in patients with chronic whiplash injury symptoms. Spine 2003;28:1725–1734.

71. *Treleaven J, Jull G, Murison R, et al*. Is the method of signal analysis and test selection important for measuring standing balance in chronic whiplash? Gait Posture 2005;21:395–402.

72. *Stapley PJ, Beretta MV, Dalla Toffola E, et al*. Neck muscle fatigue and postural control in patients with whiplash injury. Clin Neurophysiol 2006;47:610–622.

73. *Horak F, Nashner L, Diener H*. Postural strategies associated with somatosensory and vestibular loss. Exp Brain Res 1990;82:167–177.

74. *Shumway Cook A, Horak F*. Assessing the influence of sensory integration on balance. Phys Ther 1986;66:1548–1550.

75. *Nashner LM, Peters JF*. Dynamic posturography in the diagnosis and management of dizziness and balance disorders. Neurol Clin 1990;8:331–349.

76. *Allum JHJ, Bloem BR, Carpenter MG, et al*. Differential diagnosis of proprioceptive and vestibular deficits using dynamic support-surface posturography. Gait Posture 2001;14:217–226.

77. *Alpini D, Ciavarro GL, Andreoni G, et al*. Evaluation of head-to-trunk control in whiplash patients using digital CranioCorpoGraphy during a stepping test. Gait Posture 2005;22:308–316.

78. *Heikkila HV, Wenngren BI*. Cervicocephalic kinesthetic sensibility, active range of cervical motion, and oculomotor function in patients with whiplash injury. Arch Phys Med Rehabil 1998;79:1089–1094.

79. *Hildingsson C, Wenngren B, Bring G, et al*. Oculomotor problems after cervical spine injury. Acta Orthopaed Scand 1989;60:513–516.

80. *Prushansky T, Dvir Z, Pevzner E, et al*. Electro-oculographic measures in patients with chronic whiplash and healthy subjects: a comparative study. J Neurol Neurosurg Psychiatry 2004;75:1642–1644.

81. *Kelders WPA, Kleinrensink GJ, Van der Geest JN, et al*. The cervico-ocular reflex is increased in whiplash injury patients. J Neurotrauma 2005;22:133–137.

82. *Montfoort I, Kelders WPA, van der Geest JN, et al*. Interaction between ocular stabilization reflexes in patients with whiplash injury. Invest Ophthalmol Vis Sci 2006;47:2881–2884.

83. *Storaci R, Manelli A, Schiavone N, et al*. Whiplash injury and oculomotor dysfunctions: clinical-posturographic correlations. Eur Spine J 2006;15:1811–1816.

84. *Hildingsson C, Toolanen G*. Outcome after soft-tissue injury of the cervical spine: a prospective study of 93 car-accident victims. Acta Orthop Scand 1990;61:357–359.

85. *Gimse R, Bjorgen I, Straume A*. Driving skills after whiplash. Scand J Psychol 1997;38:165–170.

86. *Karlberg M, Magnusson M, Johansson R*. Effects of restrained cervical mobility on voluntary eye movements and postural control. Acta Otolaryngol 1991;111:664–670.

87. *Fattori B, Borsari C, Vannucci G, et al*. Acupuncture treatment for balance disorders following whiplash injury. Acupunct Electrother Res 1996;21:207–217.

88. *Revel M, Minguet M, Gregory P, et al*. Changes in cervicocephalic kinesthesia after a proprioceptive rehabilitation program in patients with neck pain: a randomized controlled study. Arch Phys Med Rehabil 1994;75:895–899.

89. *Hansson EE, Mansson NO, Ringsberg KAM, et al*. Dizziness among patients with whiplash-associated disorder: a randomized controlled trial. J Rehabil Med 2006;38:387–390.

90. *Herdman S*. Vestibular Rehabilitation. Philadelphia: Davis, 2000.

91. *Tee LH, Chee NW*. Vestibular rehabilitation therapy for the dizzy patient. Ann Acad Med Singapore 2005;34:289–294.

92. *Brandt T*. Cervical vertigo – reality or fiction? Audiol Neurootol 1996;1:187–196.

93. *Herdman S*. Advances in the treatment of vestibular disorders. Phys Ther 1997;77:602–617.

94. *Fitzgerald DC*. Head trauma: hearing loss and dizziness. J Trauma 1996;40:488–496.

95. *Chung YS, Han DH*. Vertebrobasilar dissection: a possible role of whiplash injury in its pathogenesis. Neurol Res 2002;24:129–138.

96. *Furman JM, Jacob RG*. Psychiatric dizziness. Neurology 1997;48:1161–1166.

97. *Ruckenstein MJ*. A practical approach to dizziness. Questions to bring vertigo and other causes into focus. Postgrad Med 1995;97:70–72, 75–78, 81.

7

# Psychological and Psychosocial Factors in Neck Pain

## Introduction

Neck pain and its associated symptoms often result in functional problems manifested by a variety of complex physical impairments. The current state of knowledge of the physical impairments associated with neck pain will be discussed in subsequent chapters. In the current multidimensional model of musculoskeletal pain, psychosocial and psychological factors must also be considered as having a role in the initiation and perpetuation of neck pain conditions. It is important for clinicians to have an understanding of the involvement of these factors, such that adaptation of treatment strategies can be made in order to account for psychological influences, to ensure that psychological disturbances may be identified and appropriate referral instituted when required. However it should be noted that the relationship between psychosocial/ psychological variables, physical impairment, and pain and disability is complex and not yet fully understood.[1] Clinicians should maintain an open mind with respect to potential interrelationships between these factors.

Investigation of psychological factors in pain and disability associated with neck pain has been relatively sparse when compared to some other musculoskeletal pain conditions, for example low-back pain. This has not prevented extrapolations being made from findings of studies on low-back pain to cervical spine pain. In some studies, psychological factors such as fear avoidance beliefs found to be important in low-back pain are automatically assumed to be relevant in neck pain without data to support these assertions. This was exemplified in a relatively recent review of psychological risk factors for back and neck pain.[2] Of the 37 studies that met the selection criteria for review, only four were studies that recruited participants with either neck pain alone or with back and neck pain. Despite this, the conclusions of the review were that there was high-level evidence that psychosocial and psychological factors are "clearly linked to the onset of back and neck pain."[2] In contrast to these assertions, it is becoming clear that such extrapolations should not be made in light of recent evidence demonstrating that the development and maintenance of neck pain probably involve psychological factors unique to this condition. It is important that such psychological factors associated with neck pain are realized to enable the development of appropriate treatment interventions. This chapter will explore the psychosocial and psychological factors associated with cervical spine pain.

## Psychological factors and chronic neck pain

There is no doubt that persistent neck pain, whether of insidious or traumatic onset, is associated with psychological distress.[3, 4] In the case of chronic whiplash-associated disorders (WAD), psychological distress may include affective disturbances, anxiety, depression, and behavioral abnormalities, as well as moderate levels of posttraumatic stress reaction (PTSR).[3, 5, 6]

Whilst the presence of psychological distress is not disputed, the direction of the relationship between psychological distress and persistent pain and disability is not clear and remains an area of vigorous debate. Do the ongoing pain and disability, characteristic of persistent neck pain, result in the patient being psychologically distressed or does the relationship occur in the opposite direction?

Whilst the exact nature of this relationship is difficult to determine, there is some evidence available which suggests that, at least in the case of whiplash injury, the psychological distress seen in the later chronic stage of the condition is most likely as a consequence of ongoing pain and disability. Gargan et al.[7] showed normal levels of psychological distress (measured with the General Health Questionnaire (GHQ-28)) in whiplash patients within a week of injury that became elevated at 3 months postinjury in association with restricted neck movement. Sterling et al.,[6] also using the GHQ-28, measured psychological responses to whiplash injury and found that at 3–4 weeks postinjury, all those experiencing a whiplash injury demonstrated psychological distress (albeit to varying degrees), irrespective of their levels of pain and disability. Psychological distress decreased by 2–3 months postinjury in those who recovered and those with lesser symptoms, seemingly paralleling decreasing levels of pain and disability (Figure 7.1). This finding of psychological distress, apparent in all whiplash-injured participants, appears to contrast with that of Gargan et al.,[7] who showed normal levels of distress a week after injury. However the different inception times of the studies should be noted. Gargan et al.[7] recruited whiplash participants within a week of injury whereas the inception time for the study of Sterling et al.[6] was 3–4 weeks. Further investigation of the development of psychological distress in this early acute stage of whiplash injury is required.

A large cross-sectional study showed an association between anxiety and depression and pain and disability in whiplash patients whose accidents occurred over 2 years previously, but not in those with acute injury, suggesting that symptom persistence is the trigger for psychological distress.[5] This view is supported by other prospective studies where delayed recovery following whiplash injury could not be predicted from psychological factors such as personality

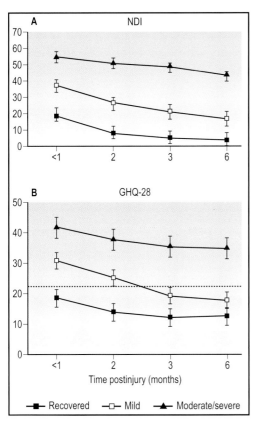

**Figure 7.1** Scores of the Neck Disability Index (NDI) and General Health Questionnaire (GHQ-28: a measure of psychological distress) in three groups of whiplash-injured participants (recovered, < 8 NDI; milder pain and disability, 10–28 NDI; moderate/severe pain and disability, > 30 NDI) at < 1 month, 2, 3, and 6 months postinjury. The dotted line indicates the threshold score for the GHQ-28.

provides some evidence that ongoing psychological distress may be dependent upon symptom persistence.

## Psychological factors in transition from acute to chronic neck pain

Since the emergence of the biopsychosocial model of pain, much research has focused on the role of psychological factors in the transition from acute to chronic pain. The most efficacious design to investigate the development or not of chronic pain following an acute pain episode is a prospective or longitudinal study design where a patient cohort is followed over time and participants developing neck pain are compared to those who do not. Most prospective studies of neck pain have investigated outcome following whiplash injury.

The seminal longitudinal study of whiplash injury was conducted in Switzerland by Radanov and colleagues.[8] One hundred and seventeen acutely injured whiplash patients were recruited and followed to 2 years postinjury. This study, although identifying some important prognostic indicators of outcome such as initial levels of pain and disability and symptomatic factors such as arm pain, failed to show that psychological factors such as personality traits (nervousness, depression, neuroticism, and passivity), self-rated well-being, or cognitive ability were predictive of outcome. However the psychological factors investigated by Radanov et al.[8] were not those perhaps more commonly acknowledged as playing a role in the transition to chronicity in other musculoskeletal conditions. Psychological factors such as fear avoidance beliefs, fear of movement/reinjury and coping strategies that are thought to play a significant role in the development of chronic low-back pain[2] were not investigated in this study.

traits or self-rated well-being but was related to initial symptom severity.[8, 9]

Wallis et al.[10] attempted to address the relationship between pain and disability and psychological distress from the opposite direction. These authors proposed that the relief or decrease of pain would allow resolution of psychological distress. They demonstrated this to be the case when psychological distress (measured with the Symptom Checklist-90 (SCL-90)) was shown to decrease following pain relief using zygapophyseal joint blocks in patients with chronic WAD. Whilst this procedure was performed in only a highly selected group of whiplash participants, it nevertheless

Fear avoidance beliefs have been hypothesized as the most important and specific psychosocial factor in predicting disability in patients with low-back pain.[11] The Fear Avoidance Model proposes that the individual's fear of pain and subsequent avoidance behavior are the most important determinants of the relationship between the sensory and emotional components of pain perception.[12] Data from several studies indicate that the relationship between fear avoidance beliefs and disability in neck pain may not be as strong in this condition as it is proposed to be in low-back pain. A cross-sectional study by George et al.[13] found that weaker relationships existed between these two factors in patients with chronic neck pain when compared to those with low-back pain. More recently, a prospective study of acute whiplash injury[6] showed that increased fears of movement and reinjury were not confined to those with a poor outcome (moderate/severe levels of pain and disability) 6 months postinjury. The participants who reported only milder residual symptoms at 6 months also demonstrated high initial scores (within a month of injury) on the Tampa Scale of Kinesiphobia (TSK), with the scores of both groups being markedly similar to those of chronic low-back pain. Interestingly, initial TSK scores of those participants left with residual milder symptoms at 6 months postinjury decreased by 2–3 months in tandem with reported symptomatic improvement. Furthermore, TSK scores of this whiplash group closely approximated those of fully recovered subjects by 2–3 months postaccident. These findings suggest that fear of movement may be justified in the acute stage of injury as a protective mechanism against further injury and to allow healing to occur, as has been proposed by some authors[14] but often overlooked when considering acute spinal pain.

The prospective longitudinal whiplash study conducted by our research group also found that fear of movement/reinjury was not a significant predictor of outcome following whiplash injury. In addition to the inclusion of measures of physical impairment, a variety of psychological measures were incorporated in an attempt to account for a broad array of psychological factors. The psychological factor found to be the strongest predictor of outcome was the presence of an early acute PTSR (measured with the Impact of Events Scale). This factor was a better predictor of outcome at both 6 months and 2 years postinjury than either TSK scores or general psychological distress (GHQ-28).[15, 16] This finding appears to be in contrast to those recently reported by Nederhand et al.,[17] who demonstrated that baseline levels of pain and disability together with TSK scores could account for 83% of the variance in pain and disability at 24 weeks post whiplash injury. However, Nederhand et al. only investigated two predictor variables (initial pain and disability and TSK scores) with no inclusion of either physical factors or additional psychological factors. Sterling et al.[15, 16] utilized both physical and psychological factors to gauge the predictive capacity of a multifactorial set of measures. In this context it was a combination of physical and psychological factors which proved to be the strongest predictors of outcome, with PTSR showing a stronger predictive capacity than both the TSK and general psychological distress measured with the GHQ-28. Inclusion of a measure of posttraumatic stress in the study of Nederhand et al. may have produced different results and highlights the necessity that a wide array of variables (including physical, psychological, and psychosocial factors) should be included in whiplash prediction studies such that a broad view of the condition is realized.

Maladaptive coping strategies such as catastrophizing have also been shown to be associated with ongoing low-back pain[18] but have been less well investigated in neck pain cohorts. Buitenhuis et al.[19] investigated the association between coping styles used by participants and the duration of neck complaints following whiplash injury. A palliative reaction or one where the patient seeks palliative relief of symptoms such as distraction, smoking, or drinking was significantly associated with a longer duration of neck symptoms at 12 months postinjury. Those participants who sought social support and shared their concerns with others showed a better outcome with less symptom duration.[19] Carroll et al.[20] also showed that passive coping strategies were associated with slower recovery following whiplash injury. They suggest that attention to the types of coping styles adopted by whiplash patients in the early stages of their condition may decrease the length of time that symptoms are reported. In contrast, Kivioja et al.[21] found no evidence that different coping styles in the early stage of injury influenced the outcome at 1 year postaccident. These studies involved different inception times. The participants of the Carroll et al.[20] study were recruited within 6 weeks of injury, with the inception time of the latter study being within hours of the injury. Thus coping strategies may vary depending on the stage of the condition or injury and this requires further investigation. Nevertheless, whilst coping styles may not be independently associated with poor recovery, improvement of the individual patient's coping mechanisms via education and assurance is recommended and in keeping with current treatment guidelines.[22, 23]

Few studies have investigated the influence of coping styles on pain and disability in insidious-onset neck pain. Two large studies have demonstrated that a passive coping style is a risk factor for pain and disability in chronic neck pain; however, the cohorts of these studies were not well described and it was likely that both whiplash and insidious-onset neck pain participants were included.[24, 25] Thus the differential effect of this psychological factor in these two neck pain conditions remains to be elucidated.

# The role of acute posttraumatic stress reaction in the whiplash injury

Whiplash injury differs from most other musculoskeletal pain syndromes, including insidious-onset neck pain, in that it is precipitated by a traumatic event, namely a motor vehicle crash. The effect of the psychological stress surrounding the crash itself as opposed to distress about neck pain complaints may have an influence on outcome.

Evidence of a diagnosis of posttraumatic stress disorder in some patients with chronic WAD has been reported.[26] In addition an acute PTSR appears to be present in some whiplash-injured individuals soon after injury, with moderate to high levels of distress (measured with the Impact of Events Scale) being demonstrated both within days of injury and within 3–4 weeks of injury.[27, 28] The presence of posttraumatic stress symptoms is associated with greater levels of pain and disability, more severe whiplash complaints, and poor functional recovery from the injury (Figure 7.2).[6, 29] Furthermore, following a motor vehicle crash, those with a diagnosis of whiplash (neck pain) are significantly more likely to have a posttraumatic stress disorder at 12 months postaccident compared to those who never reported neck pain postaccident.[26] A moderate PTSR, present within a month of injury, is a strong predictor of poor outcome at both 6 months and 2 years postinjury, being stronger than both general psychological distress (GHQ-28) and fear of movement and reinjury (TSK).[15, 16]

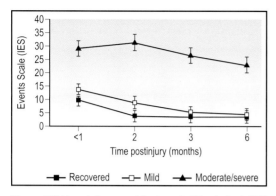

**Figure 7.2** Mean (SD) scores of the Impact of Events Scale (IES) (a measure of posttraumatic stress symptoms) in three groups of whiplash-injured participants (recovered, < 8 NDI; milder pain and disability, 10–28 NDI; moderate/severe pain and disability, > 30 NDI) at < 1 month, 2, 3, and 6 months postinjury. NDI, Neck Disability Index.

Symptoms of posttraumatic stress may include intrusive thoughts and/or images of the event (in this case the motor vehicle crash); avoidance behavior associated with the event, such as driving avoidance or avoidance via substance abuse; and hyperarousal such as panic attacks, hypervigilance, and sleep disturbance. It is not clear if any of these symptoms plays a specifically greater role than the others in whiplash pain, disability, or outcome. Our longitudinal data suggested that avoidance behavior may have a stronger influence on recovery[6] and recently Buitenhuis et al.[29] showed that a greater number of hyperarousal symptoms in the acute stage of injury was a stronger predictor of symptom persistence. Further investigation is required to determine the relative importance of the substrates of posttraumatic stress as this may provide direction for approaches to the psychological management of the whiplash patient.

In summary, the available data to date indicate that posttraumatic stress symptoms play an important role in recovery from a whiplash injury, at least in some individuals. This suggests that specific treatments directed toward these factors may be more efficacious than a broadly applied cognitive behavioral approach in the management of whiplash.

# Relationships between physical and psychological factors

The biopsychosocial model considers pain and disability as the result of multiple factors, with biomedical (physical) and psychological factors intimately intertwined. However it is not clear what the relative role of each factor may be or how they interact.

Complex sensory disturbances such as widespread mechanical and thermal hyperalgesia seem to be a feature of chronic WAD but are not so apparent in chronic neck pain of insidious origin (Chapter 2).[30] The sensory changes observed in whiplash are not only a feature of the chronic stage of the condition but are present from soon after injury in those who develop persistent pain and disability, remaining virtually unchanged from the acute to chronic stages of the condition.[31] Elevated levels of psychological distress, including general distress, PTSR, and fears of movement and reinjury, occur concomitantly with sensory hypersensitivity in whiplash-injured persons. It is recognized that psychological distress such as anxiety can have an effect on psychophysical sensory tests, particularly those measuring a threshold response.[32] PTSR may also be associated with heightened reactivity to stimuli as well as being manifested by sympathetic nervous system changes in some individuals.[33] It is likely that the co-occurrence of sensory hypersensitivity, increased muscle activity, and psychological distress in some whiplash-injured people is not merely coincidental. Potentially, these factors are related (possibly mechanistically) and knowledge of these relationships is important in order to improve understanding of processes underlying the condition.

With respect to the phenomenon of sensory hypersensitivity in whiplash, it is generally accepted that the sensory disturbances reflect alterations in the underlying neurobiological processing of pain. However, there are still those who suggest that all hypersensitive responses seen in WAD are a result of psychological factors or even malingering by the injured persons.[34, 35] Our prospective investigation of whiplash injury clearly showed that the persistent widespread sensory changes were present from early after injury in those with poor recovery but were not a feature of participants with full or fair recovery. These clear group differences remained even when the higher levels of psychological distress (GHQ-28) of the group with poor recovery were accounted for in the analysis of the group data.[31] Whilst it is acknowledged that only one aspect of psychological distress was used in this analysis, this was the first time that the relationship between sensory changes and psychological factors had been investigated in WAD. It suggests that sensory hypersensitivity does not solely occur due to anxiety and psychological distress.

There does appear to be some relationship between psychological factors and sensory disturbance. Sterling et al.[36] demonstrated moderate associations between pain thresholds (pressure and cold) at some sites, particularly at more remote sites such as in the lower limb, and both psychological distress (GHQ-28) and catastrophization (Pain Catastrophizing Scale: PCS). Notably, there was no relationship between catastrophization and the intensity of electrical stimulation required to elicit a flexor withdrawal response in biceps femoris in the same patient group (Chapter 2).[36] The latter test is a measure of spinal cord hyperexcitability requiring no cognitive response from the participant.[37] These findings indicate that psychological factors play a role in central hypersensitivity. However, they do not support the

assumption that psychological factors are the only or main factors responsible for central hypersensitivity in whiplash patients. In particular, spinal cord hyperexcitability appears not to be affected, at least significantly, by the psychological factors that were assessed.

The relationships between sensory and sympathetic changes and PTSR have also been explored. Sterling and Kenardy[38] showed that the early presence of sensory hypersensitivity (mechanical and cold hyperalgesia) was associated with persistent posttraumatic stress symptoms but that this relationship was mediated by initial pain and disability levels (in this case, Neck Disability Index scores). In contrast, early sympathetic disturbance (impaired peripheral vasoconstriction) was associated with persistent posttraumatic stress symptoms and showed no relationship with initial pain and disability levels (Figure 7.3). Although speculative, this may be an indication of a biological vulnerability in some with acute whiplash injury that could be a trigger for posttraumatic stress symptoms seen in the chronic stage of the condition.

When taken together, these findings indicate that psychological factors such as distress, catastrophization, and posttraumatic stress symptoms show some association with sensory hypersensitivity in chronic whiplash. However this relationship is not consistent for all modalities, measures, or at all body sites tested and may be mediated by levels of pain and disability. This would suggest that psychological factors are not the only or main factors responsible for central hypersensitivity in whiplash patients. Central hyperexcitability after whiplash is therefore a complex phenomenon that probably involves both neurobiological changes as well as psychological factors.

Recent models have been put forward in an attempt to provide a basis for the complex interrelationships between physical and

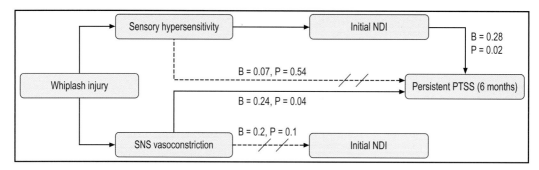

**Figure 7.3** Relationships between sensory and sympathetic disturbances and persistent posttraumatic stress symptoms (PTSS) following whiplash injury. The relationship between sensory hypersensitivity and PTSS is moderated by pain and disability (Neck Disability Index: NDI) levels. Sympathetic nervous system (SNS) vasoconstriction independently predicts persistent PTSS.[38]

psychological aspects of the whiplash condition. It has been suggested that the dysregulation of neurobiological pain processing is related to the stress response and/or sympathetic activation in the early stages following injury and this interaction may be a critical step in the development of persistent pain.[38-40]

Models such as these, which aim to integrate the physical and psychological manifestations of whiplash and neck pain, are overdue in the conceptualization and investigation of musculoskeletal pain and will provide a framework for future investigation of WAD and similar conditions. They will also provide an improved basis for the integration and appropriate timing of treatments directed toward both physical (biological) impairments and psychological factors. It is suggested that this integrated approach will be the way forward in the management of musculoskeletal pain rather than the dichotomous separation of physical and psychological factors that so often occurs in research and practice.

Only one study has explored sensory disturbances and psychological distress in insidious-onset neck pain.[30] In this study the participants with insidious-onset neck pain showed only local mechanical hyperalgesia over the cervical spine, with more widespread hyperalgesia being reserved for the whiplash patients. The local cervical spine hyperalgesia was independent of anxiety levels at the time of testing, as measured with the State Trait Anxiety Index. This study did not use more extensive measures of psychological distress and as such the relationship between these factors in insidious-onset neck pain requires further investigation.

There has been some preliminary exploration of the relationship between the motor dysfunction seen in whiplash-injured persons and fears of movement/reinjury. Fears of movement and reinjury have been associated with altered lumbar paraspinal muscle activity in chronic low-back pain.[41] Similarly, fear of pain (induced experimentally) can alter lumbar spine muscle recruitment patterns, albeit in asymptomatic subjects.[42] We have shown that motor dysfunction, including cervical range of movement loss, kinesthetic deficits, and altered cervical flexor muscle recruitment patterns, occurred independently (statistically) of TSK scores, with this relationship being consistent at both the acute and chronic stages of whiplash injury.[28] We interpreted these findings as an indication of physiological disturbances in motor function as opposed to fears of movement.[28]

In contrast to our findings, Nederhand and colleagues[43] showed that fear of movement (TSK scores) was independently associated with decreased activity in the upper trapezius in a prospective whiplash cohort. These two studies appear to provide conflicting results. However, different muscles were measured in each study, with the cervical flexors of Sterling et al.'s[28] study showing increased activity and the upper trapezius of Nederhand et al.'s study showing decreased activity. It is feasible that psychological factors such as fear of movement influence the motor system in different ways or both physiological and psychological factors are interrelating in their effects on the motor system.

There is still much to be learnt about the nexus between physical (sensory and motor) manifestations and psychological aspects of neck pain conditions. For practitioners it is important to realize the potential influence of psychological factors on the patient's physical presentation. The challenge is to disentangle these relationships in both the research environment and in the clinical situation.

## Psychosocial factors in neck pain

A recent systematic review of psychosocial risk factors for neck pain identified 29 studies that met sufficient selection criteria.[44] Many more studies were identified but most were excluded as they did not investigate neck pain alone but rather neck pain in combination with shoulder and/or arm pain.[44] Furthermore many studies were cross-sectional, a design which is methodologically problematic when the aim is to identify factors associated with symptom development[45] as both predictive factors and outcome are measured at the same time. Due to the lack of prospective data in this area, Ariens et al.[44] were forced to include cross-sectional studies in their review and this emphasizes the need for further high-quality longitudinal studies in this area. There was also variance in the types of populations studied. Some studies investigate working populations, with the types of occupation studied also varying, ranging from manual-type labor to sedentary desk workers. Other studies utilize a more general community-based cohort.

As a result, Ariens et al.[44] examined various psychosocial risk factors in predominantly working populations and grouped them into nine categories (quantitative job demands, social support, conflict at work, job control, skill discretion, job strain, job satisfaction, job security, rest break opportunities). They then determined the level of evidence for these nine categories. The results of the systematic review demonstrated some evidence for poor social (coworker) support, low job control, low skill discretion, and low job satisfaction as risk factors for higher levels of neck pain. Inconclusive evidence was found for poor supervisor support, conflicts at work, low job security, high job strain, and limited opportunity for rest breaks. Since this review was undertaken some additional prospective studies have been conducted. Viikari-Juntara et al.[6] identified age, gender, body mass index, smoking, and mental stress as being associated with radiating neck pain in forest workers. Croft et al.[47] reported that the factors of number of children, poor self-assessed health, and previous neck and back pain were associated with future episodes of neck pain.

It seems likely that interactions between various psychosocial factors will occur where a combination of factors increases the risk of neck pain and/or disability, and this has been shown in some studies.[48,49] Johnston et al.[49] for example demonstrated that interactions between job demands, decision authority, and supervisor support were associated with higher levels of pain and disability in female office workers. Such interactions may be important to consider in the initial assessment of neck pain patients, particularly office workers, but as these studies were cross-sectional in design, further longitudinal data are required to clarify their importance on long-term outcomes of work-related neck pain.

Probably what can be gained from these studies is that psychosocial factors do play a role in the development of neck pain but this may vary depending on the cohort recruited. Therefore it may then be difficult to extrapolate these findings to all neck pain patients. An example of this can be seen from the research of WAD. There has been some investigation of psychosocial and sociodemographic risk factors for recovery from whiplash injury. However when this condition is looked at in isolation from more general neck pain populations, few psychosocial factors are shown to be consistent predictors of outcome. Both recent systematic reviews of prognostic indicators for outcome following whiplash injury could not find any consistent evidence that marital status, number of dependants, income, work activities, or education influence recovery.[50, 51] This illustrates the caution that is required when trying to take the results of such studies into the clinical assessment of individual patients.

## Implications for assessment and management of neck pain

Clinicians managing patients with neck pain must be aware of the potential complexity of the condition in terms of both physical and psychological impairments. The presence of psychological disturbance will impact upon the nature of the physical treatment provided and modifications may need to be made to the particular treatment approach in order to accommodate psychological changes.[52]

Firstly the clinician must be able to recognize the presence of psychological distress in the assessment of an individual patient. This can be achieved by the administration of questionnaires designed to assess specific psychological factors (for example, GHQ-28, Short Form-36 (SF-36)). The clinician must then decide an appropriate plan of action. The decision to refer the patient to a psychologist or to continue care with physical therapies, which is inclusive of assurance and advice, can be a difficult one. As with management of physical impairments, where it appears specificity is a necessary component, the same specific approach may also be required for the management of psychological disturbance.

In whiplash injury, levels of general psychological distress have been shown to decrease with the resolution of pain and disability.[6] It could be argued, in these less complicated cases, that management alone with physical therapies will be sufficient to address both physical impairment and psychological distress. Preliminary evidence to support this argument can be found in a recent randomized controlled trial of chronic whiplash injury where a physiotherapy program of assurance, advice, manual therapy, and specific exercise was sufficient to decrease psychological distress (measured with the GHQ-28) in some patients.[53] More specifically, these were patients with a "less complicated" presentation, that is, lower levels of pain and disability and without signs of widespread sensory disturbance.

In contrast to this scenario are those neck pain patients with more severe psychological distress. In particular, some whiplash-injured patients show higher levels of PTSR in addition to their general distress levels. Longitudinal data have shown that the acute PTSR did not resolve in approximately 13% of participants of the cohort studied.[6] Furthermore a multimodal physiotherapy program including both specific exercise and spinal manual therapy failed to decrease PTSR significantly in patients with chronic whiplash.[53] These findings indicate the importance of the clinician being alert to the presence of PTSR and instituting appropriate psychological referral. However this does not imply that physical therapy treatments are abandoned. Whilst we have demonstrated that physiotherapy treatment alone failed to improve symptoms of posttraumatic stress, psychological treatment alone has likewise been shown not to have an influence on pain levels of whiplash.[54] The findings of these two clinical trials provide further evidence that complex and interrelating mechanisms underlie the whiplash condition and that cooperative multiprofessional management will be necessary in those with a "more complicated" presentation.

As mentioned previously, symptoms of posttraumatic stress may include intrusive thoughts and/or images of the event (motor vehicle crash); avoidance behavior associated with the event such as driving avoidance or avoidance via substance abuse; and intense arousal such as panic attacks, hypervigilance, and sleep disturbance. These symptoms may become apparent to the clinician during the standard patient interview or alternatively via administration of a questionnaire such as the Impact of Events Scale.[55]

The timing of psychological referral for PTSR is controversial, with some believing that a too-early referral may in fact exacerbate posttraumatic stress symptoms in those who otherwise may spontaneously recover. The general consensus indicates that an early PTSR should be allowed some time for natural recovery to occur. When this recovery is not apparent within several (3–6) weeks, guidelines suggest that psychological referral should be instigated.[23]

## Conclusion

It is clear that psychosocial and psychological factors play a role in the development and maintenance of pain and disability associated with neck pain. The direction of the relationship between pain and disability and psychological factors is unclear but, at least in the case of WAD, there is evidence to suggest that persistent higher symptomatic levels drive elevated levels of psychological distress.

Whiplash injury is further complicated by the presence, in some, of an acute PTSR and this psychological factor may need to be specifically addressed in those patients for whom this reaction is identified. There appears to be some psychological influences to both the sensory and motor disturbances that characterize the whiplash condition. Neck pain patients need to be comprehensively assessed for the presence to varying degrees of psychological and physical impairments. For some patients with a complex presentation involving interrelationships between psychological and physical factors, multiprofessional approaches to management may be the most beneficial approach.

## References

1. *Linton S*. Psychological risk factors for neck and back pain. In: Nachemson A, Jonsson E (eds) Neck and Back Pain: The Scientific Causes, Diagnosis and Treatment. Philadelphia: Lippincott Williams and Wilkins, 2000:57–78.

2. *Linton S*. A review of psychological risk factors in back and neck pain. Spine 2000;25:1148–1156.

3. *Peebles J, McWilliams L, MacLennan R*. A comparison of symptom checklist 90-revised profiles from patients with chronic pain from whiplash and patients with other musculoskeletal injuries. Spine 2001;26:766–770.

4. *Luo X, Edwards C, Richardson W, et al*. Relationships of clinical, psychological and individual factors with the functional status of neck pain patients. Value Health 2004;7:61–69.

5. *Wenzel H, Haug T, Mykletun A, et al*. A population study of anxiety and depression among persons who report whiplash traumas. J Psychosom Res 2002;53:831–835.

6. *Sterling M, Kenardy J, Jull G, et al.* The development of psychological changes following whiplash injury. Pain 2003;106:481–489.

7. *Gargan M, Bannister G, Main C, et al.* The behavioural response to whiplash injury. J Bone Joint Surg 1997;79B:523–526.

8. *Radanov B, Sturzenegger M, Di Stefano G.* Long-term outcome after whiplash injury. A 2-year follow-up considering features of injury mechanism and somatic, radiologic, and psychological findings. Medicine 1995;74:281–297.

9. *Borchgrevink G, Stiles T, Borchgrevink P, et al.* Personality profile among symptomatic and recovered patients with neck sprain injury, measured by MCMI-1 acutely and 6 months after car accidents. J Psychosom Res 1997;42:357–367.

10. *Wallis B, Lord S, Bogduk N.* Resolution of psychological distress of whiplash patients following treatment by radiofrequency neurotomy: a randomised, double-blind, placebo controlled trial. Pain 1997;73:15–22.

11. *Vlaeyen J, Linton S.* Fear-avoidance and its consequences in chronic musculoskeletal pain: a state of the art. Pain 2000;85:317–332.

12. *Slade P, Troup J, Lethem J.* The fear-avoidance model of exaggerated pain perception. Behav Res Ther 1983;21:409–416.

13. *George S, Fritz J, Erhard R.* A comparison of fear-avoidance beliefs in patients with lumbar spine pain and cervical spine pain. Spine 2001;26:2139–2145.

14. *Vlaeyen J, Kole-Snijders A, Boeren R.* Fear of movement/reinjury in chronic low-back pain patients and its relation to behavioural performance. Pain 1995;1995:363–372.

15. *Sterling M, Jull G, Vicenzino B, et al.* Physical and psychological factors predict outcome following whiplash injury. Pain 2005;114:141–148.

16. *Sterling M, Jull G, Kenardy J.* Physical and psychological predictors of outcome following whiplash injury maintain predictive capacity at long term follow-up. Pain 2006;122:102–108.

17. *Nederhand M, Ijzerman M, Hermens H, et al.* Predictive value of fear avoidance in developing chronic neck pain disability: consequences for clinical decision making. Arch Phys Med Rehabil 2004;85:496–501.

18. *Pincus T, Burton A, Vogel S, et al.* A systematic review of psychological factors as predictors of chronicity/disability in prospective cohorts of low-back pain. Spine 2002;27:E109–E120.

19. *Buitenhuis J, Spanjer J, Fidler V.* Recovery from acute whiplash – the role of coping styles. Spine 2003;28:896–901.

20. *Carroll L, Cassidy D, Cote P.* The role of pain coping strategies in prognosis after whiplash injury: passive coping predicts slowed recovery. Pain 2006;124:18–26.

21. *Kivioja J, Jensen I, Lindgren U.* Early coping strategies do not influence the prognosis after whiplash injuries. Injury 2005;36: 935–940.

22. *Scholten-Peeters G, Bekkering G, Verhagen A, et al.* Clinical practice guideline for the physiotherapy of patients with whiplash associated disorders. Spine 2002;27:412–422.

23. *Motor Accidents Authority.* Guidelines for the management of whiplash associated disorders. Sydney: Motor Accidents Authority, 2006:16.

24. *Mercado A, Carroll L, Cassidy D, et al.* Passive coping is a risk factor for disabling neck or low-back pain. Pain 2005;117:51–57.

25. *Hurwitz E, Goldstein M, Morgenstern H, et al.* The impact of psychosocial factors on neck pain and disability outcomes among primary care patients: results from the UCLA neck pain study. Dis Rehabil 2006;28:1319–1329.

26. *Freidenberg B, Hickling E, Blanchard E, et al.* Posttraumatic stress disorder and whiplash after motor vehicle accidents. In: Young G, Kane A, Nicholson K (eds). Psychological Knowledge in Court. New York: Springer, 2006:215–224.

27. *Drottning M, Staff P, Levin L, et al.* Acute emotional response to common whiplash predicts subsequent pain complaints: a prospective study of 107 subjects sustaining whiplash injury. Nord J Psychiatry 1995;49:293–299.

28. *Sterling M, Jull G, Vizenzino B, et al.* Development of motor system dysfunction following whiplash injury. Pain 2003;103:65–73.

29. *Buitenhuis J, DeJong J, Jaspers J, et al.* Relationship between posttraumatic stress disorder symptoms and the course of whiplash complaints. J Psychosom Res 2006;61:681–689.

30. *Scott D, Jull G, Sterling M.* Sensory hypersensitivity is a feature of chronic whiplash associated disorders but not chronic idiopathic neck pain. Clin J Pain 2005;21:175–181.

31. *Sterling M, Jull G, Vicenzino B, et al.* Sensory hypersensitivity occurs soon after whiplash injury and is associated with poor recovery. Pain 2003;104:509–517.

32. *Rhudy J, Meagher M.* Fear and anxiety: divergent effects on human pain thresholds. Pain 2000;84: 65–75.

33. *Harvey A, Bryant R.* Acute stress disorder: a synthesis and critique. Psychol Bull 2002;128: 886–902.

34. *Ferrari R.* Whiplash and symptom amplification. Pain 2001;89:293–294.

35. *Greve K, Bianchini K.* More on the clinical and scientific relevance of 'symptom amplification' and psychological factors in pain. Pain 2004;110:499–500.

36. *Sterling M, Pettiford C, Hodkinson E, et al.* Psychological factors are related to some sensory pain thresholds but not nociceptive flexion reflex threshold in chronic whiplash. Clin J Pain 2008; in press.

37. *Banic B, Petersen-Felix S, Andersen O, et al.* Evidence for spinal cord hypersensitivity in chronic

pain after whiplash injury and in fibromyalgia. Pain 2004;107:7–15.

38. *Sterling M, Kenardy J*. The relationship between sensory and sympathetic nervous system changes and acute posttraumatic stress following whiplash injury – a prospective study. J Psychosom Res 2006;60:387–393.

39. *McLean S, Clauw D, Abelson J, et al*. The development of persistent pain and psychological morbidity after motor vehicle collision: integrating the potential role of stress response systems into a biopsychosocial model. Psychosom Med 2005;67:783–790.

40. *Passatore M, Roatta S*. Influence of sympathetic nervous system on sensorimotor function: whiplash associated disorders (WAD) as a model. Eur J Appl Physiol 2006;98:423–449.

41. *Watson P, Booker C, Main C*. Evidence for the role of psychological factors in abnormal paraspinal activity in patients with chronic low-back pain. J Musculoskel Pain 1997;5:41–56.

42. *Moseley G, Nicholas M, Hodges P*. Does anticipation of back pain predispose to back trouble? Brain 2004;127:2339–2347.

43. *Nederhand M, Hermens H, Ijzerman M, et al*. The effect of fear of movement on muscle activation in posttraumatic neck pain disability. Clin J Pain 2006;22:519–525.

44. *Ariens G, van Mechelen W, Bongers P, et al*. Psychosocial risk factors for neck pain: a systematic review. Am J Ind Med 2001;39:180–193.

45. *Malchaire J, Cock N, Vergracht S*. Review of factors associated with musculoskeletal problems in epidemiological studies. Int Arch Occup Environ Health 2001;74:79–90.

46. *Viikari-Juntara E, Martikainen R, Luukonen R, et al*. Longitudinal study on work related and individual risk factors affecting radiating neck pain. Occup Environ Med 2001;58:345–351.

47. *Croft P, Lewis M, Papageorgio A, et al*. Risk factors for neck pain: a longitudinal study in the general population. Pain 2001;93:317–325.

48. *Leroux J, Dionne C, Bourbonnais R, et al*. Prevalence of musculoskeletal pain and associated factors in the Quebec working population. Int Arch Occup Environ Health 2005;78:379–386.

49. *Johnston V, Jimmieson N, Souvlis T, et al*. Interaction of psychosocial factors explain increased neck problems among female office workers. Pain 2007;129:311–320.

50. *Cote P, Cassidy D, Carroll L, et al*. A systematic review of the prognosis of acute whiplash and a new conceptual framework to synthesize the literature. Spine 2001;26:E445–E458.

51. *Scholten-Peeters G, Verhagen A, Bekkering G, et al*. Prognostic factors of whiplash associated disorders: a systematic review of prospective cohort studies. Pain 2003;104:303–322.

52. *Childs J, Fritz J, Piva S, et al*. Proposal of a classification system for patients with neck pain. J Orthop Sports Phys Ther 2004;34:686–696.

53. *Jull G, Sterling M, Kenardy J, et al*. Does the presence of sensory hypersensitivity influence outcomes of physical rehabilitation for chronic whiplash? A preliminary RCT. Pain 2007; 129:28–34.

54. *Blanchard E, Hickling E, Devineni T, et al*. A controlled evaluation of cognitive behaviour therapy for posttraumatic stress in motor vehicle accident survivors. Behav Res Ther 2003;41:79–96.

55. *Horowitz M, Wilner N, Alvarez W*. Impact of Event Scale: a measure of subjective stress. Psychosom Med 1979;41:209–218.

# 8

# Whiplash-associated Disorders

## Introduction

Whiplash-associated disorders (WAD) are a common, disabling and costly condition that occurs as a consequence of a motor vehicle crash (MVC). Whilst the figures vary depending on the cohort studied, the current understanding is that by 3 months approximately one-third of an inception cohort will have recovered from their initial pain and disability, approximately one-third will have persisting lower levels of pain and disability, and approximately one-third of the original cohort will have quite high levels of persisting pain and disability.[1-3] The associated cost secondary to the whiplash injury, including medical care, disability, lost work productivity, as well as personal costs, is substantial.[4,5]

Of all painful musculoskeletal conditions, whiplash is arguably one of the most controversial. This is in part due to the compensable nature of the injury and the fact that a precise pathoanatomical diagnosis is commonly not available, at least with current imaging techniques. Evidence is emerging that whiplash is a remarkably complex and varied condition involving diverse physical and psychological manifestations, with some of these factors showing an association with poor functional recovery. Evidence also suggests that whiplash shows some unique characteristics compared to other common spinal pain conditions.

The heterogeneity of the whiplash condition may explain the modest effects of treatment strategies investigated to date. Trials of treatment for acute whiplash have not demon̲s̲t̲_____ ̲s of decreasing the incidence of those who develop persistent symptoms.[6-9] This is not to suggest that little has been learnt from these randomized controlled trials. Indeed, it is apparent that maintenance of activity and sensible advice are superior to rest and prescription of a collar for most whiplash-injured people.[10] However, even in the presence of such a treatment approach, significant numbers of patients develop persistent symptoms. Furthermore, trials of treatment for the chronic stage of the condition, including various exercise forms, have shown that, although these programs were effective in decreasing pain and disability levels, only 10–20% of patients had a completely successful outcome.[11, 12]

Most trials have investigated relatively nonspecific approaches to treatment without taking the heterogeneous nature of whiplash into account. It would appear that WAD is a more complex condition than previously assumed. Recently, investigations have begun to provide insight into the characteristics of the whiplash condition, both physical and psychological, that allows speculation of potential underlying mechanisms.

This chapter will outline the whiplash injury, the possible structures involved, and the classification of WAD before discussing the burgeoning knowledge of the physical and psychological manifestations of the condition and the implications for clinical practice.

# The whiplash condition

## Symptoms

Patients may report diverse symptoms following a whiplash injury. The predominant symptom is neck pain that typically occurs in the posterior region of the neck but can also radiate to the head, shoulder and arm, thoracic, interscapular, and lumbar regions.[13] Headache, dizziness, loss of balance, visual disturbances, paresthesia, anesthesia, weakness, and cognitive disturbances such as concentration and memory difficulties are common.[13-15] The onset of symptoms may occur immediately or, in many patients, may be delayed for up to 12–15 hours.[16]

# Mechanism of injury

The majority of research has focused on eliciting the injury mechanisms associated with a rear-end impact, although other impact directions occur, including side and front-on collisions. With respect to rear-end collisions, the rather simplistic model of a flexion, hyperextension action of the head and neck has been replaced by a more sophisticated injury model as new evidence has emerged. Bioengineering studies where cadavers were subjected to simulated rear-end crashes have demonstrated perturbations in segmental movement, including inter-segmental hyperextension in the lower cervical spine, S-curve formation, and differential acceleration of the upper cervical spine.[17, 18] The cervical spine has been shown to form an S-shape shortly after impact where the lower segments extend as the upper segments are still undergoing flexion.[19] Secondary thoracic spine movement also occurs, including superiorly directed acceleration and extension/rotation of the upper thoracic spine, which has been referred to as thoracic ramping.[18] Axial and shear forces also occur, which cause intervertebral rotation and translation movements.[20] There is some evidence to suggest that muscle activation may affect head and neck responses to a greater extent in other collision directions when compared to a rear impact, thus having some protective capacity on soft tissues.[18-21]

The determination of specific injured neck structures in vivo is difficult and most likely due to the insensitivity of current imaging technology.[22] This is not to say that injuries do not occur. When combining the evidence from bioengineering studies identifying the possibility for lesions to occur[23] and cadaveric studies where clear lesions have been demonstrated in nonsurvivors of an MVC,[24] there is a reasonable argument for the presence of pathoanatomical lesions in at least some of the injured people.[25] Damaged structures may include, amongst others, zygapophyseal joints, intervertebral disks, synovial folds, vertebral bodies, and nerve tissue (including dorsal root ganglia, spinal cord, or brainstem).[26] Unfortunately for the injured person, this circumstantial in vitro evidence in the absence of a clear pathoanatomical diagnosis in vivo has been extrapolated by some to assume that there is no objective measurable tissue injury in this condition.[27] This can lead to speculation of the injured person's motives. Nevertheless, despite this skepticism, it should be remembered in the assessment of patients with whiplash that virtually any cervical structure may be involved.

Clinical studies provide some (indirect) support for the presence of peripheral structural lesions. Lord and colleagues[28] achieved significant pain relief in a proportion of patients with chronic WAD using placebo-controlled zygapophyseal joint blocks, implicating dysfunction in these joints in those patients. Clinical indication of the involvement of injured nerve tissue has also been provided with peripheral nerve tissue mechanosensitivity demonstrated with provocation testing.[29-31] Quantitative electromyography has demonstrated the presence of subtle nerve injury via altered motor unit action potentials in the upper limbs of people with chronic whiplash, with greater disturbances found in muscles innervated by C6 and C7.[32] Chien et al.[33] have shown elevated detection thresholds for vibration, electrical stimulation, and heat in people with chronic WAD. These changes were also greater in the C6 and C7 innervation zones and are suggestive of peripheral nerve fiber dysfunction.

Magnetic resonance imaging (MRI) and functional MRI have demonstrated possible lesions of the craniocervical regions in participants with chronic whiplash. Lesions have been found in the alar ligaments, transverse ligaments, tectorial membrane, and the atlanto-occipital membrane.[34-37] These studies were of patients with chronic WAD of a long-standing nature. As such they are not entirely representative of the whiplash continuum from the acute and subacute stages and the transition to persistent symptoms and more chronic stages. Thus the prevalence of craniocervical ligamentous lesions found in these studies is likely to be considerably overestimated. Nevertheless, the studies demonstrate that, at least in some individuals with whiplash, the possibility of craniocervical ligamentous injuries should be considered.

## Classification of whiplash injury

In 1995, the Quebec Task Force (QTF) put forward the Quebec Classification of WAD[38] (Table 8.1). Their aims were to facilitate the evaluation of research and to provide clinicians with useful guidelines for making decisions about therapeutic management. The QTF system classified patients with whiplash according to the type and severity of signs and symptoms observed shortly after the injury.[38]

Since its release, the QTF classification has been criticized. Much of this criticism has pointed out that, whereas the QTF review of WAD rejected many articles that did not meet rigorous scientific criteria, the guidelines themselves suffered from the same faults – they were adopted and promoted without scientific validation.[39-41] Furthermore, it was hoped that the classification system would offer some prognostic capabilities in terms of recovery or nonrecovery from the injury, but the predictive capacity of the classification criteria has been shown to be limited.[41, 42] It was recommended that a modification of grade II classification be made to distinguish between those with normal or limited range of movement, as those with less range of movement had a poorer outcome. Hartling et al.[41] have a valid point when they suggest modification of the WAD II subgroup. Sterling[43] has shown that WAD II, although exclusive of clinical findings of neurological deficit, covers a very broad range of symptoms and also a diverse array of physical and psychological impairments. This suggests that variance in outcome will be a feature when such a broad classification is used. WAD II is the most common of the four QTF classifications of whiplash and it is important that it accurately represents the whiplash subgroup it is supposed to portray.

Alternative classifications have been proposed that take account of neuropsychological and psychosocial

factors.[44, 45] However, profound physical disturbances (motor, sensorimotor control, and sensory function) have also been shown to be important in whiplash and these manifestations as well as psychological factors have been included in a proposed adaptation of the QTF classification system.[43] From the currently available evidence, Sterling[46] has argued that it is essential to consider all aspects of the whiplash condition, both biological and psychological, in classification, prognosis, assessment, and management and has proposed an adaptation of the QTF classification system (Table 8.2). This is consistent with recent proposals calling for the inclusion and understanding of biological mechanisms as well as psychological factors in the study of chronic pain development.[47]

# Physical and psychological characteristics of whiplash-associated disorders

Whilst it would be ideal for a specific structural lesion to be identified in whiplash-injured persons, the identification of the pathoanatomical source of symptoms still provides little basis for appropriate management of whiplash pain. There is now much greater knowledge and understanding of both the physical manifestations and psychological influences associated with the condition. Sterling[46] has argued that focusing the assessment and management interventions toward identified physical and psychological presentations of the condition may help to lessen the pain and disability of whiplash.

## Disturbances in motor and sensorimotor control

Disturbances in motor and sensorimotor control have been identified in both the acute and chronic stages of the whiplash condition and these disturbances are discussed in detail

**Table 8.1** The Quebec Task Force (QTF) classification of whiplash-associated disorders[38]

| QTF classification grade | Clinical presentation |
|---|---|
| 0 | No complaint about neck pain |
|   | No physical signs |
| I | Neck complaint of pain, stiffness, or tenderness only |
|   | No physical signs |
| II | Neck complaint |
|   | Musculoskeletal signs, including: |
|   | • Decreased range of movement |
|   | • Point tenderness |
| III | Neck complaint |
|   | Musculoskeletal signs |
|   | Neurological signs, including: |
|   | • Decreased/absent deep tendon reflexes |
|   | • Muscle weakness |
|   | • Sensory deficits |
| IV | Neck complaint and fracture or dislocation |

**Table 8.2** Proposed adaptation of the Quebec Task Force (QTF) classification based on identified physical and psychological factors

| Proposed classification grade | Physical and psychological impairments present |
|---|---|
| WAD 0 | No complaint about neck pain |
| | No physical signs |
| WAD I | Neck complaint of pain, stiffness, or tenderness only |
| | No physical signs |
| WAD IIA | Neck pain |
| | Motor impairment |
| | • Decreased range of movement |
| | • Altered muscle recruitment patterns (CCFT) |
| | Sensory impairment |
| | • Local cervical mechanical hyperalgesia |
| WAD II B | Neck pain |
| | Motor impairment |
| | • Decreased range of movement |
| | • Altered muscle recruitment patterns (CCFT) |
| | Sensory impairment |
| | • Local cervical mechanical hyperalgesia |
| | Psychological impairment |
| | • Elevated psychological distress (GHQ-28, Tampa) |
| WAD II C | Neck pain |
| | Motor impairment |
| | • Decreased range of movement |
| | • Altered muscle recruitment patterns (CCFT) |
| | • Increased JPE |
| | Sensory impairment |
| | • Local cervical mechanical hyperalgesia |
| | • Generalized sensory hypersensitivity (mechanical, thermal, BPPT) |
| | • Some may show SNS disturbances |
| | Psychological impairment |
| | • Psychological distress (GHQ-28, Tampa) |
| | • Symptoms of acute posttraumatic stress (IES) |

*Reproduced with permission from Sterling.[43]*

*BPPT, brachial plexus provocation test; CCFT, craniocervical flexion test; GHQ-28, General Health Questionnaire-28; IES, Impact of Events Scale; JPE, joint position error; SNS, sympathetic nervous system; WAD, whiplash-associated disorder.*

(Continued)

in Chapters 4 and 6. The most commonly researched motor deficit in WAD is that of range of cervical movement where loss of movement has been identified.[48, 49] Most prospective studies have shown that all whiplash-injured individuals have a loss of active range of cervical movement soon after injury.[50-52] Kasch et al.[51] reported that restoration of movement occurred in all individuals by 3 months postinjury, irrespective of recovery or nonrecovery. However when whiplash subjects are classified more precisely, it is evident that those with persistent moderate/severe levels

**Table 8.2** Proposed adaptation of the Quebec Task Force (QTF) classification based on identified physical and psychological factors—cont'd

| Proposed classification grade | Physical and psychological impairments present |
|---|---|
| WAD III | Neck pain |
| | Motor impairment |
| | • Decreased range of movement |
| | • Altered muscle recruitment patterns (CCFT) |
| | • Increased JPE |
| | Sensory impairment |
| | • Local cervical mechanical hyperalgesia |
| | • Generalized sensory hypersensitivity (mechanical, thermal, BPPT) |
| | • Some may show SNS disturbances |
| | Psychological impairment |
| | • Psychological distress (GHQ-28, Tampa) |
| | • Symptoms of acute posttraumatic stress (IES) |
| | Neurological signs of conduction loss, including: |
| | • Decreased or absent deep tendon reflexes |
| | • Muscle weakness |
| | • Sensory deficits |
| WAD IV | Fracture or dislocation |

of pain and disability (measured with the Neck Disability Index) continue to display active movement loss several years postinjury.[53] We were able to show that only those who had recovered or reported lesser (but still significant) pain and disability regained movement within 2–3 months of injury[54] similar to that reported by Kasch and colleagues. This demonstrates the importance of differentiating individuals with whiplash based on pain and disability levels and not regarding them as a homogeneous group.

Altered patterns of muscle recruitment in both the cervical spine and shoulder girdle regions have been clearly shown to be a feature of chronic WAD.[55, 56] Longitudinal data demonstrate that these changes are apparent very soon after injury,[54, 56] with greater deficits in those reporting higher levels of pain and disability.[54] Sterling et al.[53, 54] observed that the disturbed motor patterns persisted, not only in those with ongoing chronic symptoms, but also in those with milder pain and disability and those who

reported full recovery. They were still evident at significant time periods postinjury – up to 2 years. These persisting deficits in muscle control may leave recovered individuals more vulnerable to future episodes of neck pain, but this proposal needs to be substantiated with further investigation.[53] Nevertheless, these findings demonstrate the significant effect that the whiplash injury has on the motor function of the cervical spine and indicate that early and specific rehabilitation will likely be important in the management of all those with a whiplash injury irrespective of reported symptoms.

A recent investigation, using MRI, has shown marked structural changes to cervical spine muscles in people with chronic whiplash. Elliott et al.[57] demonstrated the presence of fatty infiltrate in both deep and superficial cervical extensor muscles compared to an asymptomatic control group (Chapter 4; Figure 4.3). Although the fatty infiltrate was generally higher in all muscles investigated for the patient group, it was highest in the deeper muscles: the rectus capitis minor/major and multifidi. The relevance of these findings in terms of pain, disability, or functional recovery and the cause of the muscle changes are not yet known but the findings illustrate the profound disturbances in motor function present in people with chronic WAD.

Dysfunction of sensorimotor control is also a feature of both acute and chronic WAD. Greater joint repositioning errors have been found in patients with chronic WAD and also in patients within weeks of their injury, particularly those with more severe pain and disability.[14, 54] Loss of balance and disturbed neck-influenced eye movement control are present in chronic WAD,[58, 59] but their presence in the acute stage of the injury is yet to be determined. It is important to note that sensorimotor disturbances seem to be greater in patients who also report dizziness or unsteadiness in association with their neck pain.[58, 59]

Many motor deficits (movement loss, altered muscle recruitment patterns) seem to be present to various degrees in whiplash injured individuals irrespective of reported pain and disability levels and rate or level of recovery.[54] These features are not unique to whiplash and have also been identified in chronic neck pain of an idiopathic (nontraumatic) nature.[55, 60] Furthermore, treatment of chronic WAD directed at rehabilitating motor dysfunction and improving general movement shows only modest effects on reported pain and disability levels.[11, 12] Together these findings suggest that motor deficits, although present, may not play the key role in the development of chronic or persistent symptoms following whiplash injury.

## Central hyperexcitability in whiplash

In contrast to the apparently consistent presence of motor dysfunction, sensory hypersensitivity (central hyperexcitability) may be a feature that could differentiate whiplash from less severe neck pain conditions and whiplash subgroupings with higher or lower levels of reported pain and disability. Whilst other chronic painful musculoskeletal conditions also demonstrate hypersensitivity to nociceptive input,[27] there appears to be a relationship between the extent of reported symptoms and sensory hypersensitivity.[61] Scott et al.[62] showed that people with chronic WAD had a more complex presentation involving lowered pain thresholds to pressure, heat, and cold stimuli in areas remote to the cervical spine which were not present in those with idiopathic (nontraumatic) neck pain. The idiopathic group also reported much lower levels of pain and disability.[62] In contrast, widespread sensory hypersensitivity is a feature of cervical radiculopathy, with this condition and whiplash reporting similar pain and disability levels.[63] This suggests that chronic whiplash and chronic cervical radiculopathy share similar underlying mechanisms but differ from idiopathic neck pain, illustrating the diversity of processes involved in various neck pain conditions.

There is now consistent evidence from numerous cohorts that demonstrates the presence of sensory hypersensitivity (or decreased pain thresholds) to a variety of stimuli (including pressure, vibration, thermal, movement provocation testing) in WAD (Chapter 2).[29, 31, 62, 64] Sensory hypersensitivity occurs at widespread body sites, including the cervical spine, upper and lower limbs and, importantly, it is present very soon after injury.[65] The importance of the sensory hypersensitivity should not be underestimated, since its early presence is associated with poor functional recovery following whiplash injury[2, 53] and a lack of responsiveness to multimodal physical therapy interventions.[12] It is generally accepted that the sensory phenomena represent augmented central pain-processing mechanisms and direct evidence of spinal cord hyperexcitability is available[66] (Chapter 2).

The reason as to why some whiplash-injured people develop a hypersensitive state is not clear. Numerous cervical spine structures are implicated as possible sources of nociception following whiplash injury. It is possible that injuries to deep cervical structures do not rapidly heal and thus become a nociceptive driver of central nervous system hyperexcitability. Although this proposal may meet opposition from those who believe injured soft tissues are healed within several weeks of injury, it is gaining support as a possible contributor to the development of chronic musculoskeletal pain, including whiplash.[67, 68] Moreover there is evidence from cadaver studies that certain lesions can persist unresolved in MVC survivors who die of unrelated causes some years later.[69] However the sensory hypersensitivity seen in whiplash is often also associated with other disturbances such as impaired sympathetic vasoconstriction[65] and stress-related factors.[70] The co-occurrence of these factors suggests that a complex interplay between various mechanisms may lead to this almost systemic response in some persons following whiplash injury. Research is now focusing on investigating such complex models which may in the future shed light on this complicated issue.[70–72]

It is essential that musculoskeletal clinicians are alert to features of a patient's clinical presentation that may indicate a propensity for the development of chronic symptoms and/or nonresponsiveness to physical interventions and for this reason assessment of sensory function in patients with whiplash injury will be important. Further details of this assessment process are presented in Chapters 2, 11, and 12.

## Psychological factors in whiplash-associated disorders

The psychological and psychosocial factors associated with neck pain are discussed in detail in Chapter 7. In brief, and with respect to WAD, it is apparent that somewhat different psychological factors may be involved when compared to conditions that do not have a traumatic onset. It seems that an acute whiplash injury leads to psychological distress, even in those reporting lesser pain and disability.[73] It is also clear that those who continue to report moderate or greater pain and disability past 2–3 months postinjury report elevated levels of psychological distress and lesser quality of life.[3, 73] Perhaps unique to WAD (when considering nontraumatic neck pain conditions) is the presence of posttraumatic stress symptomatology. Sterling et al.[2, 53] have shown that the early presence of such symptoms is predictive of poor outcome. A multimodal physical therapy approach, whilst having effects on general psychological distress, does not seem to decrease these posttraumatic stress symptoms,[12] indicating that appropriate psychological referral may be required as part of a multiprofessional approach for these patients.

In summary, most patients with acute whiplash demonstrate a fairly uncomplicated clinical presentation of mild to moderate levels of pain and disability, local hyperalgesia over the neck, mild psychological distress, and some motor dysfunction. These individuals either recover well by 2–3 months postinjury or have persisting lower levels of pain and disability.[2, 53] At the other end of the spectrum, there is the group of whiplash patients (approximately 25–30% of this cohort[2]) who demonstrate a complex clinical picture. The clinical presentation of these patients is characterized by local and widespread hyperalgesia, sympathetic nervous system dysfunction, motor and sensorimotor dysfunction, as well as (in some) posttraumatic stress symptoms.[73, 74] It is this group that demonstrate poor functional recovery at both 6 months and 2 years postinjury[2, 53] and who prove to be a challenge to currently available interventions.

# The prediction of outcome following whiplash injury

The capacity to predict outcome following a whiplash injury is important because of the need to institute appropriate early interventions for those deemed at risk of a poorer outcome and to curtail both personal and financial costs. Numerous factors have been investigated for their prognostic capability, including: sociodemographic status; crash-related variables; compensation/ litigation; and psychosocial and physical factors.[50, 75, 76] However two systematic reviews of prospective cohort studies on whiplash could agree on only high initial pain intensity as showing strong evidence for delayed functional recovery.[77, 78] Whilst knowledge of this factor may offer some assistance in identifying patients who could develop persistent symptoms, it has been shown that moderate to high initial pain and disability levels alone, although having high sensitivity, had relatively low specificity to predict those with ongoing moderate to severe symptoms at 6 months postaccident.[2] Furthermore, measurement of pain and disability levels alone is unlikely to assist in the direction of secondary and tertiary management stages of this condition. Nonetheless it will be important for clinicians to obtain a measure of reported pain and disability (for example, Neck Disability Index) in the assessment of the whiplash-injured.

Since the time of these reviews further factors have emerged as potentially useful prognostic indicators of outcome. These include physical factors of decreased range of neck movement, cold hyperalgesia or intolerance, and impaired sympathetic vasoconstriction.[2, 53, 79] The psychological domain of posttraumatic stress symptoms is emerging as a dominant factor in poor outcome following whiplash injury,[53, 80] with Buitenhuis et al.[80] demonstrating a superior predictive capacity of this variable when compared to other psychological domains.[53]

Additional psychological factors such as high catastrophizing, low self-efficacy, and palliative coping strategies have also been identified in some studies as potentially influencing recovery.[1, 81] At this stage the strongest psychosocial predictor appears to be low educational levels.[82, 83] The role of the controversial issue of compensation-related factors is inconclusive, with some studies showing it has predictive capacity[84] and others reporting no predictive capacity of this factor.[53]

# Implications for assessment of whiplash

The clinical assessment of the patient with whiplash injury should attempt to identify the physical and psychological processes shown to be involved in the condition. It is clear that a precise and thorough assessment of the whiplash-injured patient is required and is particularly important in the acute stage of injury in order to identify risk factors for chronicity that may be targeted for treatment.

The patient assessment will need to include an adequate history such as previous history of neck pain and headache as well as the possible mechanism of injury. Whilst accident-related features have not been shown to be consistent prognostic indicators of outcome,[78] they have shown some predictive capacity in certain studies.[85] Since pain and disability levels have been repeatedly shown to be a consistent indicator of prolonged recovery,[1] it is essential that a validated questionnaire, such as the Neck Disability Index, is used in the initial assessment (Chapter 11). The patient should be screened for the presence of any "red flag" condition (WAD IV – fracture/ dislocation) as well as psychosocial "yellow flags." The psychological factor of posttraumatic stress appears to be involved in the transition from the acute to chronic stages of the condition and clinicians may consider including a measure of posttraumatic stress symptoms (e.g., Impact of Events Scale) in their assessment of the whiplash-injured patient (Chapter 11).

Certain physical factors (loss of neck movement, cold hyperalgesia) are predictive of poor recovery and must be included in assessment. The identification of sensory hypersensitivity in patients with WAD is important for two reasons: (1) the association of sensory hypersensitivity with poor or delayed recovery[74]; and (2) an alert to the care that should be taken with physical interventions to avoid further provocation of central hyperexcitability and symptom exacerbation (see Chapters 2, 11, and 12). Assessment of cervical range of movement is a mainstay of assessment of whiplash due to the prognostic capacity of this measure. Assessment will also need to include muscle recruitment patterns of the cervical and shoulder girdle regions, alteration in which have been identified in both acute and chronic whiplash states. The assessment of sensorimotor control is necessary and particularly in whiplash-injured patients who report dizziness associated with their neck pain (Chapter 12).

It must be noted that, in the presence of high levels of pain and disability and sensory hypersensitivity, the examination of the whiplash-injured patient may need to be curtailed, at least in the first instance. For reasons outlined previously, it is important that symptoms and hyperalgesic responses are not exacerbated in this patient group.

## Implications for management

Currently available guidelines for the management of acute WAD promote education, assurance to the patient, the maintenance of activity levels, general and specific exercises, simple analgesics, and coping strategies.[10, 86] However the emerging multifactorial nature of WAD suggests, that although the current guidelines may benefit those whiplash patients with a less complex presentation, they are likely to be inadequate for the management of patients with a complex condition displaying both marked physical dysfunction and psychological distress. More recent clinical guidelines have recognized this group and have attempted to include recommendations for the identification of factors such as sensory disturbance and psychological distress.[86]

In focusing discussion on this group with more complex conditions, the resumption of activity is almost universally recommended in clinical practice guidelines. However the case for the avoidance of pain provocation must be clearly stated as an important aim of any physical intervention for patients demonstrating features of sensory hypersensitivity. The application of nonjudicious physical, mechanically stimulating treatments may serve to maintain and prolong this hypersensitivity and have a deleterious effect on the patient's long-term outcome. It is not suggested that these patients avoid activity, as the maintenance of activity levels opposed to rest and use of a collar has been shown to be important in the management of acute whiplash.[9] However the patient with sensory hypersensitivity should be managed with care and activity levels should be slowly increased as tolerated by the individual. Zusman[87] points out that movement (activity, exercises) should be relatively painfree to avoid long-lasting changes in neuronal synaptic memory. The old adage of activity "into pain" is not appropriate for this group of whiplash-injured patients.

It is not clear at present if physical interventions have the capacity to modulate sensory hypersensitivity in this group. Spinal manual therapy exerts a hypoalgesic effect on mechanical hyperalgesia[88] but it is not known if similar effects occur for cold hyperalgesia. Results from a preliminary randomized controlled trial of physiotherapy (exercise and manual therapy) for chronic whiplash indicate that the presence of cold and mechanical hyperalgesia mitigates against an effective reduction in pain and disability levels seen in those without these features.[12] These patients may require pharmacological intervention to achieve adequate pain relief. However the most suitable pharmacological interventions for sensory hypersensitivity are not known. Curatolo et al.[68] outline three theoretical approaches to the treatment of central hypersensitivity. These include pharmacological interventions such as nonsteroidal anti-inflammatory drugs (NSAIDs) or opioids, directed at blocking or decreasing peripheral nociceptive input; pharmacological interventions (e.g., NSAIDs, N-methyl-D-aspartic acid (NMDA) antagonists) directed at modulating spinal cord hyperexcitability, or pharmacological or psychological interventions acting at a supraspinal level and influencing descending inhibitory pathways. A recent small randomized controlled study ($n = 20$) demonstrated that drug therapy (ketamine – an NMDA receptor antagonist, remifentanil – an opioid) attenuated pain and hyperalgesia but 30% of participants were still nonresponders.[89] Furthermore the side-effects of such a treatment approach are not insignificant.[89] Further trials of pharmacological interventions for whiplash are required.

Theoretically physical interventions such as transcutaneous electrical nerve stimulation and acupuncture may also be useful in modulating sensory hypersensitivity but these have not been specifically investigated in WAD. Few studies have investigated the effects of psychologically based interventions in this condition. However Blanchard et al.[90] found that psychological intervention directed toward posttraumatic stress disorder in chronic whiplash, whilst influencing posttraumatic stress symptoms, did not have an effect on pain levels in this group.

The discussion on pharmacological, psychological, and electrophysical interventions is not to suggest that physical interventions, including exercise and manual therapy, are not indicated for those with a more complicated whiplash presentation. A combined specific exercise and manual therapy approach has demonstrated efficacy in the management of chronic cervicogenic headache (idiopathic neck pain).[91] Furthermore this treatment approach has been shown to decrease pain and disability in patients with chronic whiplash *without* the combined presence of mechanical and cold hyperalgesia.[12] A more general graded exercise program has also shown some effectiveness in this chronic patient group.[11] However, it is apparent that it will be important to identify those patients with sensory hypersensitivity (and possibly psychological distress) such that additional management can be provided, likely in the form of adequate medication for pain relief and psychological intervention, that is, a multiprofessional approach to management. Whilst this statement may appear hackneyed in the arguments for treatment approaches for this and other musculoskeletal conditions, it should be noted that many patients do not receive such a management approach until their condition is very chronic. It is time to re-evaluate this situation and provide *early* and targeted interventions to those at risk of developing chronic pain. It is not suggested that such treatment should occur in the already-overstretched multidisciplinary pain clinic environment. To the contrary, a well-integrated and cooperative approach amongst community primary care practitioners may be the most appropriate and cost-effective approach.

# Conclusion

The musculoskeletal clinician plays an important role in the assessment and management of the whiplash-injured person. It is emerging that WAD is a complex heterogeneous condition involving varying degrees of physical (motor, sensorimotor, and sensory) disturbances as well as psychological distress. Clinicians should make every attempt to examine the patient precisely and this will need to include assessment of physical and psychological factors in addition to reported levels of pain and disability. These data, together with sound clinical reasoning skills, lay the foundation for the early identification of those at risk of poor recovery and the institution of tailored and appropriate interventions for all whiplash-injured patients in order to provide optimal chance of recovery.

# References

1. *Hendricks E, Scholten-Peeters G, van der Windt D, et al*. Prognostic factors for poor recovery in acute whiplash patients. Pain 2005;114:408–416.

2. *Sterling M, Jull G, Vicenzino B, et al*. Physical and psychological factors predict outcome following whiplash injury. Pain 2005;114:141–148.

3. *Rebbeck T, Sindhausen D, Cameron I*. A prospective cohort study of health outcomes following whiplash associated disorders in an Australian population. Inj Prev 2006;12:86–93.

4. *Motor Accidents Insurance Commission*. Annual Report. Australia: Queensland Government, Brisbane 2004.

5. *Crouch R, Whitewick R, Clancy M, et al*. Whiplash associated disorder: incidence and natural history over the first month for patients presenting to a UK emergency department. Emerg Med J 2006;23: 114–118.

6. *Provinciali L, Baroni M, Illuminati L, et al*. Multimodal treatment to prevent the late whiplash syndrome. Scand J Rehabil Med 1996;28:105–111.

7. *Borchgrevink G, Kaasa A, McDonagh D, et al*. Acute treatment of whiplash neck sprain injuries. A randomized trial of treatment during the first 14 days after a car accident. Spine 1998;23:25–31.

8. *Rosenfeld M, Gunnarsson R, Borenstein P*. Early intervention in whiplash-associated disorders. A comparison of two protocols. Spine 2000;25: 1782–1787.

9. *Rosenfeld M, Seferiadis A, Carllson J, et al*. Active intervention in patients with whiplash associated disorders improves long-term prognosis: a randomised controlled clinical trial. Spine 2003;28:2491–2498.

10. *Scholten-Peeters G, Bekkering G, Verhagen A, et al*. Clinical practice guideline for the physiotherapy of patients with whiplash associated disorders. Spine 2002;27:412–422.

11. *Stewart M, Maher C, Refshauge K, et al*. Randomised controlled trial of exercise for chronic whiplash associated disorders. Pain 2007;128:59–68.

12. *Jull G, Sterling M, Kenardy J, et al*. Does the presence of sensory hypersensitivity influence outcomes of physical rehabilitation for chronic whiplash? A preliminary RCT. Pain 2007;129:28–34.

13. *Barnsley L, Lord S, Bogduk N*. The pathophysiology of whiplash. Spine 1998;12:209–242.

14. *Treleaven J, Jull G, Sterling M*. Dizziness and unsteadiness following whiplash injury – characteristic features and relationship with cervical joint position error. J Rehabil 2003;34:1–8.

15. *Radanov B, Sturzenegger M*. Predicting recovery from common whiplash. Eur Neurol 1996;36:48–51.

16. *Provinciali L, Baroni M*. Clinical approaches to whiplash injuries: a review. Crit Rev Phys Rehabil Med 1999;11:339–368.

17. *Cusick J, Pintar F, Yoganandan N*. Whiplash syndrome: kinematic factors influencing pain patterns. Spine 2001;26:1252–1258.

18. *Stemper B, Yoganandan N, Rao R, et al*. Influence of thoracic ramping on whiplash kinematics. Clin Biomech 2005;20:1019–1028.

19. *Sizer P, Poorbaugh K, Phelps V*. Whiplash associated disorders: pathomechanics, diagnosis and management. Pain Pract 2004;4:249–266.

20. *Ivancic P, Panjabi M*. Cervical spine loads and intervertebral motions during whiplash. Traffic Inj Prev 2006;7:389–399.

21. *Brolin K, Halldin P, Leijonhufvud I*. The effect of muscle activation on neck response. Traffic Inj Prev 2005;6:67–76.

22. *Ronnen J, de Korte P, Brink P*. Acute whiplash injury: is there a role for MR imaging. Radiology 1996;201:93–96.

23. *Yoganandan N, Pintar F, Cusick J*. Biomechanical analyses of whiplash injuries using an experimental model. Accid Anal Prev 2002;34:663–671.

24. *Taylor J, Taylor M*. Cervical spinal injuries: an autopsy study of 109 blunt injuries. J Musculoskel Pain 1996;4:61–79.

25. *Bogduk N*. Point of view. Spine 2002;27:1940–1941.

26. *Uhrenholt L, Grunnet-Nilsson N, Hartvigsen J*. Cervical spine lesions after road traffic accidents. A systematic review. Spine 2002;27:1934–1941.

27. *Shir Y, Pereira J, Fitzcharles M-A*. Whiplash and fibromyalgia: an ever widening gap. J Rheumatol 2006;33:1045–1047.

28. *Lord S, Barnsley L, Wallis B, et al*. Chronic cervical zygapophysial joint pain after whiplash: a placebo-controlled prevalence study. Spine 1996;21: 1737–1745.

29. *Sterling M, Treleaven J, Jull G*. Responses to a clinical test of mechanical provocation of nerve tissue in whiplash associated disorders. Man Ther 2002;7:89–94.

30. *Ide M, Ide J, Yamaga M, et al*. Symptoms and signs of irritation of the brachial plexus in whiplash injuries. J Bone Joint Surg (Br) 2001;83:226–229.

31. *Sterling M, Treleaven J, Edwards S, et al*. Pressure pain thresholds in chronic whiplash associated disorder: further evidence of altered central pain processing. J Musculoskel Pain 2002;10:69–81.

32. *Chu J, Eun S, Schwartz J*. Quantitative motor unit action potentials (QUAMP) in whiplash patients with neck and upper limb pain. Electromyogr Clin Neurophysiol 2005;45:323–328.

33. *Chien A, Eliav E, Sterling M*. Hypoaesthesia occurs with sensory hypersensitivity in chronic whiplash: indication of a minor peripheral neuropathy? Man Ther 2008; in press.

34. *Krakenes J, Kaale B, Moen G, et al*. MRI assessment of the alar ligaments in the late stage of whiplash injury – a study of structural abnormalities and observer agreement. Neuroradiology 2002;44: 617–624.

35. *Krakenes J, Kaale B, Moen G, et al*. MRI of the tectorial and posterior atlanto-occipital membranes in the late stage of whiplash injury. Neuroradiology 2003;44:637–644.

36. *Johansson B*. Whiplash injuries can be visible by functional magnetic resonance imaging. Pain Res Manage 2006;11:197–199.

37. *Kaale B, Krakenes J, Albrektsen G, et al*. WAD impairment rating: Neck Disability Index score according to severity of MRI findings of ligaments and membranes in the upper cervical spine. J Neurotrauma 2005;4:466–475.

38. *Spitzer W, Skovron M, Salmi L, et al*. Scientific Monograph of Quebec Task Force on Whiplash associated Disorders. Spine 1995;20:1–73.

39. *Freeman M, Croft A, Rossignol A*. "Whiplash associated disorders: redefining whiplash and its management" by the Quebec Task Force. A critical evaluation. Spine 1998;23:1043–1049.

40. *Teasell R, Shapiro A*. Whiplash injuries: an update. Pain Res Manage 1998;3:81–90.

41. *Hartling L, Brison R, Ardern C, et al*. Prognostic value of the Quebec classification of whiplash associated disorders. Spine 2001;26:36–41.

42. *Kivioja J, Lindgren U, Jensen I*. A prospective study on the Quebec Classification as a predictor for the outcome after whiplash injury. In: Anton H, Alien M, Blair D et al (eds) World Congress on Whiplash-Associated Disorders. Vancouver, Canada: Physical Medicine Research Foundation (publisher), 1999, pp. 131.

43. *Sterling M*. A proposed new classification system for whiplash associate disorders – implications for assessment and management. Man Ther 2004;9: 60–70.

44. *Tenenbaum A, Rivano-Fischer M, Tjell C, et al*. The Quebec classification and a new Swedish classification for whiplash-associated disorders in relation to life satisfaction in patients at high risk of chronic functional impairment and disability. J Rehabil Med 2002;34:114–118.

45. *Soderlund A, Denison E*. Classification of patients with whiplash associated disorders: reliable and valid subgroups based on the Multidimensional Pain Inventory (MPI-S). Eur J Pain 2006;10:113–119.

46. *Sterling M*. Whiplash injury pain: basic science and current/future therapeutics. Rev Analg 2007;9: 105–116.

47. *Smith B, Macfarlane G, Torrance N*. Epidemiology of chronic pain, from the laboratory to the bus stop: time to add understanding of biological mechanisms to the study of risk factors in population-based research? Pain 2007;127:5–10.

48. *Heikkila H, Wenngren B*. Cervicocephalic kinesthetic sensibility, active range of cervical motion and oculomotor function in patients with whiplash injury. Arch Phys Med Rehabil 1998;79:1089–1094.

49. *Dall'Alba P, Sterling M, Trealeven J, et al*. Cervical range of motion discriminates between asymptomatic and whiplash subjects. Spine 2001;26:2090–2094.

50. *Radanov B, Sturzenegger M, Di Stefano G*. Long-term outcome after whiplash injury. A 2-year follow-up considering features of injury mechanism and somatic, radiologic, and psychological findings. Medicine 1995;74:281–297.

51. *Kasch H, Stengaard-Pedersen K, Arendt-Nielsen L, et al*. Headache, neck pain and neck mobility after acute whiplash injury. Spine 2001;26:1246–1251.

52. *Sterling M, Jull G, Vicenzino B, et al*. Characterisation of acute whiplash associated disorders. Spine 2004;29:182–188.

53. *Sterling M, Jull G, Kenardy J*. Physical and psychological predictors of outcome following whiplash injury maintain predictive capacity at long term follow-up. Pain 2006;122:102–108.

54. *Sterling M, Jull G, Vizenzino B, et al*. Development of motor system dysfunction following whiplash injury. Pain 2003;103:65–73.

55. *Jull G, Kristjansson E, Dall'Alba P*. Impairment in the cervical flexors: a comparison of whiplash and insidious onset neck pain patients. Man Ther 2004;9:89–94.

56. *Nederhand M, Hermens H, Ijzerman M, et al*. Cervical muscle dysfunction in chronic whiplash associated disorder grade 2. The relevance of trauma. Spine 2002;27:1056–1061.

57. *Elliott J, Jull G, Noteboom T, et al*. Fatty infiltration in the cervical extensor muscles in persistent whiplash associated disorders: an MRI analysis. Spine 2006;31: E847–855.

58. *Treleaven J, Jull G, Low Choy N*. Standing balance in persistent whiplash: a comparison between subjects with and without dizziness. J Rehabil Med 2005;37:224–229.

59. *Treleaven J, Jull G, LowChoy N*. Smooth pursuit neck torsion test in whiplash associated disorders: relationship to self-reports of neck pain and disability, dizziness and anxiety. J Rehabil Med 2005;37:219–223.

60. *Sterling M, Jull G, Wright A*. Cervical mobilisation: concurrent effects on pain, sympathetic nervous system activity and motor activity. Man Ther 2001;6:72–81.

61. *Carli G, Suman A, Biasi G, et al*. Reactivity to superficial and deep stimuli in patients with chronic musculoskeletal pain. Pain 2002;100: 259–269.

62. *Scott D, Jull G, Sterling M*. Sensory hypersensitivity is a feature of chronic whiplash associated disorders but not chronic idiopathic neck pain. Clin J Pain 2005;21:175–181.

63. *Chien A, Eliav E, Sterling M*. Chronic whiplash and cervical radiculopathy share similar mechanisms. 2007; submitted for publication.

64. *Moog M, Quintner J, Hall T, et al*. The late whiplash syndrome: a psychophysical study. Eur J Pain 2002;6:283–294.

65. *Sterling M*. Sensory hypersensitivity and psychological distress following whiplash injury: is there a relationship? Melbourne: Australian Pain Society Annual Scientific Meeting, 2006.

66. *Banic B, Petersen-Felix S, Andersen O, et al*. Evidence for spinal cord hypersensitivity in chronic pain after whiplash injury and in fibromyalgia. Pain 2004;107:7–15.

67. *Vierck C*. Mechanisms underlying development of spatially distributed chronic pain (fibromyalgia). Pain 2006;124:242–263.

68. *Curatolo M, Arendt-Nielsen L, Petersen-Felix S*. Central hypersensitivity in chronic pain: mechanisms and clinical implications. Phys Med Rehabil Clin North Am 2006;17: 287–302.

69. *Taylor J, Finch P*. Acute injury of the neck: anatomical and pathological basis of pain. Ann Acad Med Singapore 1993;22:187–192.

70. *Sterling M, Kenardy J*. The relationship between sensory and sympathetic nervous system changes and acute posttraumatic stress following whiplash injury – a prospective study. J Psychosom Res 2006;60:387–393.

71. *McLean S, Clauw D, Abelson J, et al*. The development of persistent pain and psychological morbidity after motor vehicle collision: integrating the potential role of stress response systems into a biopsychosocial model. Psychosom Med 2005;67:783–790.

72. *Passatore M, Roatta S*. Influence of sympathetic nervous system on sensorimotor function: whiplash associated disorders (WAD) as a model. Eur J Appl Physiol 2006;98:423–449.

73. *Sterling M, Kenardy J, Jull G, et al*. The development of psychological changes following whiplash injury. Pain 2003;106:481–489.

74. *Sterling M, Jull G, Vicenzino B, et al*. Sensory hypersensitivity occurs soon after whiplash injury and is associated with poor recovery. Pain 2003;104:509–517.

75. *Cassidy JD, Carroll LJ, Cote P, et al*. Effect of eliminating compensation for pain and suffering on the outcome of insurance claims for whiplash injury. N Engl J Med 2000;20:1179–1213.

76. *Kasch H, Flemming W, Jensen T*. Handicap after acute whiplash injury. Neurology 2001;56: 1637–1643.

77. *Cote P, Cassidy D, Carroll L, et al*. A systematic review of the prognosis of acute whiplash and a new conceptual framework to synthesize the literature. Spine 2001;26:E445–E458.

78. *Scholten-Peeters G, Verhagen A, Bekkering G, et al*. Prognostic factors of whiplash associated disorders: a systematic review of prospective cohort studies. Pain 2003;104:303–322.

79. *Kasch H, Qerama E, Bach F, et al*. Reduced cold pressor pain tolerance in non-recovered whiplash patients: a 1 year prospective study. Eur J Pain 2005;9:561–569.

80. *Buitenhuis J, DeJong J, Jaspers J, et al*. Relationship between posttraumatic stress disorder symptoms and the course of whiplash complaints. J Psychosom Res 2006;61:681–689.

81. *Buitenhuis J, Spanjer J, Fidler V*. Recovery from acute whiplash – the role of coping styles. Spine 2003;28:896–901.

82. *Ottoson C, Nyren O, Johansson S, et al*. Outcome after minor traffic accidents: a follow-up study of orthopedic patients in an inner city area emergency room. J Trauma 2005;58:553–560.

83. *Sterner Y, Toolanen G, Gerdle B, et al*. The incidence of whiplash trauma and the effects of different factors on recovery. J Spinal Disord 2003;16:195–199.

84. *Dufton J, Kopec J, Wong H, et al*. Prognostic factors associated with minimal improvement following acute whiplash associated disorders. Spine 2006;31: E759–E765.

85. *Sturzenegger M, Radanov B, Stefano GD*. The effect of accident mechanisms and initial findings on the

long-term course of whiplash injury. J Neurol 1995;242:443–449.

86. *MAA*. Guidelines for the Management of Whiplash Associated Disorders. Sydney: Motor Accidents Authority, 2006:16.

87. *Zusman M*. Mechanisms of musculoskeletal physiotherapy. Phys Ther Rev 2004;9:39–49.

88. *Vicenzino B, Collins D, Benson H, et al*. An investigation of the interrelationship between manipulative therapy induced hypoalgesia and sympathoexcitation. J Manipul Physiol Ther 1998;21:448–453.

89. *Lemming D, Sorensen J, Graven-Nielsen T, et al*. Managing chronic whiplash pain with a combination of low-dose opioid (remifentanil) and NMDA-antagonist (ketamine). Eur J Pain 2007;11:719–732.

90. *Blanchard E, Hickling E, Devineni T, et al*. A controlled evaluation of cognitive behaviour therapy for posttraumatic stress in motor vehicle accident survivors. Behav Res Ther 2003;41:79–96.

91. *Jull G, Trott P, Potter H, et al*. A randomised controlled trial of physiotherapy management for cervicogenic headache. Spine 2002;27:1835–1843.

9

# Cervicogenic Headache: Differential Diagnosis

## Introduction

Headache is a common complaint in society, with high personal and socioeconomic impacts.[1-3] No age group is immune from the disorder and headache can present across the lifespan.[4-7] Headache has many causes.[8] It may be a primary disorder such as migraine, tension-type, or cluster headache or a secondary disorder, in other words, a symptom complex arising from another recognizable cause. Cervicogenic headache is a secondary headache, the primary pathophysiology being in the cervical structures. Patients often present to musculoskeletal practitioners for management of their headaches and, most commonly, for treatment of cervicogenic, migraine, or tension-type headaches.[9, 10] However the evidence is divided for the effect of management methods such as cervical manipulative therapy and specific therapeutic exercise for migraine and tension-type headache.[11-22] Yet there is evidence that these methods are beneficial for cervicogenic headache, the secondary headache arising from a cervical musculoskeletal disorder.[19, 23, 24]

It is a reasonable premise that if headache is to be treated with cervical manipulative therapy and specific therapeutic exercise, then impairments in the cervical musculoskeletal system should be major features of the headache syndrome. Yet migraine and tension-type headache are primary headaches whose pathogeneses do not lie in cervical musculoskeletal dysfunction. For example, the biological markers for the activation of the trigeminovascular system are present in migraine but not in cervicogenic headache.[25] This may be the obvious and simple explanation for the lack of benefit of effect for manipulative and exercise therapies for many cases of migraine and tension-type headache. Further, it has been noted that in some studies where benefits of these therapies were found, the headaches were associated with signs of cervical musculoskeletal impairment,[26] which could question the original diagnoses or subject inclusion criteria in these studies. However it might also point to basic problems in differential diagnosis of the common frequent intermittent headache types of migraine without aura, tension-type, and cervicogenic headache because of symptomatic overlap or highlight the potential for mixed headache types.[27]

This chapter will focus on cervicogenic headache and its differential diagnosis from other benign frequent intermittent headache types and will discuss some of the factors which can make this a challenging task in some patients. The evidence for the nature of cervical musculoskeletal impairment in cervicogenic headache will be presented, which also provides the basis for treatment prescription.

# The clinical diagnosis of cervicogenic headache

The history and clinical presentation of any headache contribute in a significant way to its diagnosis. The International Headache Society (IHS) has published criteria for diagnosis of all recognized headache types.[8] A summary of the main features of the three most common benign frequent intermittent headache types – migraine without aura, tension-type, and cervicogenic headache – is presented in Table 9.1 for ready comparison. In relation to cervicogenic headache, other features in the patient's history and presentation can add to its picture. For example, pain most typically starts in the neck in cervicogenic headache whereas it typically starts in the head in migraine.[28, 29] When autonomic symptoms are present,

they are not dominant features as they can be in migraine. Both migraine and cervicogenic headache are typically (although not inevitably) a unilateral headache, but migraine can change sides within or between attacks, as opposed to cervicogenic headache, which, is side-consistent.[30] There is a lack of response to drugs such as ergotomine and sumatriptan in cervicogenic headache, which however, can assist in the diagnosis of migraine.[31-33] Furthermore, cervicogenic headache has an unchanged pattern during pregnancy as opposed to migraine, which can cease temporarily.[34] However reports of headache aggravation with sustained activities such as computer work are not unique to any headache type, highlighting the similarity in some activities which aggravate the different headache types.

## Symptomatic overlap

Primary headaches such as migraine with aura and cluster headaches have distinct characteristics and are usually reasonably readily diagnosed.[8, 35] However despite having characteristic features (Table 9.1), it is well recognized that there can be difficulties in differential diagnosis between cervicogenic headache, the various temporal presentations of migraine without aura, and tension-type headaches because of the considerable symptomatic overlap between these headache types.[31, 36, 37] Even though pathophysiological processes are different, these headaches have a common pathway in the trigeminal system which goes towards explaining this symptomatic overlap.[38-42] Studies have been conducted examining the reliability of the criteria for differentially diagnosing the three headache types. Those of the IHS[8] have been used in studies for migraine and tension-type headache and those of the Cervicogenic Headache International Study Group (CHISG)[33] for cervicogenic headache. In the main, moderate agreement is in evidence in identifying the headache types.[43-46]

**Table 9.1** A summary of the symptomatic features of cervicogenic, migraine without aura, and tension-type headache

| Cervicogenic headache | Migraine without aura | Tension-type headache |
|---|---|---|
| 1. Symptoms and signs of neck involvement<br><br>  (a) Precipitation of comparable head pain by:<br>    – Neck movement or sustained awkward head postures, and/or<br>    – External pressure over the upper cervical or occipital region on the symptomatic side<br><br>  (b) Restriction of range of motion in the neck<br><br>  (c) Ipsilateral neck, shoulder, or arm pain<br><br>2. Positive response to diagnostic anesthetic blocks<br><br>3. Unilaterality of head pain, without sideshift<br><br>4. Head pain characteristics<br><br>  (a) Moderate to severe, nonthrobbing and nonlancinating pain, usually starting in the neck<br><br>  (b) Episodes of varying duration<br><br>  (c) Fluctuating continuous pain<br><br>5. (a) Nausea<br>  (b) Phonophobia and photophobia<br>  (c) Dizziness<br>  (d) Ipsilateral blurred vision<br>  (e) Difficulties on swallowing<br>  (f) Ipsilateral edema, mostly in the periocular area<br><br>**Addendum**<br>At least seven criteria should be present<br><br>Most consistent: unilateral, sidelocked headache aggravated by neck posture and movement[46] | 1. Headache attacks lasting 4–72 hours (untreated or unsuccessfully treated)<br><br>2. Headache has at least two of the following characteristics:<br><br>  (a) Unilateral location<br><br>  (b) Pulsating quality<br><br>  (c) Moderate or severe intensity<br><br>  (d) Aggravation by or causing avoidance of routine physical activity (e.g., walking, climbing stairs)<br><br>3. During headache at least one of the following:<br><br>  (a) Nausea and/or vomiting<br><br>  (b) Photophobia and phonophobia<br><br>4. Not attributed to another disorder<br><br>5. Have had at least five attacks of headache fulfilling these criteria | **Episodic**<br><br>1. At least 10 episodes occurring < 1 day per month on average (< 12 days per year) and fulfilling criteria 2–4<br><br>Frequent episodic tension-type headache<br><br>At least 10 episodes occurring on ≥ 1 but < 15 days per month for at least 3 months<br><br>2. Headache lasting from 30 minutes to 7 days<br><br>3. Headache has at least two of the following characteristics:<br><br>  (a) Bilateral location<br><br>  (b) Pressing/tightening (nonpulsating) quality<br><br>  (c) Mild or moderate intensity<br><br>  (d) Not aggravated by routine physical activity such as walking or climbing stairs<br><br>4. Both of the following:<br><br>  (a) No nausea or vomiting (anorexia may occur)<br><br>  (b) No more than one of photophobia or phonophobia<br><br>5. Not attributed to another disorder<br><br>**Chronic**<br>1. Headache occurring on ≥ 15 days per month on average for > 3 month (≥ 180 days per year) and fulfilling criteria 2–4<br><br>2. Headache lasts hours or may be continuous<br><br>3. As for episodic<br><br>4. Both of the following:<br><br>  (a) No more than one of photophobia, phonophobia, or mild nausea<br><br>  (b) Neither moderate or severe nausea nor vomiting<br><br>5. Not attributed to another disorder |

*Adapted from the criteria published by the Cervicogenic Headache International Study Group for cervicogenic headache[33] for cervicogenic headache and the International Headache Society for migraine and tension-type headache.[8]*

With the overlap in symptoms, other authors have highlighted the difficulty often encountered in diagnosis when patients present with symptoms that could be attributed to more than one headache type. They express the fact that it may not be possible to identify a particular headache type in many individuals.[47-50] The situation is further complicated if headache patients suffer a mixed headache type or more than one type of headache concurrently.[27, 51-53] Unfortunately the situation is not helped when there is no laboratory test to identify a migraine or tension-type headache cause.

## Presence of neck pain

The presence of neck pain with headache is attractive to the diagnosis of cervico-genic headache. Nevertheless, practitioners should not be misled. Neck pain is not an uncommon accompaniment of any headache type, including migraine and tension-type headache.[12, 29, 49, 54-57] It is estimated that up to 60–80% of frequent intermittent headache sufferers will report neck pain of some description in association with their headache.[56, 58] Notably the incidence of cervicogenic headache within chronic headache popu-lations has been reported at between 15 and 20% in preliminary studies,[53, 59] a far lower incidence than the occurrence of neck pain with headache. It is important to appreciate that there are bidirectional interactions between trigeminal afferents and afferents from the three upper cervical nerves in the trigeminocervical nucleus.[60, 61] Thus, as much as nociceptive activity in cervical afferents can refer pain to the head, nociceptive activity in the trigeminal afferents can refer pain into the neck. In other words, the neck pain can merely be a referred area of pain with its cause elsewhere.

## Neck trauma and headache

A history of head or neck trauma is commonly reported by patients as a precipitant of cervicogenic headache. A survey established that, within the general population, a history of neck injury in a motor vehicle crash was associated with higher odds (odds ratio: 2.09) of suffering headaches that had a moderate to severe impact on the individual's health.[62] The authors correctly cautioned against inferring a causal relationship between a whiplash injury and chronic neck pain and headaches from this association. However logical it might seem to sum automatically *neck injury + headache = cervicogenic headache*, this may be erroneous clinical reasoning. For example, Radanov et al.[63] investigated 112 patients with chronic posttraumatic headache on average 2.5 years following a whiplash injury. Neck pain was associated with headache in 93% of cases. They classified the headache on the IHS criteria and determined that 37% of the patients had tension-type headache, 27% migraine, 18% cervicogenic, and 18% of headaches were unclassifiable. Most patients reported that headaches only began following the whiplash injury. Retrospective recounts have to be accepted with caution. Nevertheless, two further prospective studies of whiplash-induced headache reported not dissimilar incidences of the three headache types.[64, 65]

The comparative low incidence of cervicogenic headache in whiplash-induced headache might seem surprising with such an apparent direct association between the neck injury, neck pain, and headache. Clinicians thus need to consider not only the physical stresses of a whiplash injury to the neck but also the psychological stress of the situation. It is possible that these psychological stressors could precipitate episodes of a primary headache type.[65]

## Musculoskeletal pain and headache

The presence of musculoskeletal pain in association with headache is not uncommon. Hagen et al.[66] surveyed 51 050 adults resident in a Norwegian county and identified a strong association between the presence of musculoskeletal pain and the occurrence of headache. Musculoskeletal symptoms could involve any region of the body. There was a strong association between both migrainous and nonmigrainous headache and musculoskeletal pain. In particular, the prevalence of frequent intermittent headache (> 14 days/month) was four times greater in those with musculoskeletal pain. Those with neck pain were more likely to have headaches than persons who suffered musculoskeletal pain in other regions of the body.

Thus the situation with headache can be complex. Neck pain is a primary feature of cervicogenic headache, but neck pain lacks specificity for cervicogenic headache. Neck trauma can precipitate cervicogenic headache but not all headaches resulting from a whiplash injury are necessarily cervicogenic. Musculoskeletal pain is strongly associated with the occurrence of headache, especially if it is located in the neck. Sjaastad and Fredriksen[67] have stressed the importance of accurately using the classification criteria for cervicogenic headache for diagnosis. No one symptom should be relied upon, rather a characteristic pattern of headache is sought. Nevertheless it is evident that further objective tests are required to identify positively a cervical cause of headache.

## Further diagnostic methods

Both the IHS and CHISG headache classifications[8, 33] mandate the use of diagnostic anesthetic nerve or joint blocks to diagnose cervicogenic headache definitely. Neither plain X-rays nor magnetic resonance imaging has been shown to be sensitive to detect relevant pathological change in the cervical spine.[68–70] Diagnostic blocks can confirm the presence of cervicogenic headache and, for an unequivocal diagnosis, it is advocated that the blocks are placebo-controlled and performed under fluoroscopic guidance.[71] They cannot be performed as office procedures.[72] It is pertinent to consider the mandatory use of diagnostic blocks for diagnosis of cervicogenic headache in the context of the high frequency of frequent intermittent headache in the community and the numbers that would have to undergo this procedure given the frequent difficulty in making a preliminary differential diagnosis.[50] If the diagnosis of cervicogenic headache cannot be made in any other way, the resources, expertise, and manpower requirements of this diagnostic procedure would make it cost- and manpower-prohibitive to diagnose the vast majority of potential cervicogenic patients. Diagnostic blocks are undoubtedly essential when surgical management such as neurotomies are being considered in management.[73–75] Such surgical procedures are usually restricted to the cervicogenic headache sufferers who have failed all attempts at conservative care.[76] They are not the first line of management for the majority of cervicogenic headache patients seen in general practice and thus other more cost-effective and noninvasive diagnostic methods must be found for this large group.

Physical examination of the cervical musculoskeletal system is the method of diagnosis used by musculoskeletal practitioners. However, the IHS[8] indicates that, to diagnose a cervicogenic headache, there must be evidence that the headache can be attributed to a neck disorder. They suggest that this could be achieved by the demonstration of clinical signs that would implicate a source of pain in the neck and the IHS calls for evidence and research in this area of diagnosis to validate this method.

# The physical examination in differential diagnosis

The criteria for physical impairment in the cervical musculoskeletal system are not defined extensively in the current classification systems. There are two criteria, those of reduced range of neck movement and pain elicited by external pressure over the occipital or suboccipital region, ipsilateral to headache.[33, 77] While these are important signs, they lack specificity. Tenderness in the occipital or suboccipital regions, although present in cervicogenic headache, is not unique to the disorder[78] and range of movement can reduce as a factor of age alone.[79] There are several studies that have shown the incidence of cervical musculoskeletal impairment in a cervicogenic headache population using a particular measure of impairment.[80-86] However if the spread in values documented for each individual measure is compared to the spread in nonheadache or other headache populations, there is overlap in values. This means that a certain absolute value of a measure could be recorded in a person with or without cervicogenic headache. Thus when physical signs (in research or clinical practice) are taken singularly, their diagnostic significance is questionable.[83, 87]

Musculoskeletal conditions when considered in their broadest context do not present with an isolated physical sign and usually present with changes in the articular and muscle systems at the least. We have recently undertaken a study in which several parameters of cervical musculoskeletal function were measured concurrently in patients presenting with frequent intermittent headaches to investigate whether or not and how well a group or pattern of physical features could distinguish cervicogenic headache.[58, 88] The measures included range of cervical movement, manual examination for symptomatic cervical segment dysfunction, the cranio-cervical flexion test (CCFT), neck flexor and extensor strength, cervical joint position error, and a measure of cross-sectional area of selected extensor muscles at the C2 level. In agreement with previous studies, all individual measures of physical function in persons reporting a single headache were found to be impaired in the cervicogenic headache group when compared to the migraine, tension-type headaches, and control groups.[58] The exception was measures of cervical joint position error where no differences were recorded. Furthermore there was the expected spread of values in each single measure which indicated the overlap in values between groups. For example, the measure for sagittal plane range of motion was $85 \pm 11.0°$ in the cervicogenic group, $100.5 \pm 14.4°$ in the migraine group, $101.1 \pm 14.1°$ in the tension-type headache group, and $98.9 \pm 15.1°$ in the control group. The between-group differences are clear but the magnitude of the standard deviations shows, for instance, that a person with 90° of sagittal plane motion could be a member of any group. Thus, of major importance, subsequent analysis revealed that three measures together most strongly separated the groups. Collectively they had 100% sensitivity and 94% specificity to distinguish cervicogenic headache. The measures were reduced range of motion (range of extension in this instance) together with the presence of painful joint dysfunction in the upper cervical joints (C0–3) and with impairment in muscle function as determined in the CCFT. That is, there was a pattern of joint, movement, and muscle impairment which typified cervicogenic headache – a pattern that similarly presents in any musculoskeletal disorder. The histories of all headache types were prolonged, which suggests that, even with time, migraine and tension headache sufferers do not automatically develop secondary neck dysfunction.

The presentation may sometimes be more difficult when a patient reports suffering two or more different types of headache. Nevertheless it was shown that this collective of reduced motion, painful upper cervical joint dysfunction, and muscle impairment in the CCFT could distinguish cervicogenic headache as one of a multiple-headache syndrome.[88] Thus patients without a cervicogenic headache as one of their multiple headache types did not have this pattern of musculoskeletal impairment in association with their headaches. They may have had an isolated measure that was in the realm of the cervicogenic headache group, but they did not have the three features of the pattern concurrently. While this collective of signs is very promising for the diagnosis of cervicogenic headache, the validity of the pattern needs to be tested in other groups of patients with frequent intermittent headache to realize its diagnostic potential.

The results of this study are nevertheless reinforced by the evidence provided in other studies that the primary headaches of migraine and tension-type are typically not associated with cervical musculoskeletal impairment such as is present in cervicogenic headache.[85, 86, 89-91] The primary headaches of migraine and tension-type may have an isolated musculoskeletal sign. They may exhibit reactions in the muscle system such as trigger points in muscles[91-93] or increased muscle activity under stressful situations.[94] However these reactions are seemingly co-occurrences and possibly manifestations of the sensitization of trigeminocervical neurons.[54, 95-97] They reveal the multiple dimensions in effect that may occur in headache syndromes but do not imply a cervical musculoskeletal cause of primary headache types.

## Other musculoskeletal impairments in cervicogenic headache

In addition to the impairments already discussed, other impairments have been identified in the cervical musculoskeletal system in cervicogenic headache. Further research is necessary to understand fully all musculoskeletal impairment in cervicogenic headache and indeed any association with other frequent intermittent headaches types. Such knowledge may further expand or strengthen the clinical signs, as called for by the IHS.[8]

### Posture

Cervicogenic headache on traditional clinical lines has been linked with a forward head posture. Nevertheless, studies measuring the craniovertebral angle (C7 to tragus) in upright standing or sitting are divided with regard to the strength of any relationship between this angle and the presence of cervicogenic headache.[81, 85, 98-100] Pertinently, no differences in craniovertebral angle were found between migraine, cervicogenic headache, and nonheadache groups[81, 85] and neither was the static angle of forward head posture predictive of responsiveness to physical therapy treatment.[101]

However, the critical feature may be the drift into a more forward head posture in work tasks that has been observed in those with neck pain (Chapter 4).[102, 103] More specific research of headache populations is required to determine if this is a differentiating feature of cervicogenic headache.

### Cervical range of movement

Reduced range of cervical movement is a criterion for cervicogenic headache[33] and there is now substantive evidence that reduced cervical range of movement is a feature of cervicogenic headache and not one of migraine or tension-type headache.[58, 81, 85, 86, 88] Some work has been conducted to investigate more specific movement restrictions. The measure of head rotation has been taken with the cervical spine in full flexion to bias the rotation to the C1–2 segment.[104, 105] It was determined that a reduced range of head rotation was highly sensitive to distinguish cervicogenic headache subjects with C1–2 joint dysfunction, determined by manual examination, from those with migraine headache and control subjects. This line of research investigating regional movement restrictions has promise and should be continued.

## Manual examination of cervical segmental joint dysfunction

The validity of manual examination as a clinical test to determine a cervical segmental source of pain is still debated.[106] Nevertheless there are now several studies conducted by physiotherapists that have demonstrated that cervicogenic headache patients can be differentiated from patients with other headache types and nonheadache control subjects through the presence of symptomatic upper cervical dysfunction detected by manual examination.[58, 81, 85, 88–90, 107, 108] The presence of dysfunction in the C0–3 segments is in accordance with the mechanism for cervicogenic headache of convergence of cervical afferents on the trigeminal sensory circuit[109] and is in line with the active cervical motion loss in these patients. Relief of cervicogenic headache with surgical procedures to the lower cervical area have been reported[110] and it is apparent from clinicians' patterns of treatment that other segments in the upper thoracic region may be dysfunctional in cervicogenic headache sufferers.[111] Thus a manual examination should consider all regions of the cervical and upper thoracic spines.

## Alterations in motor control and cervical muscle properties

There is growing evidence of impaired muscle control in cervical musculoskeletal disorders (Chapter 4). Impaired activation of the cervical flexor muscles, as measured in the CCFT, has been demonstrated in cervicogenic headache patients and was one of the three impairments that formed the set of signs that differentiated this headache from migraine and tension-type headache. Commensurate with persons with idiopathic neck pain and whiplash,[112–114] cervicogenic headache patients have been shown to have higher levels of activity in the sternocleidomastoid in the progressive stages of the test.[58, 85, 88] The performances of the migraine and tension-type headache groups in the CCFT were no different to the control groups.

There have not as yet been specific studies of the activity of the suboccipital and neck extensors in cervicogenic headache sufferers. There is preliminary evidence that the semispinalis capitis has reduced cross-sectional area at the C2 level in persons with cervicogenic headache,[58, 88] and degenerative changes (fatty infiltrate) have been shown in particularly the suboccipital and multifidus muscles in patients with chronic whiplash-associated disorders.[115] These changes highlight the need for future investigation of the extensor muscles in the cervicogenic headache patient.

The pattern of activation in the upper trapezius muscle has been investigated under the condition of a stressful task. Elevated activity was found in both cervicogenic and tension-type headache patients,[80, 94] suggesting that both patient groups react to a stressful situation in a similar way. To date, the activity of the neck flexors or extensors has not been examined under these conditions.

## Muscle strength and endurance

Cervicogenic headache sufferers demonstrate deficits in the strength of the cervical flexor and extensor muscles whereas the strength in migraine and tension-type headache groups has not been shown to be different from control subjects.[58, 81, 84, 88] Preliminary data indicate lesser endurance, albeit only studied in the neck flexor group in cervicogenic headache at this time.[81, 84, 100] One study has shown that lesser endurance was not found in patients with migraine.[81] Further research is required to investigate neck muscle strength and endurance and, more specifically, that of the craniocervical flexors and extensors now that technology is available for this purpose.[116]

## Muscle length

Tests of muscle length have been undertaken using clinical assessment methods.[82, 85, 100] Zito et al.[85] compared the incidence of muscle tightness in cervical and axioscapular muscles in persons with cervicogenic headache and migraine as well as those without neck pain and headache. The incidence of muscle tightness was significantly higher in the cervicogenic headache group (34.9% of all muscle length tests) than the migraine with aura or control groups, where the incidence was low (16.7% and 16.3% respectively). No one muscle was found to have a higher incidence. What is relevant is that many with cervicogenic headache were judged to have several muscles with normal length, similar to migraine and control subjects. This concurs with the findings of other studies[82, 100] and indicates that some muscle tightness might be present in cervicogenic headache but does not strongly characterize this headache type.

## Nerve tissue mechanosensitivity

Direct physical compromise of nerve structures can contribute to the pathogenesis of some cervicogenic headaches and nerves may become physically painful. Greater occipital nerve and C2 root allodynia may be present in cervicogenic headache.[33, 117] The dura mater of the upper cervical cord and the posterior cranial fossa receives innervation from branches of the upper three cervical nerves[109] and, as such, is capable of being a pain source in cervicogenic

headache. There are fibrous connections between the rectus capitis posterior minor and the cervical dura mater[118] and continuity has been observed between the ligamentum nuchae and the posterior spinal dura at the first and second cervical levels.[119] Such connections indicate the mechanical interdependence of neural, ligamentous, and muscular structures in movements and postures of the upper cervical spine, and increased activity in cervical muscles has been demonstrated with noxious stimulation of cervical meningeal tissues.[120] It is feasible that changes in movement and attendant pathophysiological reactions within the upper cervical region in cervicogenic headache could, in some cases, involve the upper cervical dura mater.[121]

Little is known about the sensitivity of nerve structures to movement in cervicogenic headache. Preliminary clinical observations in two cervicogenic headache populations suggest an incidence between 7 and 10%.[23, 85] These observations were made using the movement of craniocervical flexion with the patient prepositioned in straight-leg raise and brachial plexus provocation test positions respectively.[122] Further research is required in this field. Nevertheless, when cervical nerve tissues are sensitive to movement, care must be taken in treatment and especially when retraining the cervical flexor muscles, as the movement used may be provocative of pain (Chapter 14).

## Joint position error

Reduced kinesthetic sense, measured as the error in head reposition sense, has been identified in patients with neck disorders (Chapter 6). Measures of joint position error to date in groups of cervicogenic headache patients have failed to determine any significant differences from control populations.[58, 81, 85] However, these studies did not consider the influence of the presence or not of dizziness or light-headedness with headache in these patients (Chapter 6). It might be premature to rule out deficits in joint position sense as a possible impairment in at least some patients with cervicogenic headache, especially as it was shown that the presence of light-headedness was associated with lower odds of achieving long-term relief of headache[101] in the clinical trial testing the effectiveness of manipulative therapy and therapy for cervicogenic headache.[23] Further research is needed.

### Balance disturbances

To our knowledge, no studies have studied balance specifically in patients with cervicogenic headache. Nevertheless balance has been studied in patients with migraine and tension-type headache when tested under various conditions.[123, 124] Deficits have been determined in some patients with these headache types, reasoned to reflect either dysfunction in the vestibulospinal system[123] or an impairment in control of involuntary oculomotility of central origin.[124] Research is indicated in patients with cervicogenic headache.

# Conclusion

Cervicogenic headache is a distinct secondary headache associated with cervical musculoskeletal impairment. There is a pattern of symptoms that is characteristic of cervicogenic headache, but there can be symptomatic overlap with migraine without aura and tension-type headaches. If clinicians perform a skilled examination of the cervical musculoskeletal system and find a pattern of joint, movement, and muscle impairment in conjunction with the symptomatic pattern, they can be confident of confirming a diagnosis of cervicogenic headache with a high degree of certainty. They can be equally certain that if this pattern of physical impairment is not present, then the cervical musculoskeletal impairment is highly unlikely to be contributing to the cause of the patient's headache.

Knowledge of the types of musculoskeletal impairments associated with cervicogenic headache is growing and, importantly, they direct the nature of interventions required (Chapters 13 and 14). There is evidence of the effectiveness of manipulative therapy and specific therapeutic exercise for cervicogenic headache.[19, 23, 24] There are clear indications to use or not use such treatment methods in headache management when clear diagnoses of cervicogenic and migraine and tension-type headache are made. Nevertheless, the indications are not so clear when patients present with mixed headache types, with more isolated signs of cervical musculoskeletal impairment, or with painful trigger points in the neck or axioscapular muscles in association with migraine or tension-type headaches. It is possible that manual therapies might assist in headache management in a multimodal/multiprofessional approach to headache management by at least modulating input to the trigeminocervical system. However, more research needs to be conducted in this field to provide definitive directives. At the present time, such patients should be managed with regular and rigorous evaluation of treatment effect to avoid prolonged courses of ineffective therapy.

# References

1. *Leonardi M, Musicco M, Nappi G*. Headaches as a major public health problem: current status. Cephalalgia 1998;18(Suppl. 21):66–69.

2. *van Suijlekom H, Lame I, van den Berg SS, et al*. Quality of life of patients with cervicogenic headache: a comparison with control subjects and patients with migraine or tension-type headache. Headache 2003;43:1034–1041.

3. *Wiendels N, van Haestregt A, Neven AK, et al*. Chronic frequent headache in the general population: comorbidity and quality of life. Cephalalgia 2006;26:1443–1450.

4. *Anttila P, Metsahonkala L, Mikkelsson M, et al*. Muscle tenderness in pericranial and neck–shoulder region in children with headache. A controlled study. Cephalalgia 2002;22:340–344.

5. *Biondi DM*. Cervicogenic headache: mechanisms, evaluation, and treatment strategies. J Am Osteopath Assoc 2000;100 (Suppl):S7–S14.

6. *Kan L, Nagelberg J, Maytal J*. Headaches in a paediatric emergency department: etiology, imaging and treatment. Headache 1999;40:25–29.

7. *Pearce JM*. The importance of cervicogenic headache in the over-fifties. Headache Q, Curr Treatment Res 1995;6:293–296.

8. *Headache Classification Subcommittee of the International Headache Society*. The International Classification of Headache Disorders, 2nd edn. Cephalalgia 2004;24(Suppl. 1):1–151.

9. *Niere K*. Can subjective characteristics of benign headache predict manipulative physiotherapy treatment outcome? Aust J Physiother 1998;44: 87–93.

10. *Quin A, Niere K*. Development of a headache-specific disability questionnaire for physiotherapy patients. In: Magarey M (ed) Proceedings of the 12th Biennial Conference Musculoskeletal Physiotherapy Australia. Adelaide, South Australia: 2001:34–37.

11. *Astin JA, Ernst E*. The effectiveness of spinal manipulation for the treatment of headache disorders: a systematic review of randomized clinical trials. Cephalalgia 2002;22:617–623.

12. *Blau JN, MacGregor EA*. Migraine and the neck. Headache 1994;34:88–90.

13. *Boline PD, Kassak K, Bronfort G, et al*. Spinal manipulation vs amitripyline for the treatment of chronic tension-type headaches: a randomized clinical trial. J Manipul Physiol Ther 1995;18: 148–154.

14. *Bronfort G, Assendelft W, Evans R, et al*. Efficacy of spinal manipulation for chronic headache: a systematic review. J Manipul Physiol Ther 2001;24:457–466.

15. *Bronfort G, Nilsson N, Haas M, et al*. Non-invasive physical treatments for chronic/recurrent headache. Cochrane Database Syst Rev. 2004;3: CD001878.

16. *Bove G, Nilsson N*. Spinal manipulation in the treatment of episodic tension-type headache: a randomized controlled trial. J Am Med Assoc 1998;280:1576–1579.

17. *van Ettekoven H, Lucas C*. Efficacy of physiotherapy including a craniocervical training programme for tension-type headache; a randomized clinical trial. Cephalalgia 2006;26:983–991.

18. *Nilsson N, Bove G*. Evidence that tension-type headache and cervicogenic headache are distinct disorders. J Manipul Physiol Ther 2000;23:288–289.

19. *Nilsson N, Christensen HW, Hartvigsen J*. The effect of spinal manipulation in the treatment of cervicogenic headache. J Manipul Physiol Ther 1997;20:326–330.

20. *Parker GB, Pryor DS, Tupling H*. Why does migraine improve during a clinical trial? Further results from a trial of cervical manipulation for migraine. Aust NZ J Med 1980;10:192–198.

21. *Tuchin P, Pollard H, Bonello R*. A randomized controlled trial of chiropractic spinal manipulative therapy for migraine. J Manipul Physiol Ther 2000;23:91–95.

22. *Vernon H, Steiman I, Hagino C*. Cervicogenic dysfunction in muscle contraction headache and migraine: a descriptive study. J Manipul Physiol Ther 1992;15:418–429.

23. *Jull G, Trott P, Potter H, et al*. A randomized controlled trial of exercise and manipulative therapy for cervicogenic headache. Spine 2002;27:1835–1843.

24. *Schoensee SK, Jensen G, Nicholson G, et al*. The effect of mobilization on cervical headaches. J Orthop Sports Phys Ther 1995;21:184–196.

25. *Frese A, Schilgen M, Edvinsson L, et al*. Calcitonen gene-related peptide in cervicogenic headache. Cephalalgia 2005;25:700–703.

26. *Hubka MJ*. Cervicogenic dysfunction in muscle contraction headache and migraine: a descriptive study [letter]. J Manipul Physiol Ther 1993;16: 428–431.

27. *Sjaastad O, Fredriksen T, Pareja JA, et al*. Coexistence of cervicogenic headache and migraine without aura (?). Funct Neurol 2000;14:209–218.

28. *Kelman L*. Migraine pain location: a tertiary care study of 1283 migraineurs. Headache 2005;45: 1038–1047.

29. *Sjaastad O, Fredriksen TA, Sand T*. The localisation of the initial pain of attack: a comparison between classic migraine and cervicogenic headache. Funct Neurol 1989;4:73–78.

30. *Sjaastad O, Bovim G, Stovner LJ*. Laterality of pain and other migraine criteria in common migraine. A comparison with cervicogenic headache. Funct Neurol 1992;7:289–294.

31. *Antonaci F, Fredriksen T, Sjaastad O*. Cervicogenic headache: clinical presentation, diagnostic criteria and differential diagnosis. Curr Pain Headache Rep 2001;5:387–392.

32. *Bono G, Antonaci F, Dario A, et al*. Unilateral headaches and their relationship with cervicogenic headache. Clin Exp Neurol 2000;18: S11–S15.

33. *Sjaastad O, Fredriksen TA, Pfaffenrath V*. Cervicogenic headache: diagnostic criteria. The Cervicogenic Headache International Study Group. Headache 1998;38:442–445.

34. *Sjaastad O, Fredriksen T*. Cervicogenic headache: lack of influence of pregnancy. Cephalalgia 2002;22:667–671.

35. *Smetana G*. The diagnostic value of historical features in primary headache syndromes: a comprehensive review. Arch Intern Med 2000;160:2729–2737.

36. *Antonaci F, Ghirmai S, Bono G, et al*. Cervicogenic headache: evaluation of the original diagnostic criteria. Cephalalgia 2001;21:573–583.

37. *Biondi DM*. Cervicogenic headache: diagnostic evaluation and treatment strategies. Curr Pain Headache Rep 2001;53:61–68.

38. *Cecchini AP, Sandrini G, Fokin I, et al*. Trigeminofacial reflexes in primary headaches. Cephalalgia 2003;23(Suppl. 1):33–41.

39. *Milanov I, Bogdanova D*. Trigemino-cervical reflex in patients with headache. Cephalalgia 2003;23:35–38.

40. *Nardone R, Tezzon F*. The trigemino-cervical reflex in tension-type headache. Eur J Neurol 2003;10:307–312.

41. *Piovesan E, Kowacs P, Tatsui C, et al*. Referred pain after painful stimulation of the greater occipital nerve in humans: evidence of convergence of cervical afferences on trigeminal nuclei. Cephalalgia 2001;21:107–109.

42. *Weiler C, May A, Limmroth V, et al*. Brain stem activation in spontaneous human migraine attacks. Nat Med 1995;1:658–660.

43. *Granella F, D'Alessandro R, Manozi G*. International Headache Society classification: interobserver reliabilty in diagnosis of primary headache. Cephalalgia 1994;14:16–20.

44. *Leone M, Filippini G, D'Amico D, et al*. Assessment of International Headache Society diagnostic criteria: a reliability study. Cephalalgia 1994;14:280–284.

45. *van Suijlekom JA, de Vet HC, van den Berg SG, et al*. Interobserver reliability of diagnostic criteria for cervicogenic headache. Cephalalgia 1999;19:817–823.

46. *Vincent M*. Validation of criteria for cervicogenic headache. Funct Neurol 1998;13:74–75.

47. *Leone M, D'Amico D, Moschiano F, et al*. Possible identification of cervicogenic headache among patients with migraine: an analysis of 374 headaches. Headache 1995;35:461–464.

48. *Rokicki L, Semenchuk E, Bruehl S, et al*. An examination of the validity of the IHS classification system for migraine and tension-type headache in the college student population. Headache 1999;39:720–727.

49. *Solomon S*. Diagnosis of primary headache disorders: validity of the International Headache Society criteria in clinical practice. Neurol Clin 1997;15:15–26.

50. *Xiaobin Y, Cook A, Hamill-Ruth R, et al*. Cervicogenic headache in patients with presumed migraine: missed diagnosis or misdiagnosis? J Pain 2005;6:700–703.

51. *Gawel MJ, Rothbart PJ*. Occipital nerve block in the management of headache and cervical pain. Cephalalgia 1992;12:9–13.

52. *Lance JW*. Mechanism and Management of Headache. 6th edn. Oxford: Butterworth-Heinemann, 1998.

53. *Pfaffenrath V, Kaube H*. Diagnostics of cervicogenic headache. Funct Neurol 1990;5:159–164.

54. *Bartsch T, Goadsby P*. The trigeminocervical complex and migraine: current concepts and synthesis. Curr Pain Headache Rep 2003;7:371–376.

55. *Fishbain D, Cutler R, Cole B, et al*. International Headache Society headache diagnostic patterns in pain facility patients. Clin J Pain 2001;17:78–93.

56. *Henry P, Dartigues JF, Puymirat C, et al*. The association cervicalgia–headaches: an epidemiologic study. Cephalalgia 1987;7:189–190.

57. *Leone M, D'Amico D, Grazzi L, et al*. Cervicogenic headache: a critical review of current diagnostic criteria. Pain 1998;78:1–5.

58. *Jull G, Amiri M, Bullock–Saxton J, et al*. Cervical musculoskeletal impairment in frequent intermittent headache. Part 1: Subjects with single headaches. Cephalalgia 2007;27:793–802.

59. *Nilsson N*. The prevalence of cervicogenic headache in a random population sample of 20–59 year olds. Spine 1995;20:1884–1888.

60. *Bartsch T, Goadsby P*. Stimulation of the greater occipital nerve induces increased central excitability of dural afferent input. Brain 2002;125:1496–1509.

61. *Bartsch T, Goadsby P*. Increased responses in trigeminocervical nociceptive neurons to cervical input after stimulation of the dura mater. Brain 2003;126:1801–1813.

62. *Cote P, Cassidy J, Carroll L*. Is a lifetime history of neck injury in a traffic collision associated with prevalent neck pain, headache and depressive symptomatology? Acc Anal Prev 2000;32:151–159.

63. *Radanov B, Di-Stefano G, Augustiny K*. Symptomatic approach to posttraumatic headache and its possible implications for treatment. Eur Spine J 2001;10:403–407.

64. *Drottning M, Staff P, Sjaastad O*. Cervicogenic headache (CEH) after whiplash injury. Cephalalgia 2002;22:165–171.

65. *Schrader H, Stovner L, Obelieniene D, et al*. Examination of the diagnostic validity of 'headache

attributed to whiplash injury': a controlled, prospective study. Eur J Neurol 2006;13:1226–1232.

66. *Hagen K, Einarsen C, Zwart J, et al*. The co-occurrence of headache and musculoskeletal symptoms amongst 51050 adults in Norway. Eur J Neurol 2002;9:527–533.

67. *Sjaastad O, Fredriksen T*. Cervicogenic headache: the importance of sticking to the criteria. Funct Neurol 2002;17:35–36.

68. *Coskun O, Ulcer S, Karakurum B, et al*. Magnetic resonance imaging of patients with cervicogenic headache. Cephalalgia 2003;23:842–845.

69. *Fredriksen TA, Fougner R, Tangerud A, et al*. Cervicogenic headache. Radiographical investigations concerning head/neck. Cephalalgia 1989;9:139–146.

70. *Hinderaker J, Lord SM, Barnsley L, et al*. Diagnostic value of C2–3 instantaneous axes of rotation in patients with headache of cervical origin. Cephalalgia 1995;15:391–395.

71. *Lord SM, Barnsley L, Bogduk N*. Percutaneous radiofrequency neurotomy in the treatment of cervical zygapophysial joint pain: a caution. Neurosurg 1995;36:732–739.

72. *Bogduk N*. Distinguishing primary headache disorders from cervicogenic headache: clinical and therapeutic implications. Headache Curr 2005;2:27–36.

73. *Govind J, King W, Bailey B, et al*. Radiofrequency neurotomy for the treatment of third occipital headache. J Neurol Neurosurg Psychiatry 2003;74:88–93.

74. *McDonald GJ, Lord SM, Bogduk N*. Long-term follow-up of patients treated with cervical radiofrequency neurotomy for chronic neck pain. Neurosurg 1999;45:61–67.

75. *van Suijlekom JA, van Kleef M, Barendse GA, et al*. Radiofrequency cervical zygapophyseal joint neurotomy for cervicogenic headache: a prospective study of 15 patients. Funct Neurol 1998;13:297–303.

76. *Lord S, Bogduk N*. Radiofrequency procedures in chronic pain. Best Pract Res Clin Anaesth 2002;16:597–617.

77. *Sjaastad O, Fredriksen TA*. Cervicogenic headache: criteria, classification and epidemiology. Clin Exp Neurol 2000;18:S3–S6.

78. *Bovim G*. Cervicogenic headache, migraine, and tension-type headache. Pressure–pain threshold measurements. Pain 1992;51:169–173.

79. *Chen J, Solinger AB, Poncet JF, et al*. Meta-analysis of normative cervical motion. Spine 1999;24: 1571–1578.

80. *Bansevicius D, Sjaastad O*. Cervicogenic headache: the influence of mental load on pain level and EMG of shoulder–neck and facial muscles. Headache 1996;36:372–378.

81. *Dumas JP, Arsenault AB, Boudreau G, et al*. Physical impairments in cervicogenic headache: traumatic vs. nontraumatic onset. Cephalalgia 2001;21:884–893.

82. *Jull G, Barrett C, Magee R, et al*. Further characterisation of muscle dysfunction in cervical headache. Cephalalgia 1999;19:179–185.

83. *Sjaastad O, Fredriksen T, Petersen H, et al*. Features indicative of cervical abnormality. A factor to be reckoned with in clinical headache work and research? Funct Neurol 2003;18:195–203.

84. *Watson DH, Trott PH*. Cervical headache: an investigation of natural head posture and upper cervical flexor muscle performance. Cephalalgia 1993;13:272–284.

85. *Zito G, Jull G, Story I*. Clinical tests of musculoskeletal dysfunction in the diagnosis of cervicogenic headache. Man Ther 2006;11:118–129.

86. *Zwart JA*. Neck mobility in different headache disorders. Headache 1997;37:6–11.

87. *Bogduk N*. The neck and headaches. Neurol Clin North Am 2004;22:151–171.

88. *Amiri M, Jull G, Bullock-Saxton J, et al*. Cervical musculoskeletal impairment in frequent intermittent headache. Part 2: subjects with multiple headaches. Cephalalgia 2007;27:891–898.

89. *Gijsberts TJ, Duquet W, Stoekart R, et al*. Pain-provocation tests for C0–4 as a tool in the diagnosis of cervicogenic headache. Cephalalgia 1999;19:436.

90. *Gijsberts TJ, Duquet W, Stoekart R, et al*. Impaired mobility of cervical spine as tool in diagnosis of cervicogenic headache. Cephalalgia 1999;19:436.

91. *Marcus DA, Scharff L, Mercer S, et al*. Musculoskeletal abnormalities in chronic headache: a controlled comparison of headache diagnostic groups. Headache 1999;39:21–27.

92. *Calandre E, Hidalgo J, Garcia-Leiva J, et al*. Trigger point evaluation in migraine patients: an indication of peripheral sensitization linked to migraine predisposition? Eur J Neurol 2006;13:244–249.

93. *Fernandez-de-Las-Penas C, Alonso-Blanco C, Cuadrado M, et al*. Myofascial trigger points and their relationship to headache clinical parameters in chronic tension-type headache. Headache 2006;46:1264–1272.

94. *Bansevicius D, Westgaard R, Sjaastad O*. Tension-type headache: pain, fatigue, tension, and EMG responses to mental activation. Headache 1999;39:417–425.

95. *Bendtsen L*. Central sensitization in tension-type headache – possible pathophysiological mechanisms. Cephalalgia 2000;20:486–508.

96. *Matharu M, Bartsch T, Ward N, et al*. Central neuromodulation in chronic migraine patients with suboccipital stimulators: a PET study. Brain 2004;127:220–230.

97. *Olesen J*. Clinical and pathophysiological observations in migraine and tension-type headache explained by integration of vascular,

supraspinal and myofascial inputs. Pain 1991;46:125–132.

98. *Griegel-Morris P, Larson K, Mueller-Klaus K, et al.* Incidence of common postural abnormalities in the cervical, shoulder, and thoracic regions and their association with pain in two age groups of healthy subjects. Phys Ther 1992;72:425–431.

99. *Haughie LJ, Fiebert IM, Roach KE.* Relationship of forward head posture and cervical backward bending to neck pain. J Manipul Ther 1995;3:91–97.

100. *Treleaven J, Jull G, Atkinson L.* Cervical musculoskeletal dysfunction in post-concussional headache. Cephalalgia 1994;14:273–279.

101. *Jull G, Stanton W.* Predictors of responsiveness to physiotherapy treatment of cervicogenic headache. Cephalalgia 2005;25:101–108.

102. *Falla D, Jull G, Russell T, et al.* Effect of neck exercise on sitting posture in patients with chronic neck pain. Phys Ther 2007;87:408–417.

103. *Szeto G, Straker L, Raine S.* A field comparison of neck and shoulder postures in symptomatic and asymptomatic office workers. Appl Ergon 2002;33:75–84.

104. *Hall T, Robinson K.* The flexion–rotation test and active cervical mobility – a comparative measurement study in cervicogenic headache. Man Ther 2004;9:197–202.

105. *Ogince M, Hall T, Robinson K, et al.* The diagnostic validity of the cervical flexion–rotation test in C1/2-related cervicogenic headache. Man Ther 2007; 12:256–262.

106. *King W, Lau P, Lees R, et al.* The validity of manual examination in assessing patients with neck pain. Spine J 2007;7:22–26.

107. *Jull G, Bogduk N, Marsland A.* The accuracy of manual diagnosis for cervical zygapophysial joint pain syndromes. Med J Aust 1988;148:233–236.

108. *Jull G, Zito G, Trott P, et al.* Inter-examiner reliability to detect painful upper cervical joint dysfunction. Aust J Physiother 1997;43:125–129.

109. *Bogduk N.* Cervicogenic headache: anatomic basis and pathophysiologic mechanisms. Curr Pain Headache Rep 2001;5:382–386.

110. *Fredriksen T, Stolt-Nielsen A, Skaanes K, et al.* Headache and the lower cervical spine: long term, postoperative follow-up after decompressive neck surgery. Funct Neurol 2003;18:17–28.

111. *Jull G.* The use of high and low velocity cervical manipulative therapy procedures by Australian manipulative physiotherapists. Aust J Physiother 2002;48:189–193.

112. *Falla D, Jull G, Hodges P.* Patients with neck pain demonstrate reduced electromyographic activity of the deep cervical flexor muscles during performance of the craniocervical flexion test. Spine 2004;29:2108–2114.

113. *Jull G, Kristjansson E, Dall'Alba P.* Impairment in the cervical flexors: a comparison of whiplash and insidious onset neck pain patients. Man Ther 2004;9:89–94.

114. *Sterling M, Jull G, Vicenzino B, et al.* Characterisation of acute whiplash associated disorders. Spine 2004;29:182–188.

115. *Elliott J, Jull G, Noteboom J, et al.* Fatty infiltration in the cervical extensor muscles in persistent whiplash associated disorders (WAD): an MRI analysis. Spine 2006;31:E847–E855.

116. *O'Leary S, Vicenzino B, Jull G.* A new method of isometric dynamometry for the cranio-cervical flexors. Phys Ther 2005; 85:556–564.

117. *Pollmann W, Keidel M, Pfaffenrath V.* Headache and the cervical spine: a critical review. Cephalalgia 1997;17:801–816.

118. *Hack GD, Koritzer RT, Robinson WL, et al.* Anatomic relation between the rectus capitis posterior minor muscle and the dura mater. Spine 1995;20:2484–2486.

119. *Mitchell BS, Humphries BK, O'Sullivan E.* Attachments of ligamentum nuchae to cervical posterior dura and the lateral part of the occipital bone. J Manipul Physiol Ther 1998;21: 145–148.

120. *Hu JW, Vernon H, Tatourian I.* Changes in neck electromyography associated with meningeal noxious stimulation. J Manipul Physiol Ther 1995;18:577–581.

121. *Alix ME, Bates DK.* The proposed etiology of cervicogenic headache: the neurophysiologic basis and anatomical relationship between the dura mater and rectus posterior capitis minor muscle. J Manipul Physiol Ther 1999;22:534–539.

122. *Jull G.* Management of cervical headache. Man Ther 1997;2:182–190.

123. *Ishizaki K, Mori N, Takeshima T, et al.* Static stabilometry in patients with migraine and tension-type headache during a headache-free period. Psychiatry Clin Neurosci 2002;56: 85–90.

124. *Rossi C, Alberti A, Sarchielli P, et al.* Balance disorders in headache patients: evaluation by computerized static stabilometry. Acta Neurol Scand 2005;111:407–413.

# 10

# Differential Diagnosis of Cervicobrachial Pain

## Introduction

The presence of concomitant upper-quadrant pain and other symptoms in association with cervical spine pain is common and often causes a diagnostic dilemma to musculoskeletal clinicians. One reason for confusion surrounding pain in this body area is the nonuniform terminology used to describe its presence. Cervicobrachial pain, nonspecific arm pain, neck/arm syndrome, repetitive strain injury, work-related upper-limb disorder are a few of the nomenclature used to describe upper-quadrant pain that may involve structures including the cervical spine, shoulder, arm, hand, upper back, and upper chest, with some authors also suggesting that headache may be an associated symptom.[1] The arm pain is often described as aching, burning, or paroxysmal.[2] In addition, sensory symptoms such as paresthesia, hypoesthesia, hyperesthesia, vasomotor changes, and weakness may also be reported.[3]

The proportion of patients who report upper-quadrant pain in association with their neck pain has not been extensively reported. Barnsley et al.[4] noted a frequent occurrence of these symptoms in chronic whiplash subjects and this is supported by our findings where approximately 60% of chronic whiplash subjects with symptoms longer than 3 months' duration also reported the presence of arm pain.[5] Daffner et al.[6] compared the impact of concomitant arm and neck symptoms versus neck pain alone on overall health status. Accounting for age and gender, individuals with additional arm symptoms were more disabled and showed lower levels of general health and well-being than those individuals with only neck pain. These findings applied to both the physical and mental health components of the Short Form-36 (SF-36) instrument. This is the first study demonstrating that the presence of arm pain in addition to neck pain has a greater effect on patients' disability levels and has implications for the management, rehabilitation, and possible outcomes of these patients.

There are several potential causes of cervicobrachial pain, including somatic pain referral from pathological cervical spine structures, the involvement of peripheral nerve tissue ranging from irritation or sensitization of nerve tissue to radiculopathy or nerve root compression, as well as potential involvement of neurovascular tissue. More sinister pathology such as a Pancoast tumor may also be a cause of neck and arm pain[7] and practitioners of manual therapy must be alert to clues present in the assessment of such patients suggestive of a nonmusculoskeletal cause of symptoms and ensure appropriate medical referral.

This chapter will outline the possible mechanisms that may underlie the presence of cervicobrachial pain. The differential diagnosis of arm and neck pain and the effectiveness of current management strategies will be discussed.

# Mechanisms underlying cervicobrachial pain

## Pain of somatic referral

The presence of arm pain in association with neck pain often leads the clinician to assume the involvement of peripheral nerve tissue as contributing to the patient's symptoms. However arm pain may result as a consequence of referred pain from nonneural cervical structures with essentially any structure that receives a nerve supply being a possible source of nociception. Experiments in both healthy control subjects and those with neck pain have demonstrated that neck muscles, zygapophyseal joints, and

intervertebral disks may refer pain into the upper limb,[8, 9] with C5–6, C6–7, and C7–T1 being the implicated segmental levels.[10] Referred pain is usually perceived as a dull, poorly localized ache.[11] Areas of somatic referred pain are not uncommonly encountered by clinicians in their patients presenting with neck disorders. Details of possible mechanisms underlying referred pain are discussed in Chapter 2.

## Neuropathic pain

Arm pain may involve peripheral nerve tissue and is thus termed a "neuropathic" pain condition. The International Association for the Study of Pain (IASP) defines neuropathic pain as pain resultant from a primary lesion or dysfunction in the peripheral or central nervous systems.[12] Alternative terminology such as neurogenic pain (primary lesion, dysfunction, or transitory perturbation in the peripheral or central nervous system) and neuritis (pain where an inflammatory cause is thought to be present) are also used seemingly interchangeably. It has been suggested that the more general term "neuropathic pain" be used to encapsulate the often multiple mechanisms that may be at play with pain originating from nerve tissue.[13] It also avoids the situation where a specific mechanism is implied from the terminology used but, as often occurs in the clinical situation, the exact underlying mechanisms are far from clear. For these reasons the term "neuropathic pain" will be used in this chapter to refer to pain arising from the involvement of nerve tissue.

The quandary that confronts the clinician is being able to determine whether the pain is in fact neuropathic in nature when, in many cases presenting to the clinician, a neuropathy is difficult to determine. An example of this scenario occurs when a patient presents with a cervical radiculopathy where clinical neurological assessment manifests sensation loss, decreased muscle power, and decreased tendon reflexes. This clinical example clearly implicates impaired peripheral nerve conduction as a diagnosis of the patient's condition. However pain arising from nerve tissue may not always be associated with nerve conduction loss[14] and thus makes diagnosis difficult and opens the door to skeptical interpretation of patients' condition and their motives for reporting continuing arm pain.[15] Furthermore, there is no "gold-standard" diagnostic tool that allows the diagnosis of peripheral nerve tissue pathology as a contributor to a patient's arm symptoms.[16] Electrophysiological testing such as nerve conduction tests is often considered to be a test to determine the presence of peripheral nerve dysfunction. However it has several drawbacks that impede its usefulness in determining the presence of minor peripheral nerve lesions. The fascicles within the nerve may be affected heterogeneously with the large myelinated fibers being relatively unaffected (the target of nerve conduction tests) or affected to varying degrees, thus the conduction velocity and latency will remain normal.[17] Furthermore, electrophysiology testing is not useful for pathology involving the brachial plexus because of the potential difficulty in localizing the lesion, a requirement for accurate result.[18]

Recent animal models of nerve injury have provided evidence demonstrating the presence of painful symptoms where only minor nerve injury has been induced. The two animal models of nerve tissue pain that appear to be most relevant to cervicobrachial pain syndromes seen in musculoskeletal practice are the chronic constrictive injury (CCI) and the neuritis models. Other animal models involving nerve ligation or transection have been explored but these are characterized by gross sensory and motor deficits and are not part of the topic discussed in this chapter.

## Animal models of nerve injury

CCI is created when ligatures are tightened around the peripheral nerve trunk and blood flow is impeded but the nerve is not transected.[19] Induction of CCI in the rat sciatic nerve produces spontaneous ectopic discharge at the lesion site which may be associated with spontaneous pain, hyperalgesia, and allodynia[20]; these changes are apparent within 2 days of injury, peaking at 10–18 days, and lasting for up to 2 months.[19] A few days after CCI, primary afferent nerve fibers fire spontaneously, the discharge originating in the dorsal root ganglia.[21] Most of the activity is seen in the A-beta and A-delta fibers with C-fiber activity occurring at a later time postinjury.[22] In addition to spontaneous activity, morphological changes also occur with a significant loss of peripheral afferent fibers, particularly A-beta fibers, although axonal loss may not be uniform and may not occur across all fascicles.[14]

The CCI model of nerve injury involves both axonal damage and periaxonal inflammation. The presence of inflammation alone is also of interest, particularly in musculoskeletal conditions, where the presence of sensitized nerve tissue is often sought.[23] Eliav et al.[13] used inflammatory agents to produce an experimental neuritis in the sciatic nerves of rats (known as the neuritis model). In this animal model, where inflammation of the nerve sheath occurs with no axonal damage to the nerve, neuropathic-like symptoms, including mechanical and heat hyperalgesia as well as mechanical and cold allodynia, were present and persisted for several days after the experiment.[13] The neuropathic pain sensations occurred not only at the inflammation site but also in a distant region, in this case the ipsilateral hind paw. Later studies by this group showed additional responses of spontaneous ectopic activity from the nerve trunk affected by inflammation[24] and that these responses occurred in both lower-limb nerve trunks as well as in orofacial nerves.[25]

Clinical observation of pain felt along the nerve trunk is not new[26] and has been proposed to occur as a result of sensitization of the nervi nervorum (the nociceptive innervation of the nerve sheaths).[23, 27] However this hypothesis has been disputed for several reasons. The amount of nociceptor activity generated from the nervi nervorum is quite small because the sheath's innervation is relatively sparse and therefore unlikely to be sufficient to generate the pain symptoms seen.[13] Denervation of the nervi nervorum with alcohol does not alter the pain responses seen in the neuritis model animals.[13] An alternative hypothesis is suggested for the neuropathic pain responses demonstrated with induced neuritis. Pain is considered to be as a result of a neuro-immune interaction in the endoneurial compartment.[13] These authors propose that infiltration of immune cells and fibroblasts into the endoneurium expose the A-delta and C fibers to other proinflammatory cytokines, thus producing ectopic discharge both toward the spinal cord (orthodromically) and toward the periphery (antidromically). The orthodromic discharge leads to central hypersensitivity in the spinal cord and the antidromic activity results in the release of neuropeptides such as substance P into peripheral tissues.[13]

Extrapolation of data from investigation of these two animal models to human clinical presentations suggests that sensory symptoms seen in patients with arm pain but without signs of nerve conduction loss, such as hyperalgesia, allodynia, and cold sensitivity, as well as the often highly irritable nature of the pain, may be as a consequence of nerve inflammation and sensitization as well as some or partial axonal damage, as occurs with the CCI model. Since traditional methods of assessing nerve fiber conduction in the clinic such as the neurological examination and even nerve conduction testing are unlikely to detect the more subtle changes that occur with the sorts of nerve injuries described, the development of quantitative methods to identify changes such as fiber sensitization and A-beta fiber loss in humans is paramount.

## Evidence of minor nerve injury in humans

Investigation of the neuritis model of neuropathic pain has commenced in human subjects. Recent studies have utilized electrocutaneous stimulation to investigate the sensitivity of large-diameter A-beta fibers. Inflammation around nerve trunks results in increased sensitivity (reduced detection threshold) of the A-beta afferents mediating touch sensation of the innervated organ.[28] These altered detection thresholds can be assessed using weak electrical stimuli that preferentially activate the A-beta fibers themselves by bypassing the terminal receptors.[29, 30] Reduced electrical detection thresholds are present in patients with neuritis of oral nerves and the sensory changes were apparent at an early stage even before the onset of symptoms.[28]

In an attempt to explore the usefulness of electrical detection thresholds in neck pain conditions, Chien et al.[31] recently utilized this methodology in participants with chronic whiplash. In contrast to the findings of Eliav et al.,[28] our study showed increased (hypoesthesia), not decreased, detection thresholds (hypersensitivity) in this patient group regardless of the presence of arm pain (Figure 10.1).[31] However our participants reported a chronic condition (> 3 months) where inflammatory responses that were initially present may now have led to nerve damage and thus hyposensitivity. Barbe et al.[32] propose from their results of animal studies that persistent inflammation leads to fibrosis and compression of nerve tissue, affecting conduction in some fibers, which

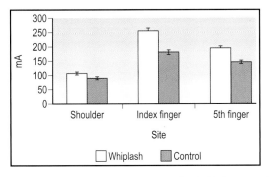

**Figure 10.1** Electrocutaneous detection thresholds (mean ± SE) tested at three sites at a frequency of 2000 Hz. All $P < 0.01$.

then presents as hyposensitivity. Benoliel et al.[33] have also demonstrated hypersensitivity to electrical detection threshold testing in an acute inflammatory state compared to the opposite findings (increased thresholds or hyposensitivity) in the chronic stages.

Altered A-beta fiber function has also been investigated using vibratory stimuli (Figure 10.2). In these studies increased vibration detection thresholds of upper-limb nerve trunks (particularly the median nerve) were shown to be present in office workers with nonspecific arm pain and patients with nonspecific arm pain.[34, 35] Greening and Lynn[34] propose that the findings represent minor nerve compression as a result of postural abnormalities. In keeping with their argument, decreased transverse and anteroposterior movement of the median nerve at the wrist with wrist movement was demonstrated with both ultrasound and magnetic resonance imaging in this patient group.[36, 37] This reduced movement is hypothesized to occur as a result of postural adaptations that consequently may result in nerve irritation and impedance of endoneurial blood flow.[37]

We have found similar elevated vibration detection thresholds in the hands of patients with chronic whiplash (Figure 10.3).[31] As is usually the case with this condition, the changes were generalized across the innervation zones of the three upper-limb nerve trunks. The hyposensitivity to

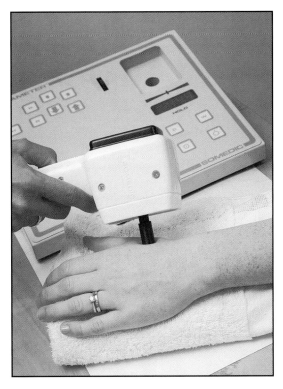

**Figure 10.2** Measurement of vibration detection thresholds over the dorsum of the hand using a Vibrametre (Somedic, Sweden).

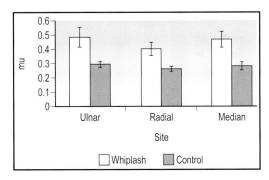

**Figure 10.3** Mean (± SE) vibration thresholds measured at the hand innervated by ulnar, radial, and median nerves. All $P < 0.05$.

vibration occurred regardless of whether or not the participant reported arm pain and this raises an interesting issue. These findings could be perceived as unusual where some arm pain or other symptoms would be expected in the presence of a neuropathy. However Greening et al.[38] have shown that asymptomatic office workers manifest similar nerve dysfunction to patients with cervicobrachial pain, that is, elevated vibration detection thresholds. Together these studies suggest a possible subclinical presentation that may be present in asymptomatic office workers and our whiplash cohort without arm symptoms. Whether or not the asymptomatic office workers develop pain or the localized symptoms of the patients with chronic whiplash become more widespread remains to be seen. Alternatively it is known that neural damage does not cause pain in all patients. Only 20% of diabetics with peripheral neuropathy have neuropathic pain. The reason for this apparent selectivity of the presence of pain is not known but is suspected to be as a result of subtly different underlying mechanisms.[17]

Additional evidence of nerve tissue involvement associated with cervico-brachial pain has been provided. C-fiber dysfunction has been demonstrated by a reduced flare area to both capsaicin and histamine stimulation of forearm and hand areas of subjects with cervicobrachial pain.[38, 39] Altered sympathetic nervous system activity has also been shown to be present, manifested by decreased sympathetic vasoconstrictive responses[38] and thermographic disturbances.[40]

The presence of irritated or sensitized nerve tissue may occur as a direct consequence of primary nerve tissue injury. Cadaveric studies of persons who sustained neck injuries as a result of a motor vehicle crash have demonstrated nerve tissue pathology, including nerve root injuries, bleeding into the dorsal root ganglia, and spinal cord damage.[41, 42] It could be argued that postmortem analysis of traffic accident victims is not representative of whiplash injury and extrapolations to survivors of such accidents should not be made. However it is generally acknowledged that the concurrence of evidence from postmortem, biomechanical, and clinical studies suggests the involvement of such structures, at least in some whiplash-injured persons.[43] Alternatively it is possible that irritation of nerve tissue may occur as a secondary phenomenon. Inflammatory processes in neighboring structures such as the zygapophyseal joints and intervertebral disks could also affect adjacent nerve structures, rendering them highly mechanosensitive and giving rise to neuritis-evoked neuropathic pain.[44] The profound effect that inflammatory mediators have on nerve tissue has been outlined above.[13, 24]

## Involvement of vascular tissues

In addition to the involvement of peripheral nerve tissues, some patients present with symptoms suggestive of vascular compromise. These may include color changes or cyanosis in the periphery, edema, and impaired capillary refill[45] in addition to arm pain, sensory loss, and/or weakness. This condition has been referred to as thoracic outlet syndrome as the tissue compromise is thought to occur within the thoracic outlet. However it is suggested that, if physiotherapists are to be encouraged to consider neck pain conditions from a more mechanisms-based diagnosis approach, terminologies such as this should be avoided as they tend to label a symptom set without clear and sound clinical reasoning as to processes underlying the reported symptoms.

The astute clinician will be alert to signs of vascular compromise via the patient's reported symptom. Examination may also include specific physical tests but the validity and reliability of these are uncertain.[46] Signs of severe vascular compromise indicate that immediate medical referral is mandatory. Further details of this condition are available in the review of Huang and Zager.[45] The differential diagnosis of nerve tissue involvement without vascular compromise will be discussed below.

# Clinical differential diagnosis of cervicobrachial pain

The main aim of clinical assessment of the patient presenting with cervicobrachial arm pain should be to determine the involvement or otherwise of a neuropathic component to the condition. This will influence the management of the patient's condition in several ways. It will allow accurate treatment prescription, including both physical therapy treatments and the likely use of medication. It will provide some indication of the clinical course of the condition, as those with a neuropathic component may be more recalcitrant to intervention. Importantly, the presence of mechanosensitive nerve tissue dictates that physical treatments should be undertaken with care so as not to provoke the patient's symptoms further.[5, 47]

The determination of a nerve tissue dysfunction as contributing to a patient's neck and arm pain cannot be made lightly and a thorough clinical examination is required.

## Patient-reported symptoms

It has been suggested that clinical differentiation of somatically referred arm pain from nerve tissue pain can be made on the patient's reported symptoms. Referred pain may be felt as a deep ache, with radicular pain being sharp, shooting, or lancinating in nature.[11] This may be true in the case of a cervical radiculopathy with nerve conduction loss, but pain arising from a minor peripheral nerve injury without conduction loss may not present with such definitive symptoms. Rasmussen et al.[48] attempted to differentiate three groups of patients by their reported symptoms. The patient groups included: (1) those with a definite neuropathic pain condition (for example, peripheral neuropathy); (2) those with possible neuropathic pain (including some patients with musculoskeletal pain); and (3) those with unlikely neuropathic pain. Considerable overlap of the symptoms reported was found between the three groups, including symptoms often ascribed to neuropathic pain such as burning and shooting pain. Bouhissera and Attal[49] demonstrated improved differentiation between neuropathic pain and other somatic pain using patient-reported descriptors of symptoms (burning, electric shocks, cold pain) in conjunction with nonpainful symptoms such as paresthesia, numbness, tingling, and itching. The findings of these studies would suggest that a thorough patient interview should be conducted in order to gain an appreciation of the patient's painful complaint, the nature of the pain, as well as the presence (or not) of additional nonpainful symptoms. A combination of these factors together may imply the presence of peripheral nerve tissue dysfunction that can be further confirmed or denied during the physical examination of the patient.

There are several neuropathic pain-screening questionnaires available that aim to detect pain that is principally neuropathic as opposed to nociceptive pain.[50] The present difficulty for musculoskeletal clinicians is that most of these questionnaires were formulated and validated in populations with a relatively clearcut neuropathic condition such as diabetic neuropathy. Their usefulness to detect a neuropathic component (perhaps more subtle) to painful musculoskeletal conditions commonly managed by clinicians is unclear. However, Sterling[51] recently demonstrated that 30% of patients with acute whiplash likely have a neuropathic pain condition as per responses to the self-report version of the Leeds Assessment of Neuropathic Symptoms and Signs (S-LANSS) questionnaire, suggesting that such an instrument should be included in the assessment of neck and/or arm pain where neuropathic pain is suspected.

## The physical examination

Practitioners of manual therapy will be well aware of the brachial plexus provocation test (BPPT) or upper-limb tension test (ULTT) which was developed in order to assess for sensitized nerve tissue involvement in the patient's pain syndrome (Figure 10.4).[52, 53] These tests are also often referred to as "neurodynamic" tests.[54] The BPPT has been shown to stimulate mechanically various neural components of the upper limb and cervical spine.[52] The examiner assesses for changes in resistance throughout the range of movement of the test: these changes are proposed to be an indication of the onset of muscle activity recruited in order to protect the nerve tissue from further provocation.[23] The onset of resistance or of muscle activity should coincide with the patient's report of symptom onset.[23]

Neural provocation tests have been criticized for being nonspecific in terms of the structures they provoke.[55] Certainly in some cases interpretation of findings from these tests is difficult. In the case of chronic whiplash-associated disorders, generalized responses to the BPPT have been demonstrated.[5] In this study, participants with chronic whiplash showed bilateral loss of elbow extension with the BPPT (compared to healthy controls) irrespective of whether they reported the presence of arm pain or not. It was proposed that these nonspecific responses reflect hypersensitive flexor withdrawal responses as a consequence of altered central nervous system pain-processing mechanisms.[5] This is in contrast to responses to the BPPT in persons with confirmed cervical radiculopathy. These participants respond to the BPPT in the clinically expected manner, that is, their loss of elbow extension was confined to their symptomatic side and coincided with the reproduction of their pain.[56] The contrasting responses to the BPPT illustrated by these two studies demonstrate that factors other than the isolated involvement of nerve tissue can influence the responses and interpretation of findings from nerve provocation tests.

However what is often not realized is that the BPPT, used alone, is insufficient to make a diagnosis of nerve tissue involvement and that a range of physical tests is required in order to clarify the clinical scenario.[23, 47] The

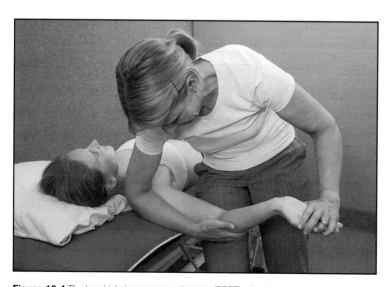

**Figure 10.4** The brachial plexus provocation test (BPPT), also known as upper-limb tension test or upper-limb neurodynamic test.

physical signs of sensitized peripheral nerve tissue should include: (1) the presence of antalgic posture indicative of a strategy to protect irritated nerve tissue – in the case of cervicobrachial pain, shoulder girdle elevation, shoulder adduction, and elbow flexion are often seen; (2) active movement dysfunction that equates with irritated nerve tissue, for example a painful limitation of cervical lateral flexion away from the side of the pain; (3) passive movement dysfunction that parallels the active movement dysfunction present; (4) mechanical allodynia to palpation of specific nerve trunks; (5) evidence of a local cause of the sensitized nerve tissue in conjunction with adverse responses to nerve tissue provocation tests.[23 47] The validity of this examination algorithm for cervicobrachial neuropathic pain has not been determined mainly because there is no gold standard for the assessment of minor peripheral nerve injury that can be compared to the physical examination algorithm. However it is a logical starting point for the assessment of mechanosensitive nerve tissue and toward preventing clinical reasoning errors based on the results of a single test alone.

Recently, Jepsen et al.[57] investigated the agreement between two skilled examiners in identifying and localizing upper-limb neuropathy in patients with nonspecific upper-limb pain using manual muscle testing, sensibility to light touch, pinprick, and vibration and the presence of allodynia of peripheral nerve tissue, including the brachial plexus and nerve trunks. There was high interrater agreement (kappa = 0.75) between the examiners in determining the presence of a neuropathy. Interestingly, based on the specific nature of the findings, the authors proposed the dominant site of "injury" to be at the cord level of the brachial plexus. In a later study, these authors demonstrated significant correlations between physical examination findings (including detailed muscle testing, sensibility

to pinprick, vibration, and nerve trunk mechanosensitivity with palpation) and upper-limb pain severity.[58] These studies demonstrate the importance of skilled clinical assessment using a range of physical tests in order to elucidate a neuropathic component to a patient's arm pain. It also illustrates that clinicians will be required to move past the usual clinical neurological examination that is performed (decreased light touch sensation, gross muscle power, and tendon reflexes) to include more specific testing as outlined by Jepsen and colleagues[57] in order to detect the more subtle signs manifested by nerve injury without frank conduction loss. Whilst it could be argued that this approach is time-consuming, it seems that it may be necessary if an accurate clinical diagnosis is to be made.

As has been discussed previously, both vibration and electrical detection thresholds show potential to detect A-beta fiber irritation or damage but their development is in its infancy. Similarly, ultrasound evaluation of nerve trunk movement may show potential for diagnostic purposes, although it too needs to be developed further. At present the clinical diagnosis of a neuropathic component to cervicobrachial pain relies on thorough and precise clinical examination and interpretation of examination findings.

The diagnosis of radiculopathy is somewhat less obtuse. Findings from electrodiagnostic testing (needle electromyography and nerve conduction studies) of participants with cervical radiculopathy have been shown to correlate with responses to clinical tests, including the BPPT, cervical range of movement, cervical distraction test, and clinical neurological examination.[56] Interestingly, the BPPT was shown to be the most useful test to rule out cervical radiculopathy.[56] These findings indicate that a combination of physical examination tests are required to make a clinical diagnosis of cervical radiculopathy and reinforces the need for thorough and thoughtful assessment of neck pain conditions. Similar investigation of relationships between quantitative sensory tests, including vibration and electrical stimulation and clinical examination, is necessary for cervicobrachial conditions where nerve conduction remains intact.

If there is no evidence of nerve conduction loss or mechanosensitive peripheral nerve tissue, the clinical assumption is that the basis of the patient's arm pain is via somatic referral. However it should be noted that studies are yet to be conducted to validate this assumption.

# Conservative management of cervicobrachial pain

There have been several studies investigating the effect of various physical therapies on neck and upper-limb pain. The difficulty with interpretation of such studies is the heterogenic nature of the cohorts investigated. As has been highlighted, precise diagnosis of cervicobrachial pain is difficult and this inherent problem then extends into subject inclusion and exclusion criteria when investigating this condition. A systematic review of multidisciplinary biospsychosocial rehabilitation for neck and shoulder pain found little evidence of effectiveness for this form of management, with the authors noting that the number of randomized controlled trials in this area is lacking.[59]

Few studies have specifically investigated the effects of treatment in patients with mechanosensitive nerve tissue as an inclusion criterion. Since there is no gold-standard method of categorically identifying patients with this phenomenon, clinical diagnosis was established using the criteria recommended by Elvey.[47] Coppieters et al.[60] showed that an immediate significant reduction in pain occurred following manual therapy, involving a contralateral lateral glide technique to the cervical spine when compared to ultrasound therapy. Allison et al.[1] investigated the same manual therapy technique in a similar patient cohort but utilized an 8-week treatment program combined with home exercises aimed at mobilizing nerve tissue. They compared the lateral glide technique (neural treatment group) to manual therapy directed toward the glenohumeral joint and thoracic spine (articular treatment group) and controls who received no physiotherapy treatment. Both the neural and articular manual therapy groups showed significant but modest improvements in pain and disability when compared to controls, with the neural manual therapy group showing significantly lower pain at the 8-week assessment point.[1] The apparent overlap between the two types of manual therapy approach is difficult to determine in this study due to its small sample size and other methodological flaws acknowledged by the researchers.[1] It would appear that manual therapy aimed at mobilizing peripheral nerve tissue does induce some relief of pain and improvements in disability but its relative superiority to other forms of manual therapy is not known at present. A recent animal study indicated that the effects of manual therapy on inflamed nerve tissue warrant further development and investigation. Song et al.[61] found that spinal manual therapy reduced pain severity and duration in rats with induced dorsal root ganglia inflammation. In addition electrophysiological and pathological manifestations of inflammation were reduced.

One reason for the lack of effective interventions for cervicobrachial pain is that knowledge of the underlying mechanisms and pathology remains poorly understood. In this chapter a clinical approach to determine the presence of a neuropathic versus somatic referred component to neck/arm pain has been outlined. However there is argument to suggest that clinical differentiation of neuropathic and inflammatory pain may not be possible.[17] Clinicians should be aware of these arguments and take care in their diagnosis of such patients. Attal and Bouhissera[62] put forward an interesting concept: it may be possible to have varying neuropathic components to some conditions. In other words the condition may be "more or less" neuropathic. Following this model, clinical assessment could aim to detect whether or not there is evidence of a neuropathic component to the patient's condition, perhaps in combination with a nociceptive or inflammatory component. This approach may be particularly useful in the assessment of musculoskeletal conditions, including neck pain where a neuropathic component may be less obvious, as compared to a more definite neuropathic condition such as a peripheral neuropathy.[63]

Whilst the evidence for efficacy of manual therapy interventions for neuropathic cervicobrachial pain is limited, it should be remembered that there is little evidence that other management approaches, such as pharmacology, are any more beneficial. As has been pointed out in relation to pain research, it may well be that the underlying physiological mechanisms of the condition of interest may need to be better understood such that specific treatments directed toward these mechanisms can be developed.[17] The complexities of neuropathic pain conditions suggest that integration between physical, pharmacological, and cognitive approaches may be the way forward but much research is still required to determine the optimum nature and timing of these intervention strategies.

## Conclusion

Cervicobrachial pain is a disabling condition that requires careful assessment and diagnosis. Clinical assessment should be directed toward differentiating somatic referred pain from dysfunction in the cervical spine from a neuropathic condition. There is evidence from animal studies that minor nerve injury, including inflammation of the nerve, can give rise to symptoms commonly seen in patients with cervicobrachial pain such as hyperalgesia and allodynia. Evidence is now accumulating from human studies which demonstrate that minor peripheral nerve injury without nerve conduction loss may be detected using quantitative sensory testing, including electrical and vibration testing. Clinical diagnosis of a neuropathic component to cervicobrachial pain relies on a thorough patient interview detailing symptoms both painful and nonpainful and a detailed physical assessment. The diagnosis cannot be made from a single test but rather from findings and clinical reasoning processes from a range of tests in association with the patient's reported symptoms. There are few studies investigating the efficacy of physical therapy interventions for cervicobrachial pain of a neuropathic nature but preliminary evidence indicates that specific manual therapy techniques show some promise for treatment of this condition. It is likely that a combined physical therapy, pharmacological, and cognitive approach may be optimal.

# References

1. *Allison G, Nagy B, Hall T*. A randomised clinical trial of manual therapy for cervicobrachial pain. Man Ther 2002;7:95–102.

2. *Quintner J, Bove G*. From neuralgia to peripheral neuropathic pain: evolution of a concept. Reg Anesth Pain Med 2001;26:368–372.

3. *Cohen M, Arroyo J, Champion G, et al*. In search of the pathogenesis of refractory cervicobrachial pain syndrome. Med J Aust 1992;156:432–436.

4. *Barnsley L, Lord S, Bogduk N*. Clinical review. Whiplash injury. Pain 1994;58:283–307.

5. *Sterling M, Treleaven J, Jull G*. Responses to a clinical test of mechanical provocation of nerve tissue in whiplash associated disorders. Man Ther 2002;7:89–94.

6. *Daffner S, Hilibrand A, Hanscorn B, et al*. Impact of neck and arm pain on overall health status. Spine 2003;28:2030–2035.

7. *Villas C, Collia A, Aquerreta J, et al*. Cervicobrachialgia and pancoast tumour: value of standard anteroposterior cervical radiographs in early diagnosis. Orthopedics 2004;27:1092–1095.

8. *Bogduk N, Aprill C*. On the nature of neck pain, discography and cervical zygapophyseal joint blocks. Pain 1993;54:213–217.

9. *Bogduk N*. The anatomical basis for spinal pain syndromes. J Manipul Physiol Ther 1995;18:603–605.

10. *Fukui S, Ohseto K, Shiotani M, et al*. Referred pain distribution of the cervical zygapophyseal joints and cervical dorsal rami. Pain 1996;68:79–83.

11. *Bogduk N*. The neck. Baillière's Clin Rheumatol 1999;13:261–285.

12. *Merskey H, Bogduk N*. IASP pain terminology. In: Merskey H, Bogduk N (eds) Classification of Chronic Pain. Seattle: IASP Press, 1994:209–214.

13. *Eliav E, Herzberg U, Ruda M, et al*. Neuropathic pain from an experimental neuritis of the rat sciatic nerve. Pain 1999;83:169–182.

14. *Greening J, Lynn B*. Minor peripheral nerve injuries: an underestimated source of pain. Man Ther 1998;3:187–194.

15. *Ferrari R*. From railway spine to whiplash – the recycling of nervous irritation. Med Sci Monit 2003;9:HY27–HY37.

16. *Katz J, Stock S, Evanoff B, et al*. Classification criteria and severity assessment in work related upper extremity disorders: methods matter. Am J Ind Med 2000;38:369–372.

17. *Bennett G*. Can we distinguish between inflammatory and neuropathic pain? Pain Res Manage 2006;11(Suppl. A):11–15.

18. *Dellon A*. Pitfalls in interpretation of electrophysiological testing. In: Gelberman R (ed) Operative Nerve Repair and Reconstruction. Philadelphia: Lippincott, 1991:185–196.

19. *Bennett G, Xie Y*. A peripheral mononeuropathy in rat that produces disorders of pain sensation like those seen in man. Pain 1988;35:87–107.

20. *Tal M, Eliav E*. Abnormal discharge originates at the site of nerve injury in experimental constriction neuropathy (CCI) in the rat. Pain 1996;64:519–526.

21. *Study R, Kral M*. Spontaneous action potential activity in isolated dorsal root ganglion neurons from rats with a painful neuropathy. Pain 1996;65:235–242.

22. *Eliav E, Tal M*. Electrophysiological properties of experimental neuropathy (CCI) in rats. Abstr Soc Neurosci 1994;20:761.

23. *Hall T, Elvey R*. Nerve trunk pain: physical diagnosis and treatment. Man Ther 1999;4:63–73.

24. *Eliav E, Benoliel R, Tal M*. Inflammation with no axonal damage of the rat saphenous nerve trunk induces ectopic discharge and mechanosensitivity in myelinated axons. Neurosci Lett 2001;311:49–52.

25. *Benoliel R, Wilensky A, Tal M, et al*. Application of a pro-inflammatory agent to the orbital portion of the rat infraorbital nerve induces changes indicative of ongoing trigeminal pain. Pain 2002;99:567–578.

26. *Ashbury A, Fields H*. Pain due to peripheral nerve damage: an hypothesis. Neurology 1984;34:1587–1590.

27. *Bove G, Light A*. The nervi nervorum. Missing link for neuropathic pain? Pain Forum 1997;6:181–190.

28. *Eliav E, Teich S, Benoliel R, et al*. Large myelinated nerve fiber hypersensitivity in oral malignancy. Oral Surg Oral Med Oral Pathol 2002;94:45–50.

29. *Eliav E, Gracely R*. Sensory changes in the territory of the lingual and inferior alveolar nerves following lower third molar extraction. Pain 1998;77:191–199.

30. *Sang C, Max M, Gracely R*. Stability and reliability of detection thresholds for human A-beta and A-delta sensory afferents determined by cutaneous electrical stimulation. J Pain Sympt Manage 2003;25:64–73.

31. *Chien A, Eliav E, Sterling M*. Hypoaesthesia occurs with sensory hypersensitivity in chronic whiplash: indication of a minor peripheral neuropathy? Man Ther 2008; In press.

32. *Barbe M, Barr A*. Inflammation and the pathophysiology of work-related musculoskeletal disorders. Brain Behav Immun 2006;20:423–429.

33. *Benoloiel R, Biron A, Quek S, et al*. Trigeminal neurosensory changes following acute and chronic paranasal sinusitis. Quintessence Int 2006;37:437–443.

34. *Greening J, Lynn B*. Vibration sense in the upper limb in patients with repetitive strain injury and a group of at-risk office workers. Int Arch Occup Environ Health 1998;71:29–34.

35. *Tucker A, White P, Kosek E, et al*. Comparison of vibration perception thresholds in individuals with

diffuse upper limb pain and carpal tunnel syndrome. Pain 2007;127:263–269.

36. *Greening J, Smart S, Leary R, et al.* Reduced movement of the median nerve in carpal tunnel during wrist flexion in patients with non-specific arm pain. Lancet 1999;354:217–218.

37. *Greening J, Lynn B, Leary R, et al.* The use of ultrasound imaging to demonstrate reduced movement of the median nerve during wrist flexion in patients with non-specific arm pain. J Hand Surg 2001;26:401–406.

38. *Greening J, Lynn B, Leary R.* Sensory and autonomic function in the hands of patients with non-specific arm pain (NSAP) and asymptomatic office workers. Pain 2003;104:275–281.

39. *Helme R, LeVasseur S, Gibson S.* RSI revisited: evidence for psychological and physiological differences from age, sex and occupation matched control group. Aust NZ J Med 1992;22:23–29.

40. *Sharma S, Smith E, Hazlman B, et al.* Thermographic change in keyboard operators with chronic forearm pain. Br Med J 1997;314:118.

41. *Jonsson H, Bring G, Rauschning W, et al.* Hidden cervical spine injuries in traffic accident victims with skull fractures. J Spinal Disord 1991;4:251–263.

42. *Taylor J, Taylor M.* Cervical spinal injuries: an autopsy study of 109 blunt injuries. J Musculoskel Pain 1996;4:61–79.

43. *Bogduk N.* Point of view. Spine 2002;27:1940–1941.

44. *Peng B, Wu W, Li Z, et al.* Chemical radiculitis. Pain 2007;127:214–220.

45. *Huang J, Zager E.* Thoracic outlet syndrome. Neurosurgery 2004;55:897–902.

46. *Gillard J, Perez-Cousin M, Hachulla E, et al.* Diagnosing thoracic outlet syndrome: contribution of provocative tests, ultrasonography, electrophysiology and helical computed tomography in 48 patients. J Bone Spine 2001;68:416–424.

47. *Elvey R.* Physical evaluation of the peripheral nervous system in disorders of pain and dysfunction. J Hand Ther 1997;10:122–129.

48. *Rasmussen P, Sindrup S, Jensen T, et al.* Symptoms and signs in patients with suspected neuropathic pain. Pain 2004;110:461–469.

49. *Bouhissera D, Attal N.* Novel strategies for neuropathic pain. In: Villannueva L, Dickensen A, Ollat H (eds) The Pain System in Normal and Pathological States. Seattle: IASP Press, 2004; 290–310.

50. *Bennett M, Attal N, Backonja M, et al.* Using screening tools to identify neuropathic pain. Pain 2007;127:199–203.

51. *Sterling M, Pedler A.* A Neuropathic component is common in acute whiplash and associated with a more complex clinical presentation. (submitted for publication).

52. *Elvey RL.* Brachial plexus tension test and the pathoanatomical origin of arm pain. In: Glasgow E, Twomey L (eds) Aspects of Manipulative Therapy. Lincoln: Institute of Health Sciences, 1979:105–110.

53. *Butler D.* Mobilisation of the Nervous System. Melbourne: Churchill Livingstone, 1991.

54. *Shacklock M.* Improving application of neurodynamic (neural tension) testing and treatments: a message to researchers and clinicians. Man Ther 2005;10:175–179.

55. *Di Fabio R.* Neural mobilization: the impossible. J Orthop Sports Phys Ther 2001;31:224–225.

56. *Wainner R, Fritz J, Irrgang J, et al.* Reliability and diagnostic accuracy of the clinical examination and patient self report measures for cervical radiculopathy. Spine 2003;28:52–62.

57. *Jepsen J, Laursen L, Hagert C, et al.* Diagnostic accuracy of the neurological upper limb examination 1: inter-rate reproducibility of selected findings and patterns. BMC Neurol 2006;6:1–11.

58. *Jepsen J, Thomsen G.* A cross-sectional study of the relation between symptoms and physical findings in computer operators. BMC Neurol 2006;6:1–12.

59. *Karjalainen K, Malmivaara A, van Tulder M, et al.* Multidisciplinary biopsychosocial rehabilitation for neck and shoulder pain among working adults. Spine 2001;26:174–181.

60. *Coppieters M, Stappaerts K, Wouters L, et al.* Aberrant protective force generation during neural provocation testing and the effect of treatment in patients with neurogenic cervicobrachial pain. J Manipul Physiol Ther 2003;26:99–106.

61. *Song X-J, Gan Q, Cao J-L, et al.* Spinal manipulation reduces pain and hyperalgesia after lumbar intervertebral foramen inflammation in the rat. J Manipul Physiol Ther 2006;29:5–13.

62. *Attal N, Bouhissera D.* Can pain be more or less neuropathic? Pain 2004;110:510–511.

63. *Niv D, Devor M.* Refractory neuropathic pain: the nature and extent of the problem. Pain Pract 2006;6:3–9.

# 11

# Clinical Assessment: The Patient Interview and History

## Introduction

Multiple factors are considered in the examination of the neck pain patient, including physical, psychological, psychosocial, occupational, and activity-related features. The expected outcomes of the clinical assessment are a thorough understanding of patients, of the impact that the disorder is having on their working and social life as well as their general well-being. Importantly for the clinician, the examination should reveal the psychophysical processes underlying the patient's neck disorder and prognostic indicators. Such information provides the basis for the development of a management program.

It is increasingly recognized that there is a need for alternative systems of diagnosis and classification of neck pain as a definitive pathoanatomical diagnosis is not possible in the majority of neck pain patients. As illustrated in previous chapters, research is being directed towards understanding the pathophysiology of neck pain, its associated symptoms, as well as the presence and effects of any psychological features. The direction is towards developing a "processes or mechanisms"-based diagnosis that has the potential to direct specific multimodal interventions, which may include multiprofessional strategies to enhance the patient's function and quality of life. This approach fits well with the clinical reasoning model used by physiotherapists and other musculoskeletal clinicians in their clinical examination and management of the neck pain patient.

The elements and processes of clinical reasoning for musculoskeletal therapists have been well described in the text by Jones and Rivett[1] and readers are referred to this work. This chapter will present an overview of the patient interview and history of the disorder and the following chapter will present a more detailed description of the physical examination. Collectively these two chapters provide a scheme for the clinical examination with examples to assist the clinical reasoning process in the evaluation of the patient presenting with neck pain as a basis for diagnosis, management planning, and delivery.

As an introduction to the examination, two important factors will be discussed, the first relating to recognition of "red flags" and the second to the use of questionnaires in the assessment process.

## "Red flags"

The clinical examination must serve to identify any potential "red flags" that may indicate either serious underlying musculoskeletal pathology such as fractures or nonmusculoskeletal pathologies. In essence, the clinician listens for a history, presenting features, and behaviors of symptoms which are consistent with a "mechanical" musculoskeletal disorder. Fortunately the occurrence of more serious conditions such as tumors[2] is not common in patients presenting primarily with posterior neck pain without other neurological or systemic symptoms.[3] Nevertheless, the presentation of vascular disorders such as aneurysms of the vertebral or carotid arteries may be that of acute neck pain, often in association with acute-onset headache.[4–6] When the clinician has any indication or suspicion of serious underlying pathology, immediate referral for medical investigation is necessary.

The clinician is always aware and respectful of patients presenting with neck pain who also have inflammatory arthropathies such as rheumatoid arthritis

or ankylosing spondylitis. Neck pain presents in either condition.[7,8] Upper cervical involvement is not uncommon in rheumatoid arthritis and may result in atlantoaxial subluxation and impaction.[8,9] Vertebral and ligament anomalies of the upper cervical spine are well documented in congenital conditions such as Down's, Morquio, or Grisel syndromes.[10–12] Such conditions would contraindicate manipulative therapy procedures but do not necessarily mitigate against other physical therapy care. Nevertheless, any treatment must proceed with due care and safety.

## Questionnaires: outcomes and diagnostic indicators

Validated questionnaires or scales should be used to assist both the diagnostic and the outcome evaluation process. In the first instance they can provide some quantification of the impact of pain and disability and any other symptoms such as dizziness or unsteadiness on the patient's activity and lifestyle. They can assist in the recognition of neuropathic pain states as well as any psychological features that may be present. Such quantification of the condition at the initial assessment can provide the baselines on which treatment effects can be monitored and evaluated. A representative sample of the types of questionnaires that might be used in assessment of a patient presenting with a neck disorder is presented in Table 11.1. Indications for their use are suggested and the clinician can choose those most relevant to the individual patient. Importantly, their use provides the clinician with information about the disorder from the patient's perspective and provides a comparison between the patient's self-assessed pain and disability level and the clinician's own interpretation of this level.

A formal measure of the patient's self-reported pain and disability should be a routine part of the initial assessment. This may be any one of the many structured questionnaires designed for neck disorders as relevant to the presentation of the particular patient (Table 11.1). The patient should complete any structured questionnaire independently, ideally before or if necessary after the initial assessment. Interestingly, linear relationships are emerging between self-reported pain and disability levels and the magnitude of impairment in the motor, sensory, and psychological systems in neck pain patients, which reinforces their value in the overall clinical assessment.[13, 14] As indicated, the use of such structured questionnaires provides suitable outcome measures. Research has been conducted to determine what is the change required to be clinically important. This varies between questionnaires, depending on their construct. For example, at least a 20% change from the baseline score is required when using the Neck Disability Index (NDI),[15–18] a 25% reduction in the baseline score in conjunction with patients reporting that they are at least better is an acceptable clinical outcome on the basis of the Northwick Park Neck Pain Questionnaire,[19] whereas a change score of 36% is required when using the Bournemouth Questionnaire.[20]

As an alternate, or in addition to structured questionnaires, there is some argument for the use of the Patient-Specific Functional Scale (PSFS) in the clinical setting.[21, 22] The formal structured questionnaires consist of set questions about neck pain and function. Some questions may not be relevant to the individual patient and the activity which is most worrisome may not be listed. Nevertheless these questionnaires have the advantage that they give a standard that allows direct comparison between patients or patient groups. The advantage of the PSFS in the clinical setting is that it allows patients to nominate and score their particular individual activities most affected by the neck disorder, rather than scoring the generic questions of the structured questionnaires. Patients nominate three activities which are most affected by their disorder and rate their ability on a 0–10 scale, where 0 is unable to perform the activity and 10 is fully able to perform the activity. The mean of the three activity scores should change by a factor of two for a clinically relevant change. The

**Table 11.1** A sample of scales and questionnaires for neck pain disorders

| Indication | Tools |
| --- | --- |
| Rating of pain intensity | Numerical pain rating scale[33] |
| Self-rating of pain and disability | Patient-Specific Functional Scale (PSFS)[22] |
| | Neck Disability Index (NDI)[41] |
| | Northwick Park Neck Pain Questionnaire[42] |
| | Whiplash Disability Questionnaire[43] |
| | Bournemouth Questionnaire[44] |
| Rating of overall improvement | Global rating of change scale[45] |
| Investigation of a neuropathic pain state | Self-report version of the Leeds Assessment of Neuropathic Symptoms and Signs (S-LANSS) questionnaire[23] |
| The presence of dizziness or unsteadiness | Dizziness Handicap Inventory[37] |
| The presence of general distress | General Health Questionnaire-28 (GHQ 28)[39] |
| | Short Form-36 (SF-36)[46] |
| The presence of posttraumatic stress symptoms | Impact of Events Scale (IES)[40] |
| Fear avoidance behaviors | Tampa Scale of Kinesophobia (TSK)[47] |

PSFS has been shown to have better reliability, construct validity, and responsiveness than the NDI at least in patients with cervical radiculopathy.[15]

Other questionnaires may be applied at the completion of the patient interview to help the clinician understand and clarify processes underlying or associated with the patient's neck pain disorder. These could include the relevant application of a neuropathic pain questionnaire[23] or the selected use of specific psychological questionnaires (Table 11.1) when the patient interview indicates that such features could be contributing to the neck pain state. The various psychological questionnaires provide the clinician with more substantive information about a potential disorder rather than relying on the clinician's subjective opinion. Changes in questionnaire scores can again be monitored in response to treatment or the outcome or score on the questionnaire may provide indications for referral to a health psychologist.

## Communication

From the outset, the value of well-developed communication skills cannot be over-estimated in gaining patients' confidence as well as their active participation in and contribution to their management. During the interview, the clinician aims to recognize patterns or develop hypotheses towards making a provisional diagnosis appreciating physical, psychological, and social/work features of the disorder. This knowledge directs the nature and extent of the physical examination and provides initial indications for management. The clinician develops an understanding of the patient and his or her goals as well as an indication of prognosis of the disorder for subsequent collaborative management plans.

The general nature of the disorder is established in the first instance to provide initial information about the subcategory of the disorder. For example, the patient may be presenting with a primary complaint of headache, a neck disorder following a whiplash injury, neck and arm pain, or isolated neck pain. This knowledge assists the clinician in guiding the patient's narrative of the neck disorder and helps the clinician organize thoughts about the type of information required in the subsequent interview towards generating diagnostic, management, and prognostic hypotheses.

## History of the disorder

The first information required in the history includes the nature of onset and time course of the disorder. This establishes whether the condition is acute, recurrent, or chronic in nature and whether onset was traumatic or insidious. In instances of trauma such as a motor vehicle crash, sporting or work injury, details of the injury and immediate management are sought as well as initial symptoms and their progress since that time. For example, initial high levels of pain and disability reported by a patient following a whiplash injury should alert the clinician as it is one of a collection of features that may predict a poorer prognosis.[24–26] In cases of insidious-onset neck pain, the patient is asked to provide information about factors that provoked the initial onset and any subsequent bouts of pain. This may provide information towards introducing appropriate preventive strategies in, for example, workplace design or work practices. Knowledge of the disorder over time determines whether or not the disorder is progressing, unchanging, or regressing. This may provide insight into possible perpetual aggravating factors, specific pathophysiological processes, or progressive pathology and may have prognostic relevance.

In cases of headache, the onset and temporal pattern over time can be valuable in characterizing the headache type.[27] For instance, a headache which is recurrent and episodic in nature with painfree intervals between headache attacks is initially suggestive of migraine. Persistent headache originally precipitated by a whiplash injury could suggest a cervicogenic headache. However, it is pertinent to remember that Radanov et al.[28] found an incidence of only 18% for cervicogenic headache in 112 patients with chronic headache following a whiplash injury (Chapter 9). This latter example highlights the importance of not relying on any one feature but rather establishing a pattern of symptoms and signs in formulating diagnostic hypotheses.

Information regarding the type and effects of any previous treatments for the condition might provide directions for management. Additionally, it may dismiss a focus on certain treatment modalities, due to their past lack of any substantive beneficial effect in the long term. This might be powerful information which can be used later in the patient education process. For instance, if the patient has been largely a passive recipient of previous treatment, it may help emphasize the need for active participation and perhaps modification of work or lifestyle practices for more long-term relief. It may also underpin education on the need for exercise to improve movement and muscle control with the aim of preventing recurrent episodes of pain.

## Presenting symptoms

### Pain and other sensory symptoms

In the clinical reasoning process, the clinician strives to understand the underlying processes involved in the patient's pain and any sensory symptoms, as well as the regional and possibly segmental structural source of pain. Nevertheless it will take several pieces of information synthesized from the interview and physical examination to make an informed decision.

The description of the nature, quality, and intensity of local neck and any referred pain should be carefully sought and the distribution mapped on a body chart. Any other symptoms such as paresthesia, anesthesia, hyperesthesia, hyperalgesia, or allodynia, and other sensations such as feelings of arm heaviness, burning, cold, or metallic tastes should also be recorded. For a complete picture of symptoms from the outset, it is pertinent to check at this point for the presence of other symptoms such as dizziness, light-headedness, unsteadiness, nausea, or visual disturbances. Suggestion of this broader scope of symptoms often encourages description of other symptoms which the patient may not have thought relevant to report.

Studies have been undertaken to map areas of local and referred pain from the cervical disks, zygapophyseal joints, and cervical nerve roots.[29-32] Reasonably regular distributions of pain locally in the neck and referred pain to the head, trapezius, upper thoracic, thoracoscapular region, or arm have been recorded from stimulating the respective cervical segments and structures. Knowledge of the pain distributions can assist decision making for a possible segmental source of symptoms. Nevertheless, there is overlap in pain areas from different segments and sources, which needs to be considered in interpretation. It is difficult to imply a certain structural source from pain mapping alone. Whilst the presence of referred pain infers involvement of central pain-processing mechanisms (Chapter 2), some patients seem to develop a greater state of central hyperexcitability, probably involving a loss of descending inhibitory control (Chapter 2). These patients report more widespread pain over greater regions of the neck, shoulder girdle, chest, and upper limbs. The presence of augmented central pain-processing mechanisms in the patient's neck pain syndrome may be further explored by testing the sensory responses to light touch and mechanical and thermal stimuli in the physical examination.

A description of the intensity, nature, and quality of pain and other sensations is attained. A numerical pain-rating scale can be used for self-rating of pain intensity.[33] Pain referred into the arm or head calls for differentiation of a somatic or possibly neuropathic source. As previously discussed, this may not be as straightforward a process as previously thought as there can be overlap in symptoms reported from the two sources (Chapter 10). Somatic referred pain is traditionally described as a deep, diffuse ache while radicular pain is characterized more as a sharp, burning, shooting, or lancinating pain. However these are only basic guides as, for instance, descriptors such as burning and shooting have been recorded in cases of pain of a somatic origin.[34] A combination of pain descriptors (burning, electric shocks, cold pain) together with the presence of other sensory symptoms such as paresthesia or anesthesia, tingling, and itching have been shown to differentiate better neuropathic from somatic pain.[35]

A neuropathic pain diagnostic questionnaire may assist the clinician in decision making (Table 11.1)[23]; however their usefulness in musculoskeletal pain conditions such as neck pain is not yet well understood. Initial interpretations of pain processes from the descriptions of pain and other sensory symptoms direct the clinician to further tests of the nervous system in the physical examination to help to clarify the likely somatic or peripheral nerve tissue source of pain. These include a clinical neurological examination and tests of nerve tissue mechanosensitivity. They also alert the clinician to the need to restrict the physical examination to essential tests to avoid provocation of any pain.

In cases of headache, descriptions of the quality of pain contribute to headache classification criteria (Chapter 9). Cervicogenic headache is usually of an aching quality, which is commonly of moderate intensity. It can be severe if the headache pathogenesis is neuropathic in nature.[36] In contrast a description such as a headache attack of throbbing or pulsating pain, building to a severe intensity, is suggestive of migraine. The pain of tension-type headache is characterized by the description of a band-like headache of pressing or tightening quality of a mild to moderate intensity.

## Associated symptoms

Reports of symptoms such as dizziness, light-headedness, or unsteadiness require differentiation between cervicogenic, vestibular, vertebral artery, or possibly psychogenic causes such as anxiety in the physical examination. A clear description of symptoms, their relationship or not to neck pain and movement, as well as other provocative and easing factors can assist the clinical reasoning process, but are not always definitive (see Table 6.1 for the characteristics of symptoms from the different sources). Such symptoms direct the clinician to formal tests of sensorimotor control (joint position sense, oculomotor control, and balance), the vertebral artery, and possibly the vestibular system in the physical examination to try to identify their source. Completion of the short-form Dizziness Handicap Inventory questionnaire[37] will provide some quantification of the impact of dizziness on the patient's life and serves as a suitable outcome measure (Table 11.1).

The patient may report other symptoms such as visual disturbances and difficulty with reading or driving. This may be a symptom of disordered cervical afferent input (Chapter 6) and directs the physical examination to both the upper cervical musculoskeletal structures as well as to tests of oculomotor control and balance.

# Behavior of symptoms

Careful questioning about how the symptoms behave in response to movement, postures, and loading in functional activities throughout the day serves several purposes. At a basic level, symptoms provoked by mechanical loads and eased by certain postures or positions give confidence that the condition is likely to be a mechanical musculoskeletal disorder. At a deeper level, the clinician needs to analyze provocative activities and postures and establish if and how much the patient is exposing the neck to these provocateurs in daily activities. Patients may initially have difficulty identifying specific provoking activities and it may be helpful to set them the task of identifying aggravating factors in their daily life so that they can help develop neck care strategies. It is as important to explore with the patient activities, movements, and postures that are not provocative or are used to ease symptoms. This type of information can be used in designing treatment strategies and in advice to patients about self-management strategies in daily function to lessen adverse stresses on the cervical region.

The symptomatic response to provocative activities may also add information to help understand pain processes. An uncomplicated peripheral nociceptive mechanism may be suspected when neck pain is precipitated by a certain movement or posture and is relieved when the provocative stress is removed. At the other extreme, when higher levels of lasting pain are precipitated by trivial movements or activities, hypotheses about the presence of augmented pain processing in the central nervous system in the patient's pain syndrome or a neuropathic pain state may be strengthened. This is not uncommonly encountered in the more severe acute whiplash injury, in those with chronic whiplash-associated disorders with at least moderate persistent symptoms, as well as those with any neuropathic pain state. It cannot be overstressed that in the presence of abnormal pain processing or sensitization of the central nervous system, the physical examination and management must not be provocative of symptoms.

The clinician requires a good understanding of the patient's occupation and recreational or sporting pursuits. It is mandatory to have a full awareness of the relationship between these pursuits and the neck disorder and an appreciation of how the neck disorder is affecting work and activity and the impact of their disorder on these pursuits and quality of life. Workplace ergonomic analysis may be required.

The clinician must listen to and observe how patients describes symptoms, their reactions to pain, and any way in which they might have limited activities and work. It may give the clinician some insight into the presence of any psychological health features such as depression, anxiety, general distress, fear avoidance behaviors, poor coping strategies, or, in the case of a whiplash injury, symptoms of posttraumatic stress. As previously discussed (Chapter 7), many of these psychological reactions may be normal responses to an acute or chronic pain state. As shown in our studies of the whiplash-injured patient, many features resolve as the neck pain decreases and the disorder improves, at least in those with lesser pain and disability.[38] In whiplash, it has been shown, however, that moderate levels of posttraumatic stress symptoms in conjunction with higher levels of pain and other sensory and motor features are predictors of poor outcome. Symptoms of posttraumatic stress did not resolve spontaneously in those with persistent moderate to severe symptoms.[25, 26] The clinician should be alert to such symptoms that may include intrusive thoughts and/or images of the event (motor vehicle crash); avoidance behaviours associated with the event, such as driving avoidance or avoidance via substance abuse; and intense arousal such as panic attacks, hypervigilance, and sleep disturbance. Any psychological health features should be appreciated by the clinician as they may modify the examination and treatment approach. Questionnaires such as the General Health Questionnaire-28 (GH-28),[39] the Impact of Events Scale,[40] or other relevant questionnaires may be useful to help identify psychological features of concern (Table 11.1).

## General medical features

The clinician needs to understand the patient's neck disorder in the context of the patient's general health, the presence of any other comorbidities, or past history of illnesses in order to manage the patient safely. The results of X-rays or any other tests should be viewed. It is essential to document any medications that the patient is taking for this or any other medical disorder and responses to the medications.

## Clinical reasoning at the conclusion of the patient interview

At the conclusion of the patient interview, the clinician should be in possession of two or three hypotheses on the nature of the disorder and impact on the patient's functional status. These can shape and direct the physical examination and help prioritize testing as well as inform on appropriate interventions. They can also direct the clinician to caution in the physical examination as required by the pain state.

## References

1. *Jones M, Rivett D*. Clinical Reasoning for Manual Therapists. Edinburgh: Butterworth-Heinemann, 2004.

2. *Zimmermann M, Wolff R, Raabe A, et al*. Palliative occipito-cervical stabilization in patients with malignant tumors of the occipito-cervical junction and the upper cervical spine. Acta Neurochir 2002;144:783–790.

3. *Bogduk N*. Regional musculoskeletal pain. The neck. Baillières Best Practice & Research Clinical Rheumatology 1999;13:261–285.

4. *Lee V, Brown Jr RB, Mandrekar J, et al*. Incidence and outcome of cervical artery dissection: a population-based study. Neurol 2006;67:1809–1812.

5. *Silbert P, Makri B, Schievink W*. Headache and neck pain in spontaneous internal carotid and vertebral artery dissections. Neurol 1995;45:1517–1522.

6. *Sturzenegger M*. Headache and neck pain: the warning symptoms of vertebral artery dissection. Headache 1994;34:187–193.

7. *Holden W, Taylor S, Stevens H, et al*. Neck pain is a major clinical problem in ankylosing spondylitis, and impacts on driving and safety. Scand J Rheumatol 2005;34:159–160.

8. *Kim D, Hilibrand A*. Rheumatoid arthritis in the cervical spine. J Am Acad Orthop Surg 2005;13:463–474.

9. *Neva M, Kotaniemi A, Kaarela K, et al*. Atlantoaxial disorders in rheumatoid arthritis associated with the destruction of peripheral and shoulder joints, and decreased bone mineral density. Clin Exp Rheumatol 2003;21:179–184.

10. *Cornejo VF, Martinez-Lage J, Piqueras C, et al*. Inflammatory atlanto-axial subluxation (Grisel's syndrome) in children: clinical diagnosis and management. Childs Nerv Syst 2003;19:342–347.

11. *Frost M, Huffer W, Sze C, et al*. Cervical spine abnormalities in Down Syndrome. Clin Neuropathol 1999;18:250–259.

12. *Hughes D, Chadderton R, Cowie R, et al*. MRI of the brain and craniocervical junction in Morquio's disease. Neuroradiol 1997;39:381–385.

13. *Johnston V, Jull G, Souvlis T, et al*. Neck movement and muscle activity characteristics in office workers with neck pain. 2007 submitted for publication.

14. *Sterling M, Jull G, Vicenzino B, et al*. Characterisation of acute whiplash associated disorders. Spine 2004;29:182–188.

15. *Cleland J, Fritz J, Whitman J, et al*. The reliability and construct validity of the Neck Disability Index and patient specific functional scale in patients with cervical radiculopathy. Spine 2006;31:598–602.

16. *Peolsson A*. Investigation of clinically important benefit of anterior cervical decompression and fusion. Eur Spine J 2007;16:507–514.

17. *Stratford PW, Riddle DL, Blinkley JM, et al.* Using the Neck Disability Index to make decisions concerning individual patients. Physiother Can 1999;51:107–112.

18. *Vernon H*. The Neck Disability Index: Patient assessment and outcome monitoring in whiplash. J Musculoskel Pain 1996;4:95–104.

19. *Sim J, Jordan K, Lewis M, et al.* Sensitivity to change and internal consistency of the Northwick Park Neck Pain Questionnaire and derivation of a minimal clinically important difference. Clin J Pain 2006;22:820–826.

20. *Bolton J*. Sensitivity and specificity of outcome measures in patients with neck pain: detecting clinically significant improvement. Spine 2004;29:2410–2417.

21. *Stratford P, Gill C, Westaway M, et al.* Assessing disability and change in individual patients: a report of a patient specific measure. Physiother Can 1995;47:258–63.

22. *Westaway MD, Stratford PW, Blinkley JM*. The patient-specific functional scale: validation of its use in persons with neck dysfunction. J Orthop Sports Phys Ther 1998;27:331–338.

23. *Bennett M, Smith B, Torrance N, et al.* The S-LANSS score for identifying pain of predominantly neuropathic origin: validation for use in clinical and postal research. J Pain 2005;6: 149–158.

24. *Scholten-Peeters G, Verhagen A, Bekkering G, et al.* Prognostic factors of whiplash-associated disorders: a systematic review of prospective cohort studies. Pain 2003;104:303–322.

25. *Sterling M, Jull G, Vicenzino B, et al.* Physical and psychological predictors of outcome following whiplash injury. Pain 2005;114:141–148.

26. *Sterling M, Jull G, Kenardy J*. Physical and psychological factors maintain long term predictive capacity following whiplash injury. Pain 2006;122:102–108.

27. *Lance JW*. Mechanism and Management of Headache. 6th ed. Oxford: Butterworths-Heinemann Ltd, 1998.

28. *Radanov B, Di-Stefano G, Augustiny K*. Symptomatic approach to posttraumatic headache and its possible implications for treatment. Eur Spine J 2001;10:403–407.

29. *Dwyer A, Aprill C, Bogduk N*. Cervical zygapophyseal joint pain patterns: a study in normal volunteers. Spine 1990;15:453–457.

30. *Fukui S, Ohseto K, Shiotani M, et al.* Referred pain distribution of the cervical zygapophyseal joints and cervical dorsal rami. Pain 1996;68:79–83.

31. *Slipman C, Plastaras C, Patel R, et al.* Provocative cervical discography symptom mapping. Spine J 2005;5:381–388.

32. *Tanaka Y, Kokubun S, Sato T, Ozawa H*. Cervical roots as origin of pain in the neck or scapular regions. Spine 2006;31:E568–573.

33. *Jensen M, Karoly P, Braver S*. The measurement of clinical pain intensity: a comparison of six methods. Pain 1986;27:117–126.

34. *Rasmussen P, Sindrup S, Jensen T, et al.* Symptoms and signs in patients with suspected neuropathic pain. Pain 2004;110:461–469.

35. *Bouhassira D, Attal N, Fermanian J, et al.* Development and validation of the Neuropathic Pain Symptom Inventory. Pain 2004;108: 248–257.

36. *Poletti C, Sweet W*. Entrapment of the C2 root and ganglion by the atlanto-epistrophic ligament: clinical syndrome and surgical anatomy. Neurosurg 1990;27:288–291.

37. *Tesio L, Alpini D, Cesarani A, et al.* Short form of the Dizziness Handicap Inventory. Am J Phys Medical Rehabil 1999;78:233–241.

38. *Sterling M, Kenardy J, Jull G, et al.* The development of psychological changes following whiplash injury. Pain 2003;106:481–489.

39. *Goldberg D*. Manual of the General Health Questionnaire. Windsor: NFER-Nelson, 1978.

40. *Horowitz M, Wilner N, Alvarez W*. Impact of Event Scale: a measure of subjective stress. Psychosom Med 1979;41:209–218.

41. *Vernon H, Silvano M*. The Neck Disability Index: A study of reliability and validity. J Manipulative Physiol Ther 1991;14:409–415.

42. *Leak AM, Cooper J, Dyer S, et al.* The Northwick Park Neck Pain Questionnaire, devised to measure neck pain and disability. Br J Rheumatol 1994;33:469–474.

43. *Willis C, Niere K, Hoving J, et al.* Reproducibility and responsiveness of the Whiplash Disability Questionnaire. Pain 2004;110: 681–688.

44. *Bolton J, Humphreys B*. The Bournemouth Questionnaire: a short-form comprehensive outcome measure. II. Psychometric properties in neck pain patients. J Manipulative Physiol Ther 2002;25:141–148.

45. *Jaeschke R, Singer J, Guyatt G*. Measurement of health status. Ascertaining the minimal clinically important difference. Control Clin Trials 1989;10:407–415.

46. *Ware J, Snow K, Kosinski M, et al.* SF-36 Health Survey: manual and interpretation guide. Boston, MA: The Health Institute, 1993.

47. *Kori S, Miller R, Todd D*. Kinesphobia: a new view of chronic pain behaviour. Pain Manag 1990: Jan/Feb 35–43.

# 12

# Clinical Assessment: Physical Examination of the Cervical Region

## Introduction

The physical examination is a continual process of evaluation, intervention, re-evaluation, and reflection.[1] Four outcomes are sought from the physical examination. First is a physical diagnosis gained from the impairments presenting in the cervical articular and muscle systems, abnormal sensory features and disturbances in sensorimotor control, and their relationship to the patient's symptoms and functional impairment. Second is an understanding of how postures, movement, and activity impact on the patient's neck disorder in terms of both aggravating and relieving sensory symptoms. Third is a practical understanding of how work practices and the work environment, sport, and/or activities of daily living could be contributing to the disorder. Fourth is the attainment of outcome measures on which to evaluate and progress treatment. Such knowledge guides the selection of relevant interventions within a multimodal management approach and facilitates understanding of relationships between physical impairments, the pain syndrome, and function.

Potentially, the physical examination may produce a mass of information. Practically, two guidelines are helpful in the clinical reasoning process. The first is the relevance of an examination finding. Many differences from the so-called ideal can be observed in a neck pain patient. There is marked variability in any physical measure even in an asymptomatic population. A certain clinical observation may lie within the normal range and thus might have no real relevance. The clinician must recognize both relevant and potentially irrelevant findings. The second, which may help with decision making of the relevance of a finding, is to "make the pattern fit" between the symptomatic complaint and the physical findings. As a simple example, joint pathology and pain in any region of the body are always associated with reactions in the muscle system. Thus a basic expectation in order to diagnose a cervical musculoskeletal disorder is a pattern of at least movement and muscle dysfunction. Similarly, the presence of nerve tissue mechanosensitivity is confirmed when there is a pattern of antalgic postures, related cervical movement restriction, positive responses to a nerve tissue provocation test, and mechanical allodynia to palpation of specific nerve trunks (Chapter 10). Confidence in making the physical diagnosis increases when "the pattern fits." There is no certainty that a sign in isolation is relevant. Rationales for treatment directions also become stronger when the pattern of symptoms and impairments fit. One word of caution, in the enthusiasm to "make the pattern fit," is potential errors in clinical reasoning, such as confirmation bias or considering too few hypotheses.

Another clinical pointer is to try to demonstrate to the patient the link between symptoms, functional behavior, and a specific impairment. This can be a powerful tool in helping the patient understand both the condition and the rationale for treatment as well as the need for patient commitment to address the features that may be contributing to the neck pain. In the examination approach, re-evaluating a painful test movement and showing a positive change in response to a changed postural position or exercise intervention is a powerful educative tool.

Table 12.1 presents a pro forma for a physical examination of a patient presenting with neck pain. It is presented in a sequence that is used in the clinical setting, rather than a separate examination protocol for each system. We have chosen this method of presentation to highlight the clinical reasoning process in understanding the relationship of impairments within and between systems and their influence on symptoms and function. The protocol is guided by patient positioning, which also facilitates an efficient examination. The clinical reasoning process that began during the patient interview is continued into the physical examination and directs the nature and extent of the assessment. Many physical tests have been described for the cervical region. Not all tests are required for all patients. Rather, the tests are the clinician's tools to be applied when and as required in the problem-solving process of the physical examination. The examination should be regarded as a flexible and progressive process guided by the patient's pain and response to treatment. Probably the greatest challenge to clinicians is not so much to know when to expand the physical examination but when to curtail it. This is particularly important in the acute or moderate to severe pain states. As a general rule, there has been an error in judgment if a patient's neck symptoms are exacerbated by the examination or any treatment provided.

# The examination in standing

## Assessment of static posture

Assessment of static posture conventionally includes the evaluation and classification of the position of the pelvis, the shape of the postural curves, the position of the head and shoulder girdles, as well as inspection of muscle shape. There is considerable variation in static postures between individuals. The challenge is to determine the relevance of a patient's posture to the presenting signs and symptoms. In the nonacute situation, there is not strong evidence for an association

**Table 12.1** Schema of physical examination of the cervical region

| Position | Assessment | Factors assessed |
|---|---|---|
| Standing | Postural assessment | • Shape of spinal postural curves and head position |
| | | • Muscle form and resting scapular position |
| Sitting | Dynamic postural analysis | • Ability to assume an upright neutral postural position |
| | | • Dynamic analysis of scapular muscle control in posture and movement |
| | Analysis of cervical motion | • Range, pain, pattern of control of movement |
| | Vertebrobasilar insufficiency tests | • Tests for the effect on dizziness of sustained rotation and extended head positions |
| Supine | Nervous system | |
| | Neurological examination | • Patients presenting with arm pain and other sensory symptoms, tests of sensation, muscle strength, and reflexes |
| | Nerve tissue provocation tests | • Pain and protective muscle response to an ordered sequence of arm and neck movements |
| | Nerve palpation | • Allodynia of nerves |
| | Sensory tests | • Pressure pain thresholds |
| | | • Thermal pain thresholds (cold and heat) |
| | Manual examination | • Examination of passive physiological intervertebral movements of the cervical and cervicothoracic regions |
| | | • Craniocervical ligament tests |
| Prone | Manual examination | • Examination of passive accessory intervertebral movements of the cervical, cervicothoracic, and thoracic regions |
| | Tests of scapular muscles | • Analysis of pattern of control in holding the scapula on the chest wall |
| | | • Tests of static holding capacity |
| | Retest manual examination | • Determine the effect of reciprocal relaxation on positive "joint signs" |
| Supine | Craniocervical flexion test | • Analysis of ability to perform a staged test of craniocervical flexion |
| | | • Tests of static holding capacity |
| | Retest active extension: range, pain, pattern | • Determine the effect of activation of the deep neck flexors on eccentric and concentric control of cervical extension |
| | Muscle length tests | • Tests of length of cervical and cervicoscapular muscles as indicated |
| Four-point kneeling | Closed chain test of scapular stability – serratus anterior | • Test of strength and holding capacity of the serratus anterior |
| | Test of cervical extensors | • Test pattern of craniocervical and cervicothoracic extension |
| | Test of axial rotators | • Test pattern of craniocervical axial rotation |

*(Continued)*

**Table 12.1** Schema of physical examination of the cervical region — cont'd

| Position | Assessment | Factors assessed |
| --- | --- | --- |
| Sensorimotor control | | • Joint position sense |
| | | • Balance |
| | | • Oculomotor control |
| Muscle strength and endurance | Strength | • Tests of strength of craniocervical flexors and extensors |
| | | • Tests of strength of cervicothoracic flexors and extensors |
| | Endurance | • Tests of endurance of craniocervical and cervicothoracic flexors and extensors at progressive contraction intensities |
| Examination of work tasks | | • Ergonomic assessment of workplace and work tasks |
| | | • Dynamic analysis of posture and muscle control in a sedentary work task |
| | | • Dynamic analysis of posture and muscle control in an active work task |

between neck pain and structural shape. For example, studies are divided and have not produced convincing evidence for a robust association between the static measure of the forward head posture and neck pain or neck pain and headache.[2-6] Thus information gained from an assessment of static posture alone in the clinical setting may have limitations. Recent studies suggest that with sedentary work at a computer, the head subtly drifts into a more forward position and the thoracic curve subtly increases over time in persons with neck pain, but not in those without neck pain (Chapter 4).[7, 8] Altered recruitment patterns of cervical extensor and upper trapezius muscles have been measured in association with these postural changes.[9]

In light of this evidence, we favor a more dynamic analysis of control of posture in the assessment of posture. The analysis may be performed in standing but is more commonly relevant to neck pain patients when performed in sitting. A dynamic assessment of posture permits an initial observation of the patient's muscle control strategies and determines if adequate mobility is present in other spinal regions to achieve a neutral spinal posture. The assessment may be modified to replicate a patient's individual work demands better.

# The examination in sitting

## Dynamic analysis of posture

### Assessment of the upright neutral posture

The patient's unsupported sitting posture is observed to determine if he or she sits with a desired "neutral" pelvic-spinal posture or an undesirable extended or, conversely, slumped/flexed lumbopelvic posture. The lumbopelvic posture is corrected and the patient's ability to replicate and sustain

the upright neutral posture is analyzed. In the common instance of a flexed lumbopelvic posture, an appropriate pattern is observed when the pelvis rolls up into a neutral position, restoring the normal lumbar lordosis (with evident use of the lumbar multifidus), the kyphosis forms in the thoracic region with the scapulae sitting flush on the chest wall, and there is a neutral head-on-neck posture. In contrast, a poor pattern is commonly seen when an upright posture is attained with dominant use of the thoracolumbar extensors. The lordosis is formed in the thoracolumbar or the lower thoracic region and the lumbopelvic region remains in a flexed position (Figure 12.1), which is considered to signify a poor pattern of control in the lumbar region.[10]

The ability to attain a correct neutral spinal posture has a direct impact on cervical muscle function. Studies in our laboratory have confirmed that there is greater activity in both the deep cervical flexor and lumbar multifidus muscles when sitting posture is specifically facilitated with the restoration of the lumbar lordosis compared to an instruction merely to sit up straight.[11] This research points to the need for precision in re-educating the neutral upright pelvic-spinal postural position to achieve optimal postural muscle function. This research also begins to give some insight into the interplay between key trunk muscles for active support of the spine, supporting clinical observations of the interplay between neck and low-back pain.[12]

### Dynamic analysis of scapular muscle control in posture and movement

The position of the scapulae is observed during the assessment of the ability to assume an upright neutral posture. The "ideal" position of the scapulae is such that the superior angles are level with the T2 or T3 spinous process, the spines of the scapulae are level with the T3 or T4 spinous process, and the inferior angles are level with the

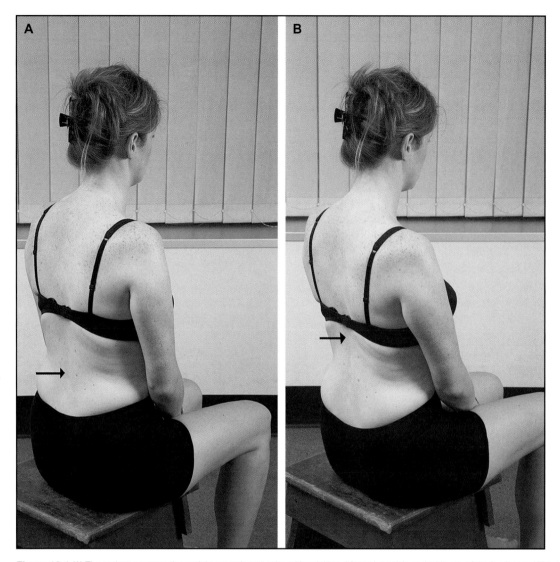

**Figure 12.1** (A) The patient assumes the upright neutral postural position, initiated from the pelvis and with use of the lumbar multifidus, with the formation of natural lumbar lordosis. (B) The thoracolumbar erector spinae are used in the postural correction strategy with formation of a thoracolumbar lordosis. The pelvis and lumbar spine remain in flexion.

T7–9 spinous process.[13] The spine of the scapulae and clavicles should have a slight superolateral orientation and the scapulae should sit flush against the chest wall in both the sagittal and transverse planes. Variations in scapular orientation are common. An inferolateral orientation of the spine of the scapula and clavicle (usually associated with scapular protraction) may indicate poor control of scapular upward rotation. Winging of the medial border may indicate

excessive internal scapular rotation. A prominence of the inferior angle may indicate excessive anterior tilt.

Alterations in scapular orientation and any lack of active scapular stability may become more obvious when the scapulae are loaded. This can be achieved by either the patient performing small arm movements (< 30–40° of motion), ranges at which the orientation of the scapulae should remain relatively stable (Chapter 3), or by having the patient perform isometric contractions of the shoulder against mild resistance. Specific small ranges of shoulder movement or isometric contractions may expose a loss of scapular control in a particular direction due to torque imposed by scapulohumeral muscles. Gently resisted isometric shoulder abduction will expose an inability to maintain an upward rotation orientation of the scapula, resisted flexion, an inability to maintain posterior tilt and resisted external rotation, an inability to rotate the scapula externally. Control of the scapula is also assessed through the full range of upper-limb elevation during which the scapula should progressively upwardly rotate, posteriorly tilt, and externally rotate (Chapter 3).

It is difficult to assign blame to any single muscle as a cause of scapular dysfunction as a complex interaction of muscle actions controls the mobile scapula three-dimensionally at any moment. Nevertheless, impairment of the trapezius and serratus anterior muscles would certainly reduce the capacity of the scapula to rotate upwardly, posteriorly tilt, and externally rotate (Chapter 3). Overactivity or altered resting tone of muscles such as the levator scapulae, rhomboids, and pectoralis minor is also implicated in a downwardly rotated and protracted scapular position. Details of tests of specific muscle performance associated with other alterations in scapular orientation have been well described by Sahrmann[14] and readers are referred to this text.

A dynamic approach is used in the assessment of the relationship between scapular orientation and the patient's symptoms. In the presence of an abnormally oriented scapula, the clinician manually assists the scapula to a neutral position, ensuring that translatory and rotary components are corrected. The patient's ability to maintain this position actively is tested. Patients are then asked to relax and reposition the scapula themselves. The clinician observes the muscle strategy used to achieve this position, which will guide the rehabilitation strategy for correction. The effect of the scapular correction on neck pain is also assessed to determine its immediate relevance to any symptom relief. Patients compare the pain in the manually corrected scapular position to that in their usual position. Some patients will note a decrease in pain in the corrected position; others will not notice a change until the support of the scapula is released. A second strategy is to retest a previously established painful cervical movement to determine if the range and pain response have changed by the scapular repositioning. A third strategy is to palpate the tension and tenderness in axioscapular muscles such as levator scapulae and upper trapezius before and after correction of position. This frequently results in a dramatic decrease in palpable tenderness. These strategies not only confirm the immediate relevancy of the abnormal scapular orientation and muscle control to the neck disorder but also make a convincing link between relief of pain and appropriate muscle control which the clinician may use in patient education and for motivation for exercise and self-help strategies.

An elevated scapular position may also be protective in nature. It is commonly found in association with nerve tissue mechanosensitivity and gives warning that the examination should be undertaken with due care and be nonprovocative in nature. The scapula will be elevated, albeit sometimes slightly, and may coincide with an apparent subtle lateral shift of the mid to lower cervical region towards the side of the mechanosensitivity. In the clinical reasoning process of the physical examination, this protective posture will be associated with four other physical signs to "make the pattern fit" for the diagnosis of nerve tissue mechanosensitivity (Chapter 10).

## Analysis of cervical motion

Examination and measurement of the active range of cervical motion and pain response are fundamental assessment tools. Deficits in cervical range of motion have been shown to distinguish patients with neck disorders from asymptomatic subjects.[2, 15-17] The assessment of active movement provides a quantitative outcome measure of range and a qualitative measure of the pain response as well as control of motion. Several inclinometers are commercially available to measure range of cervical movement, and reliability for these measures has been found to be acceptable.[18]

Active cervical movements test the integrity of articular, muscle, and neural systems as well as patient volition or fear of movement. The tests are a potent tool for determining the relationship between systems. Movement dysfunctions need to be interpreted on a multidimensional basis. Patterns of movement restriction are interpreted on kinematic and mechanical bases (Chapter 3). The pain response to movement can confirm a cervical origin of pain and provide very basic indicators of its likely structural source (for example, articular or nerve tissues). Patterns of movement restriction provide indications for treatment movement directions[19] and the pain response also provides guidance for the intensity of treatment dosage. These aspects are well described in orthopedic and manual therapy texts.[1, 20] To broaden interpretative processes, aspects of muscle control will be highlighted in the description of active movement evaluation.

As a point of technique in examination of active movements, advantage should be taken of the central and reflex connections between the visual system and neck muscles.[21, 22] The patient should be instructed first to look in the direction of the movement as a facilitation procedure.

## Cervical flexion

The patient is instructed to look down to flex the head and neck together. The extensor muscles firstly work eccentrically and then concentrically to return the head to the upright posture. The pattern of return should be initiated from the lower cervical region with the head in a neutral position. Use of excessive craniocervical extension (poked chin) on the return from the flexed position may signal dominance by superficial extensors such as semispinalis capitis with some loss of control of the craniocervical flexor muscles which may not be able to limit the unwanted craniocervical extension action of semispinalis capitis. The semispinalis capitis muscles can be observed as longitudinal ridges on the back of the neck. An apparent hypertonicity of these muscles during control of cervical flexion is commonly noted in neck pain sufferers and may signal a protective response to limit movement into flexion or altered control of the deeper cervical extensor muscles. The prominence of these muscles is often asymmetrical.

In differential assessment of cervical flexion, the lack of preparedness to maintain craniocervical neutral/flexion could be protective of nerve tissue mechanosensitivity. This can be explored further with a discrete examination of craniocervical flexion repeated with and without the sensitizing position of straight-leg raise.

## Cervical extension

The patient is requested to look towards the ceiling and follow the ceiling back with the eyes as far as possible. Cervical extension is often a painful active movement as it compresses the posterior articular structures and narrows the intervertebral foramen. Extension requires eccentric control of the flexor muscles, the weakest of all the cervical muscles. The flexors control the weight of the head into a position behind the frontal plane of the shoulders, before returning the head to the upright position with a concentric contraction. As the cervical spine extends, greater contribution may be expected from the deep cervical flexor muscles due to the reducing moment arms of the large superficial cervical flexors[23] and their inability to control the craniocervical region (Chapter 3). In the presence of poor eccentric control of the deep cervical flexors, two characteristic patterns of movement are evident:

- The patient is unwilling to allow the center of gravity of the head to move posteriorly behind the frontal plane of the shoulders, thus minimizing the effects of gravity. There is a dominant craniocervical spine extension pattern with minimal movement of the head posteriorly (Figure 12.2). This can be mistaken for a good cervical extension effort, particularly when an individual has ample range of upper cervical extension. When the movement is corrected so that the head moves backwards in extension, loss of control is evident and the movement often induces pain.

- The head moves backwards but the flexor muscles cannot control the effects of gravity/head weight. The head reaches a point of extension and then appears to drop or translate backwards, loading the osteoligamentous structures. This is often quite uncomfortable and, when control is poor, patients often wish to return immediately to the upright position, occasionally with the help of their hands. Patients may describe a feeling of loss of

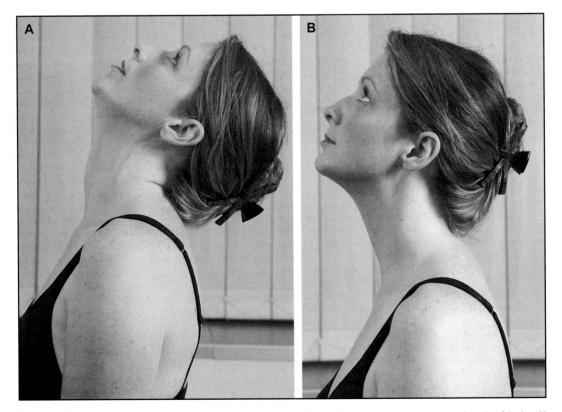

**Figure 12.2** Assessment of cervical extension. (A) A normal pattern of cervical extension in which the center of gravity of the head is moved and controlled posteriorly behind the frontal plane of the shoulders. (B) The patient performs cervical extension with predominantly extension in the craniocervical region to minimize the effects of gravity. This is a common strategy to mask weakness in the deep cervical flexors.

control, such as "my head was going to fall off the back of my shoulders."

The return from a fully extended position to a neutral upright position demands a coordinated concentric contraction of the craniocervical and cervical flexors. The dominant poor pattern is initiation of the movement from extension with the sternocleidomastoid and anterior scalene muscles, resulting in cervical flexion but not craniocervical flexion. In this poor pattern, recovery from the craniocervical extension is last, rather than the leading element of the movement.

## Craniocervical flexion and extension

Flexion and extension of the craniocervical region are assessed separately to the typical cervical region by having the patient perform the head-nodding action through its available range. The patient's ability to perform and control the motion while maintaining the typical cervical region still is assessed.

## Cervical rotation

The patient rotates the head to look over the shoulder and the motion that occurs in the upper and lower regions of the cervical spine is assessed. Patients with restricted upper cervical rotation will appear to carry the head and upper neck around using only the lower cervical spine. Upper cervical rotation can be assessed in some isolation from cervical rotation by testing the movement with the cervical spine in flexion.[24, 25] This has been found to be a sensitive test to determine impairment in patients with cervicogenic headache with joint dysfunction at C1–2.[25, 26]

Individuals with restriction in the lower cervical spine will appear to spin their head on their neck adequately but will fail to complete the rotation. Limited motion of the neck may also result from inadequate motion at the cervicothoracic junction or the upper thoracic spine. Often loss of motion from this region presents as loss of end-of-range cervical motion.

## Cervical lateral flexion

Restriction of motion in lateral flexion may be relatively discrete and reflect a segmental restriction. In contrast, hypertonicity of the scalene muscles may restrict motion en bloc to C2, with motion occurring more in the upper cervical spine. Hypertonicity or shortness of the scalenes may reflect an upper costal breathing pattern or a compensation for reduced support of the deep neck flexors,[27] or be a protective response to mechanosensitive nerve tissue. To fit the pattern of nerve tissue mechanosensitivity, the range of lateral flexion motion and pain response should be altered when lateral flexion is repeated with the arm prepositioned in various components of the brachial plexus provocation test (BPPT). Any suspicion of nerve tissue mechanosensitivity signals the need for caution and lessens any notion to include scalene stretches in a treatment program.

Of interest, lateral flexion appears to be the movement least affected in terms of range in neck disorders of long standing. Several studies have shown that neck extension and rotation range distinguish persons with persistent neck pain, while range of lateral flexion did not differ significantly from control subjects.[15, 17, 28]

## Motion of the cervicothoracic junction and upper thoracic spine

Adequate mobility in the cervicothoracic and thoracic spinal regions is vital for normal range of movement in the cervical spine and shoulder complex.[29, 30] In the sitting position, movement of these regions may be examined during both active movement of the cervical spine and arm movement. Unilateral arm movement induces lateral flexion and axial rotation in the cervicothoracic region[30] and full bilateral arm elevation induces thoracic extension.[29] Often areas of segmental hypomobility in these regions are observed with cervical spine movement and arm elevation. Loss of upper thoracic segmental movement can be confirmed by manually palpating the movement of the thoracic spinous processes during neck movements, with loss of segmental movement providing an indication for treatment.

## Additional tests

The active movement examination can be modified or progressed according to the patient's presentation. Movements can be examined in combination to determine provocative or easing combinations for purposes of technique direction selection.[19] Gentle passive pressure may be applied to the end of range of active movements to determine if active and passive ranges are similar or end ranges provoke pain.[1] Specific tests such as Spurling's compression test or the neck distraction test may be used where indicated in cases of suspected cervical radiculopathy, noting that, although these tests have high sensitivity, they have low to moderate specificity, indicating that, for example, painful cervical joints may be affected by the tests.[31]

### Tests for vertebral artery insufficiency

The symptom of dizziness or light-headedness is not uncommonly reported by persons following a whiplash injury and, to a lesser extent, those with cervicogenic headache. There are many origins to the symptom of dizziness, which could be relevant to a patient presenting with a cervical disorder. The common origins include vestibular, disturbed cervical afferentation (cervical vertigo), and anxicty (Chapter 6). Practitioners of manipulative therapy have a healthy regard for dizziness that could signal the possibility of vertebrobasilar insufficiency (VBI). Although VBI is probably a less likely cause of dizziness in neck pain patients with no other symptoms and signs of ischemia in areas of the brain supplied by the basilar artery (for example, drop attacks, dysarthria, dysphagia, diplopia, visual field defects), responsible caution is always required. Tests of the vertebral artery should be conducted on persons who present with dizziness and in those for whom manipulation is considered in management. The basic tests, which can be performed in sitting or supine lying, include sustaining the cervical movements of particularly rotation and extension, as well as the manipulation position with the aim of symptom provocation. Clinical guidelines have been developed for premanipulative testing of the vertebral artery.[32] There is still debate about the appropriateness of the tests with respect to their sensitivity and specificity for VBI.[33]

## The examination in supine lying

### Examination of the nervous system

The examination of the nervous system adds to information gained from the patient interview towards differentiating the possible origin of a patient's cervicobrachial pain or neck pain and headache. Four categories of tests are used: (1) a clinical neurological examination; (2) nerve tissue provocation tests; (3) palpation of nerve trunks; and (4) quantitative sensory testing. As discussed in Chapter 10, the clinician needs to consider symptomatic features in conjunction with results of the physical examination in the clinical reasoning process towards a diagnosis of nerve tissue dysfunction in a patient's pain syndrome.

### Neurological examination

A clinical neurological examination may be performed as a routine screening procedure in the examination of the neck pain patient.

It is indicated in those patients with referred pain or other sensory symptoms in the upper limb to assist in determining the presence or not of a cervical radiculopathy. The conventional clinical tests are tests of sensation (pinprick, light touch, vibration), muscle strength, and spinal reflexes. These tests are unlikely to detect minor peripheral neuropathies (Chapter 10) but are more likely to be positive in overt cases of impaired peripheral nerve conduction.

Nevertheless one study has shown that the clinician should not rely on the conventional clinical neurological examination alone to diagnose a cervical radiculopathy and that other tests in the clinical setting may contribute to a greater extent to this diagnosis. Wainner et al.[34] tested the diagnostic accuracy of the conventional tests of the clinical neurological examination in conjunction with selected symptom descriptors and behaviors, the Spurling (A and B), Valsalva, shoulder abduction, distraction, and brachial plexus provocation (median and radial nerve bias) tests, and ranges of cervical motion. They found that the conventional tests of the neurological examination in the main had acceptable diagnostic accuracy. However, in investigating which cluster of tests had greatest diagnostic potential, these conventional tests did not feature in the final equation. The strongest cluster was a positive BPPT (median nerve bias), range of cervical rotation less than 60° and positive Spurling (A) and distraction tests, which gave a 90% probability that the patient had a cervical radiculopathy.

## Nerve tissue provocation tests

Indications of the presence of peripheral nerves' sensitivity to movement, which were gained from the patient interview and analysis of posture and cervical movement, are further investigated with formal nerve tissue provocation tests.[35,36] The conventional BPPT, which biases the median nerve, consists of gentle shoulder girdle fixation in a neutral position, followed by shoulder abduction and lateral rotation, elbow extension, forearm supination, and wrist extension. The sequence of test movements may be altered and the test is often performed with wrist extension preceding elbow extension, so that one angle, elbow extension, can be measured in assessment. Cervical contralateral lateral flexion can be added to provoke the brachial plexus and median nerve further. As the test also involves non neural structures, test movements such as cervical lateral flexion or wrist extension, may be added or subtracted to enhance or reduce any pain elicited by the test towards structural differentiation. Furthermore the sequence and directions of test movements can be changed to bias the stress on the ulnar or radial nerves as directed by the patient's presentation.[35]

When stress is placed on the nervous system via nerve tissue provocation tests, protective muscle activity is elicited in both symptomatic and asymptomatic states.[37-40] This muscle guarding must be appreciated and respected during performance of any test. Production and reproduction of pain as well as reduced range of motion of the final test movement component are important criteria. Such elements have been shown to be reliable in test–retest studies in controlled and clinical environments.[41] A classical positive test result of the BPPT is reproduction of the patient's symptoms accompanied by a restriction in range of movement (e.g., elbow extension) on the symptomatic side as compared to the asymptomatic side.

When interest is centered on upper cervical structures, for example in cases of cervicogenic headache, craniocervical flexion is used as the principal movement to induce a cranial movement of neural structures. The dura mater is attached to the foramen magnum and to the body of the C2 vertebra and there are also fibrous connections between the rectus capitis posterior minor and the ligamentum flavum in this region.[42, 43] Thus craniocervical flexion acts as a primary movement to tension neural structures in this region. To differentiate clinically neural from any muscle or articular tissue contributions to a restriction of craniocervical flexion, craniocervical flexion is first performed passively and the range, resistance, and pain response are assessed. The movement is repeated with the nerve tissues pretensioned in each of left and right straight-leg raise and the BPPT positions.[44] A change in resistance with production of neck or head pain warns of neural tissue mechanosensitivity. This test is mandatory prior to conducting the craniocervical flexion muscle test to avoid any exacerbation of symptoms of a neuropathic origin.

While the nerve tissue provocation tests have been shown to have high sensitivity to detect cervical radiculopathy, their specificity is low,[31] indicating that the test may be positive in other conditions. This was well illustrated in our study of chronic whiplash patients[45] where, in general, there was a bilateral decrease in range of elbow extension. It was concluded that this feature represented a generalized hyperalgesic response to the BPPT in this patient group, possibly reflecting central nervous system hyperexcitability (Chapter 10).

Thus clinicians require a cautious approach in use of nerve tissue provocation tests both in their application in the presence of a sensitized peripheral and/or central nervous system as well as in the interpretation of test results. The low specificity of the tests highlights the need for the clinician to consider all elements of the patient's history and physical examination in the clinical reasoning process for diagnostic decision making. In cases where sensitized peripheral and/or central nervous systems are a probable feature, treatment approaches should be nonprovocative in nature.

## Nerve palpation

A further component of the assessment of nerve tissues is palpation of the trunks of the brachial plexus and peripheral nerves. These include the median, ulnar, and radial nerves in cases of cervicobrachial pain and the C2 root and greater and lesser occipital nerves in cases of cervicogenic headache. In the presence of sensitized peripheral nerve tissue, the nerves are tender or painful to gentle palpation; that is, they exhibit mechanical allodynia. Such findings reinforce the necessity for the physical examination and physical treatments to be undertaken with care so as not to provoke the patient's symptoms further.

## Sensory tests

Recent research has identified sensory disturbances that may be associated with neck pain of insidious and notably traumatic origins (whiplash) which may be present locally or be more widespread. This occurrence has implications for the presence of augmented neurobiological processing of pain within the central nervous system in some patients' neck pain disorders (Chapter 2).

In the clinical setting, use of quantitative sensory testing is challenged by the absence of equipment which is available in a research setting as well as an absence of comparative findings on which to interpret findings. Nevertheless, measures of mechanical pain thresholds can be made with commercially available, simple pressure algometers. Local sites in the neck and more remote sites in the upper and lower limbs should be tested. Thermal sensitivity (heat and cold pain thresholds) could be examined with thermorollers which can be set at predetermined temperatures.[46] At the least, clinicians may need to identify the nexus between patients' symptomatic complaints and any hyperalgesic response which may be evident in their manual handling of the patient. Further development of clinically valid and useful measures of sensory disturbances is vital for the recognition and understanding of sensory disturbances in the neck pain patient.

## Manual examination of the cervical segments

Techniques of manual examination of the cervical segments are well described in manipulative therapy texts and the reader is referred to such texts for detailed technique descriptions.[1, 47] Manual examination of segmental motion is a qualitative assessment and not an absolute measure. Tissue compliance and pain provocation are assessed in attempts to identify the symptomatic and dysfunctional segment(s). From a scientific viewpoint, a recent systematic review[48] rigorously evaluated studies of cervical manual examination using the Quality Assessment of Diagnostic Accuracy Studies (QUADAS) tool.[49] While several of the studies reviewed pointed to the diagnostic potential of manual examination to detect cervical symptomatic joint dysfunction, several methodological inadequacies were identified. One recommendation for improvement in future studies was the use of a valid reference standard to test the outcome of manual examination such as diagnostic joint blocks.[50, 51] Humphreys et al.[52] used subjects with a congenital fusion as a reference standard for manual examination in a study to investigate the validity of detecting major segmental hypomobility. These researchers determined moderate sensitivity and high specificity with inexperienced examiners. Clearly more studies are required with designs fulfilling the criteria of the QUADAS tool to rate scientifically and position manual examination as a clinical assessment tool. Not withstanding the future challenges, manual examination of the cervical segments continues to be used in clinical practice to gain information about the pain response to manual provocation as well as the tissue compliance to induced motion in the primary physiological or combined planes of motion of each segment.

Manual examination in the supine position includes palpation of the soft tissues of the anterior neck as well as passive tests of motion at the cervical segmental level. In relation to soft-tissue palpation, note is made of any increased tension in the scalene muscles, which is not uncommonly observed clinically in neck pain patients, especially those with chronic or recurrent neck pain. At least three possibilities could be considered in the clinical reasoning process with this finding: (1) the scalenes may be being used excessively to compensate for poor contractile capacity of the deep neck flexors; (2) they are reacting to nerve tissue mechanosensitivity; or (3) their overuse is related to a poor upper-chest breathing pattern. A combination of these factors may be present. The results of the craniocervical flexion test (CCFT), the BPPT, and observation of the relaxed breathing pattern will help make the pattern fit in the clinical decision-making process.

In the supine position, the physiological movements of each cervical segment from occiput to C7 are examined passively in each plane of movement.[1] Each segment can also be stressed using an anterior to posterior glide directed to the segment via the anterior surface of the transverse process with movement produced in line with the facet plane. The patient is positioned in side lying to test sagittal plane glide in the cervical segments (C2–7) (Figure 12.3) and physiological motions in the cervicothoracic joints (C7–T4). The clinician seeks any abnormal quality of tissue compliance and motion as well as any reproduction of pain at a segmental level to detect symptomatic segmental dysfunction to add to the picture of the patient's clinical presentation in the clinical reasoning process.

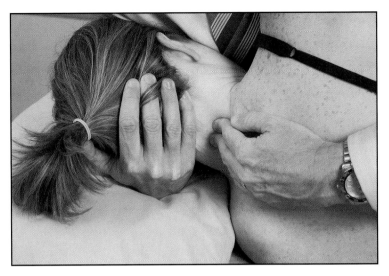

**Figure 12.3** Manual tests of sagittal plane glide. The test is used to test the C2–7 motion segments progressively.

Tests of the craniocervical ligament complex may be indicated in certain patients presenting with neck pain. Frank instabilities can occur in inflammatory arthritides such as rheumatoid arthritis and ankylosing spondylitis or conditions such as Down's syndrome.[53-55] Of more relevance, trauma from a motor vehicle crash may also precipitate injury to such structures as the craniocervical ligament complex,[56, 57] which must be considered in whiplash patients, especially those with high levels of pain and disability.[58] The current argument centers on the incidence of such injuries. There is still debate about how reliably a strain or rupture of an alar ligament can be imaged with magnetic resonance imaging techniques.[59-61]

Clinical tests of the craniocervical ligaments have been described,[62] but their reliability is questionable.[63, 64] Thus, in this state of uncertainty, the clinician is encouraged to undertake the ligament tests when indicated, but to interpret results with caution. Again, reliance must be placed on the total presentation of the patient. Those presenting with high levels of neck pain and disability, marked dizziness, and muscle guarding following trauma need to be managed with care and respect despite negative findings for fractures or ligament ruptures on magnetic resonance imaging.

## The examination in prone lying

### Manual examination

The manual examination is continued in prone lying. The posterior soft tissues are gently palpated. The bulk of the cervical extensor muscles can be shifted medially so that the clinician can palpate the deeper extensors over the laminae of the zygapophyseal joints (Figure 12.4). Discrete muscle "thickening" can often be palpated over a symptomatic zygapophyseal joint. The deep craniocervical muscles can also be palpated: the rectus capitis posterior major muscle between the C2 spinous process and the occiput and the obliquus capitis inferior muscle between the C2 spinous process and the transverse process of C1. The muscles are commonly felt to be thickened in patients with upper cervical disorders.

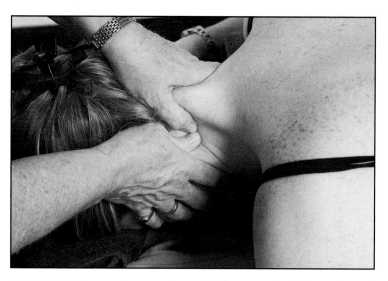

**Figure 12.4** The deeper extensor muscles overlying the zygapophyseal joints can be gently palpated using a lateral approach by first shifting the more superficial extensors medially.

Each segment in the cervical and upper thoracic regions is then gently moved in a posteroanterior direction using direct pressure through the spinous processes and laminae to bias stress over the central intervertebral and the facet joints respectively. The perceived resistance to motion and pain response is assessed. This form of manual examination can be regarded as a discrete pain provocation test. Again, the quality of tissue compliance, pain response, and reactions of the muscles overlying the segment to the pressure provocation are assessed to determine the dysfunctional segment. The patient is asked to rate the pain felt on manual examination of the symptomatic segment(s) on a 0–10-scale for reassessment purposes.

## Scapular holding test

The ability of the patient to position and maintain the scapula in an orientation that mimics its position in an upright posture is assessed against gravity using an adaptation of a conventional grade 3 muscle test for the lower trapezius.[65] The test is performed without arm load, the arm being left to rest by the patient's side. In the test, the clinician first passively positions the scapula in a neutral position on the posterior chest wall and asks the patient to hold the position (Figure 12.5). Two aspects are assessed. The first is the pattern of muscle activity that the patient uses to hold the scapular position and the second is the assessment of the muscles' holding capacity under these low-load conditions, a task akin to their functional role in holding the scapular position in upright postures. In circumstances where nerve tissues have displayed marked mechanosensitivity in the BPPT, this test might be delayed, especially if upper trapezius muscle activity is observed to be guarding the nerve tissues.

In the test, the clinician observes for activity in the lower and middle trapezius and a "balance" of activity from other contributing muscles. The patient may substitute with a variety of inappropriate muscle actions, including dominance by the latissimus dorsi (arm and scapular depression), dominance by rhomboids or levator scapulae (elevation of the scapular border and downward rotation), and even seeming dominance by the infraspinatus/

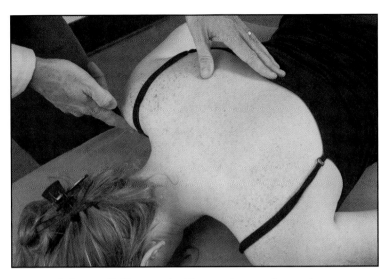

**Figure 12.5** The test of holding capacity of the scapular supporting muscles.

teres minor muscles as the patient attempts to hold the position by raising the elbow and externally rotating the arm. The clinician repeats the action passively with the instruction to lift the shoulder gently to draw the shoulder blade across the chest wall to assist the patient's learning. The patient is requested actively to reposition the scapula so that the clinician can assess the learning of the correct action.

The second aspect of the test assesses the holding capacity of the muscles under these low-load conditions. The patient is requested to hold the scapular position for approximately 10 seconds and the test is repeated up to five times until the clinician has a good appreciation of the test result. Impaired muscle activation may be observed when the patient cannot hold the position and the scapula slides towards an outer range position, the muscles develop a fatigue tremor, or the patient resorts to using another muscle strategy to hold the position.

Another clinically useful aspect of this test is the reciprocal relaxation effect it appears to have on the scapular elevators (in particular levator scapulae) and their attachments to the cervical spine. The activation of the lower trapezius muscles during this test appears to relax the levator scapulae muscle and deload its cervical attachments. It is not uncommon to detect a change in tenderness with posteroanterior palpation of the painful cervical segments immediately following the scapular holding test. This response can again make a convincing link between relief of pain and appropriate muscle control for patient motivation for exercise and training of posture.

# Continuation of the examination in supine lying

## Craniocervical flexion test

Our research has highlighted the association between impairment in the deep neck flexors and neck pain in both acute and chronic states (Chapter 4). These muscles are tested via the CCFT. The test is low-load and can be performed in the initial assessment in the vast majority of patients with either acute or chronic conditions. The clinical test has been shown to be able to differentiate neck pain patients from controls and is a suitable outcome measure, being sensitive to change as a result of a training program.[66–69]

Before commencing the test, the patient's range of craniocervical motion is assessed. This familiarizes the patient with the test movement and it allows the clinician to gain an appreciation of the patient's range of craniocervical flexion as a baseline for the analysis of the movement in the formal test. The presence of any nerve tissue mechanosensitivity with the movement must be appreciated and this is achieved by repeating the movement with the nerve tissues preset with a straight-leg raise or BPPT position. If neck or head pain is produced in these pretensioned positions, the CCFT is delayed and management of sensitive nerve tissues becomes a priority – about 10% of cervicogenic headache patients.[68, 70]

The CCFT is performed in supine crook lying with the neck in a neutral neck position (no pillow) such that the line of the face is horizontal and a line bisecting the neck longitudinally is horizontal to the testing surface. Layers of towel may need to be positioned under the head to achieve a neutral position if the head is observed to lie in slight extension (Figure 12.6). This occurs in patients with a marked cervicothoracic or thoracic kyphosis. The towel is aligned with the base of the occiput so that the upper cervical region is free for positioning of the pressure biofeedback device (Stabilizer, Chattanooga, USA). Some patients rest in a position of cervical flexion that is often associated with palpable tension in the scalene muscles. Such patients usually perform poorly in the CCFT and clinically often offer a greater challenge in rehabilitation.

Once a neutral cervical position is achieved, the uninflated pressure biofeedback device is placed behind the neck so that it abuts the occiput to monitor most effectively the change in shape of the

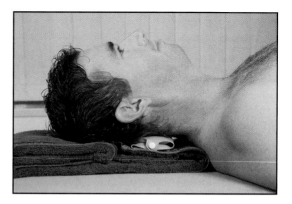

**Figure 12.6** The craniocervical and cervical regions are positioned in a neutral position using layers of towel as necessary. The pressure biofeedback unit is positioned behind the neck and is abutted against the occiput.

curve as it flattens with the contraction of the deep cervical flexors.[71] The pressure sensor is inflated to a baseline pressure of 20 mmHg, a standard pressure sufficient to fill the space between the testing surface and the neck but not push the neck into a lordosis. The pressure should be stabilized before testing commences.

Careful instruction should be given to the patient that the test is not one of strength but rather one of precision and control. From our studies the test appears to have both contractile and proprioceptive components.[72] The patient is instructed to perform a head-nodding action (as if saying "yes") to target sequentially five 2-mmHg progressive pressure increases from the baseline of 20 mmHg to a maximum of 30 mmHg as well as hold the position steady in a low-load endurance test. The movement should be performed gently and slowly and the patient instructed to feel the back of the head slide up the bed, to avoid the temptation to lift the head. The patient practices the movement without feedback prior to formal testing.

## Formal test procedure

The formal test is conducted in two stages.
Stage 1: Movement analysis of the five progressive stages of the craniocervical flexion action.

Stage 2: Testing of isometric capacity of the deep neck flexors at test stages that the patient is able to achieve with the correct craniocervical flexion action.

In the movement analysis of stage 1, the patient is provided with the feedback from the pressure sensor, and is requested to nod the head slowly to elevate the target pressure from 20 to 22 mmHg and to hold the position for 2 or 3 seconds before relaxing. This process is repeated through each of the four remaining stages of the test (Figure 12.7). The stage of the test that the patient can achieve and momentarily hold with the correct craniocervical flexion action provides quantification of performance in this stage of the test. The clinician observes two factors. The first is the motion of the head during craniocervical flexion. The second is the muscle activity in the superficial flexors.

The motion of the head should be a rotation action whose range increases through progressive stages of the test.[73] The expected incremental increases in range are gauged by the clinician from the previous assessment of range of passive craniocervical flexion. Several abnormal patterns may be observed in neck pain patients. There may not be a progressive increase in craniocervical flexion range. The patient changes the movement strategy and performs more a head retraction action to attain the progressive pressure increments required in the task.[74] Alternately, the patient may lift the head in attempts to reach the target pressures or perform the movement with speed, that is, flick the head into flexion, usually to mask weakness. Others cannot perform all test stages regardless of strategy. This is rarely encountered in asymptomatic persons.

In relation to the superficial flexor muscles, some activity has been recorded in the sternocleidomastoid and anterior scalene muscles in asymptomatic subjects but there

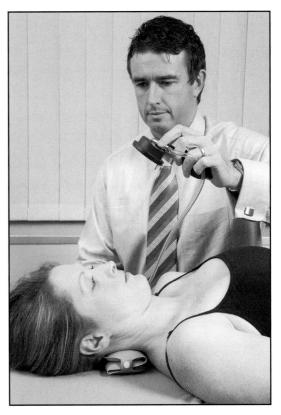

**Figure 12.7** The patient performs a head-nodding action to target the progressive pressure increments. The clinician analyzes the head rotation action of craniocervical flexion and observes for or palpates inappropriate activity of the superficial flexor muscles.

is not dominant activity of the superficial flexors. It is significantly less than that measured in neck pain patients regardless of the insidious or traumatic origin of the neck pain.[74-76] In the clinical situation this activity can be observed or palpated by the clinician. If the patient is an upper costal breather, the test should be performed during slow expiration to minimize overactivity in the anterior scalene muscles.[77] Another substitution strategy is the attempted use of the hyoid muscles to augment the contraction of the deeper muscles. The patient may use one of two strategies. One is to clench the jaw and the other is to perform craniocervical flexion with jaw opening. These strategies should likewise be corrected as required by requesting the patient to adopt a rest position of the mandible. That is, the patient is asked to place the tongue lightly on the roof of the mouth, lips together with teeth slightly apart before and when repeating the test action.

Two other situations in which an aberrant sign may be observed involve the return to the resting position. The first is that, on return from a designated pressure, the biofeedback device registers less pressure than the baseline of 20 mmHg. This may occur if the pressure in the chamber has not been adequately stabilized before testing begins, but negating this occurrence, it may indicate a deficit in proprioceptive acuity with the patient overshooting the neutral head position on return from the movement (Chapter 6). Likewise, on return to the starting position the dial may read a pressure greater than 20 mmHg. Again this may indicate a deficit in proprioceptive acuity with the patient undershooting the neutral head position but it more likely indicates an inability to relax the muscles following a contraction (Chapter 4), which holds the neck in some flexion. This is often readily appreciated with palpation of the scalene muscles where tension will be felt. Lifting the chin to neutral will result in return of the needle on the dial to 20 mmHg as well as a softening/relaxation of the scalenes.

The analysis of performance during stage 1 of the test is documented. It provides directives for stage 2 of the examination as well as for strategies that may be used in the re-education of the flexor synergy.

Stage 2 tests the isometric contraction capacity of the deep cervical flexors at low load. This stage is conducted when the patient can perform the correct craniocervical flexion action, even if they cannot reach all target pressures. This stage of the test is delayed in patients who use substitution movements (for example, head retraction) in stage 1 of the test. There is little purpose in testing the holding capacity of an incorrect muscle and movement strategy. The movement strategy requires re-education in the first instance before endurance is addressed.

The low-load endurance capacity of the deep neck flexors is tested by determining the pressure level that the patient can hold steady for 10 seconds, with minimal superficial muscle activity. The test is commenced at the lowest level (22 mmHg) and, if 10 repetitions of 10-second holds are achieved, the test is progressed to the next pressure target. The clinician must continue to observe the movement strategy that the patient uses to ensure that it remains a craniocervical rotation. Poor performance in the test is in evidence when the patient cannot hold the pressure steady at the designated test level and it falls away (even though the patient seems to be holding the head in the flexed position). Poor performance is also signaled when the superficial flexors are overtly recruited or when the pressure level is held but it is with a jerky action. The latter suggests that the patient is searching for a muscle strategy to hold the pressure level, and most likely indicates weakness or fatigue in the deep cervical flexors.

There is variability in performance of the holding test in persons without neck pain,[67, 75] but it can be expected that most asymptomatic individuals can successfully perform the test to at least the third or fourth stages (26–28 mmHg). However neck pain patients often do not achieve more than the first or the second levels of the test.[67, 68] The test stage that the patient can achieve becomes the stage at which training commences.

### Retest of active cervical extension and manual palpation

Active cervical extension is retested in sitting following the CCFT to determine the effect of activation of the deep neck flexors on eccentric and concentric control of cervical extension. Often there is an immediate improvement in extension range with a reduction in pain. Alternately, the manual segmental examination in prone lying may be repeated. We have recently shown that there is decreased tenderness following the CCFT,[78] probably again reflecting a reciprocal relaxation effect. These reassessments further illustrate to the patient the association between activation of specific muscles and pain relief to encourage compliance with exercise.

## Muscle length tests

Altered muscle length–tension relationships may have been observed in the examination of neck posture as well as that of scapular orientation, movement, and the scapular holding test. These observations can be confirmed with formal muscle length tests.[79, 80] We are nevertheless reserved about conducting muscle length tests, especially in patients with a moderate to severe pain syndrome and for those muscles whose muscle shortness may be protective of nerve tissue mechanosensitivity (scalene, suboccipital extensors, and upper trapezius muscles).

# The examination in four-point kneeling

## Closed-chain test of scapular stability

The patient is positioned in four-point kneeling so that the hips and arms are at right angles to the trunk and the curves of the spine are in a neutral position. Patients are encouraged to let the ribcage sink between the scapulae. They are then requested to push through their arms to raise their ribcage back towards their scapulae until the scapulae assume a position that mimics their upright postural position and then hold the position. This tests the capacity of the axioscapular muscles to fix the scapula to the chest wall in a neutral postural position under load. Substantial winging of the medial border of the scapula is an indication of poor axioscapular muscle control, particularly of the serratus anterior muscle. The serratus anterior may also be further tested through its inner range by raising the ribcage further, causing the scapulae to protract around the chest wall. A compensatory strategy for shoulder protraction that is not uncommonly used is trunk flexion (Figure 12.8). This aberrant action should be corrected to evaluate better the action of serratus anterior.

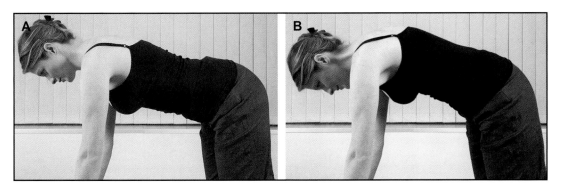

**Figure 12.8** The four-point test for the scapular muscles. The correct (A) and incorrect (B) trunk positions in the test of the serratus anterior.

## Cervical extensor muscles

All cervical extensor muscles contribute to supporting the weight of the head against gravity as well as extending the head and neck in the four-point kneeling position (or alternately, the prone-on-elbows position). It is known that structural changes occur in the extensor muscles with neck pain with most change in the suboccipital muscles, the segmental multifidus, and semispinalis cervicis.[81, 82] In this phase of the examination of the extensor muscles, emphasis is placed on testing and facilitating the posterior craniocervical muscles and the deep typical cervical extensors in respect of their important roles as cervical proprioceptors (Chapter 5) and for support of the cervical joints and lordosis (Chapter 3).

The first test biases the suboccipital extensors (rectus capitis major and minor) and suboccipital rotators (obliquus capitis superior and inferior). The therapist gently stabilizes the C2 vertebra to assist in the localization of the movement to the upper cervical region. The patient is instructed to imagine that the axis of motion passes through the ear and performs alternating small ranges of craniocervical extension and flexion (nodding action) while maintaining the cervical spine in a neutral position to assess the concentric and eccentric action of these craniocervical extensor muscles. The patient is also instructed to perform small ranges of head rotation (C1–2 rotation, no greater then 40°) such that the movement is a pure spin of the head on the neck (Figure 12.9). An aberrant feature of these tests of the craniocervical extensors and rotators is the patient's inability to perform a smooth and coordinated action and excessive motion of the typical cervical spine occurs.

The second cervical extension test biases the deeper cervical extensors (semispinalis cervicis/multifidus group) rather than the more superficial muscles such as the splenius and semispinalis capitis. The patient now

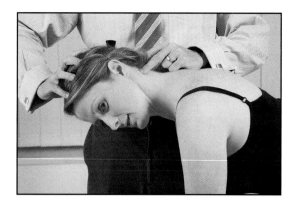

**Figure 12.9** Facilitation of the obliquus capitis superior and inferior with craniocervical rotation. C2 is stabilized to facilitate motion at C1–2.

visualizes the axis of rotation as passing through the C7 vertebra. The aim is for the patient to perform cervical extension (a rotation and not a retraction action) while keeping the craniocervical region in a neutral position. In the learning process, the patient focuses on the clinician's manual contact and facilitation on C2. Firstly, the patient is encouraged to curl the neck gently into flexion (eccentric action) followed by a curl of the neck into extension (concentric action). This action will extend the entire cervical spine but care is taken to maintain the craniocervical region in neutral to lessen any dominance in the action of splenius and semispinalis capitis muscles. In the phase from flexion to the neutral position, impairment is indicated by a loss of the neutral craniocervical position and excessive use of the semispinalis capitis muscles indicated by their marked prominence. In the phase from neutral to end-range extension, some craniocervical extension can be expected but impairment is indicated if it is excessive and the patient is unable to extend the typical cervical region into or towards the full cervical extension position. In most instances this is a painfree test, even in patients who might have pain with cervical extension in sitting. If the test does provoke pain, it can be performed within the painless range (e.g., from a flexion position to neutral). Conversely, in patients with mild pain and impairment, this action may be repeated several times or occasionally light load may need to be added to the head to challenge this large extensor muscle group adequately.

# Assessment of disturbances in sensorimotor control

When patients complain of dizziness, light-headedness, or feelings of unsteadiness in association with their neck disorder, this directs the clinician to examine features which reflect impairments in the postural control system. A legitimate argument could be raised to incorporate these tests routinely in all patients with neck pain as deficits in tests of the postural control system have been found in those not overtly complaining of these symptoms (Chapter 6). Three sets of measures are included: tests of cervical joint position sense, balance, and oculomotor control. There is always the challenge of attempting to differentiate a cervical from a vestibular origin of any impairment detected, especially in the case of balance (Chapter 6).

## Cervical joint position sense

The measure commonly used to assess cervical kinesthetic sense in the clinical setting is the person's ability to relocate the natural head posture whilst vision is occluded.[83] The joint position error (JPE) is the angular difference between the starting natural head postural position and that assumed following a neck movement. Errors are commonly measured following return from cervical extension, and rotation to the left and right, although return from flexion and lateral flexion can also be assessed. Accuracy in relocating selected points in range[84] and tracing pictorial patterns[85] have also been used to assess cervical kinesthesia. Although moderate deficits can be judged visually in the clinical situation, JPEs as little

as 3–4°[86, 87] indicate a deficit in cervical joint position sense and may be difficult to judge visually. A simple quantitative measure is preferable and is more valuable as an outcome measure on which to reassess effects of management. A simple measure can be achieved through the use of a laser pointer or pencil torch mounted on to a light-weight head band, as used by Revel et al.[83] (Figure 12.10). The patient sits such that the laser pointer is 90 cm away from a wall and the starting position is projected by the laser on to the wall and marked. After performance of a test movement, the final position is marked and the difference between the two marked points is measured in centimeters as a negative or positive value, reflecting undershoot or overshoot of the target. Alternately, a gravity-dependent goniometer may be used as a measuring instrument.

Abnormal kinesthetic sense may also be indicated clinically if the patient demonstrates jerky movements, uncertainty or searching for the initial position, overshooting the initial position, reproduction of dizziness, or when there is a noticeable difference between movement patterns when performed with the eyes closed compared to eyes open.

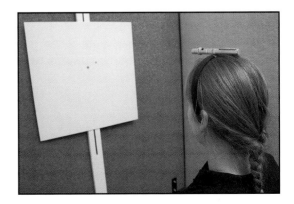

**Figure 12.10** Test of joint position sense using a laser pointer. A measure of joint relocation error is gained from measuring the distance between the return and starting positions. The average of three attempts is measured.

## Standing balance

The standard sensory organization test is used clinically to measure a person's ability to maintain equilibrium. The test systematically changes the sensory selection process by altering the environmental information and visual inputs available to the somatosensory system.[88]

In the clinical examination of standing balance, the patient is progressed through tasks that increasingly challenge the postural system by altering foot position, visual input, and the supporting surface. Balance in comfortable and subsequently narrow stance is assessed with the patient standing on a firm and then a soft surface such as a piece of 10-cm-dense foam (Figure 12.11). The tests should be performed both with the eyes open and then closed. It is reasonable to expect that a person under the age of 60 years can maintain stability for up to 30 seconds in comfortable and narrow stance tests. Large increases in sway, slower responses to correct sway, or rigidity to prevent excessive sway, as well as an inability to maintain balance are abnormal responses. The test level and response are recorded.

For increasing challenge, the patient can be tested in tandem and then single-leg stance on a firm surface with eyes open and closed. Patients under 45 years should be able to complete these more challenging tests.[89] Patients with neck pain of either insidious or traumatic origin, and especially those complaining of dizziness or unsteadiness, have been shown to have greater difficulty in completing the tandem stance tasks on a firm surface than control subjects.[89, 90]

The relationship between postural stability tests and more dynamic and functional tasks has not been investigated in patients with neck disorders. However clinicians may consider dynamic tests such as reach and step and external perturbations

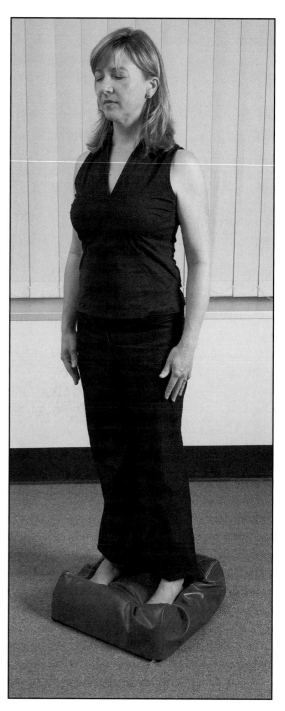

**Figure 12.11** Testing balance in comfortable stance, with eyes closed on a soft surface.

as performed with neurological or aged patients, particularly for neck pain patients complaining of dizziness, unsteadiness, or loss of balance. Tests such as the functional step test,[91] the timed 10-metre walk, Singleton's test,[92] or the Dynamic Gait Index[93] could be easily conducted in the clinical setting to provide measures of functional dynamic balance.

## Oculomotor assessment

The visual postural system consists of three eye movement systems: the smooth-pursuit, saccadic, and optokinetic systems. The smooth-pursuit system ensures stable images of a moving target with slow eye-follow movements, the saccadic system allows rapid eye movements to change a point of fixation, and the optokinetic system allows fixation of a target when a person is moving, as in walking. Several reflex mechanisms are involved in these processes (Chapter 5).

Input from cervical afferents influences the visual system and can also alter the function of the other systems.[94] Thus oculomotor assessment incorporates assessment of all aspects of eye movement. The tests include:

1. The ability to maintain gaze while moving the head – gaze stability
2. Eye follow while keeping the head still – smooth-pursuit
3. Maintaining gaze when the eyes and head are moving: eye–head coordination

The tests are usually performed with the patient in sitting. Depending on the patient's presentation, the starting position may be regressed (supine lying) or progressed in the initial and subsequent treatment sessions. Tests can be progressed to sitting with neck torsion (which will bias cervical afferent influence) and standing in various stance positions. Speed of the movement will also challenge the oculomotor system. The level of assessment required will depend on the patient's presenting symptoms and overall physical findings. Abnormal test responses include a difficulty or inability in performing the task, reproduction of symptoms, and jerky or nonfluent head and/or eye movements. Generally patients with neck-related oculomotor disturbances do not present with nystagmus at rest or during these tests. Its presence may be more indicative of vestibular pathology.

### Gaze stability

Gaze stability is assessed by asking the patient to keep the eyes focused on a target while actively moving the head into flexion,

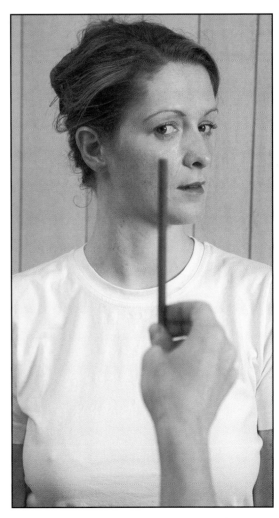

**Figure 12.12** Testing gaze stability during head rotation.

extension, and rotation to the left and right (Figure 12.12). For patients with marked symptoms, it may be necessary for the clinician to move the head passively, with the patient in supine lying. Pertinent findings are an inability to maintain focus on the target or reproduction of symptoms such as dizziness, blurring of vision, or nausea. The test can be progressed by asking patients to fix their gaze on the target and then perform the movement while the eyes are closed. They open their eyes after the head movement to check that they have maintained a stable gaze on the target. This is called imaginary gaze.[92]

## Eye follow

Eye follow is tested using the elements of the smooth-pursuit neck torsion test.[95] The patient is asked to keep the head still and follow a moving target with the eyes as closely as possible (Figure 12.13). The target is moved slowly from side to side and up and down and the test is progressed to following an H pattern. The clinician closely

monitors the patient's ability to follow well and notes any jerky or catch-up eye movements or reproduction of symptoms. The patient then rotates the trunk up to 45° or to a point just short of pain, while the clinician keeps the head still. This position of relative neck rotation (torsion) biases the cervical receptors whilst vestibular receptors are unchanged. The patient then repeats the eye-follow task keeping the head still. The trunk is then rotated to the opposite side and the test repeated. The positive sign indicating a cervical rather than, for example, a vestibular origin of symptoms is a difference in eye follow (increased saccades) or symptom reproduction in the neck torsion position compared to the neutral position. The starting position, speed, and focus point can be altered to challenge the oculomotor system.

## Eye–head coordination

Eye–head coordination is assessed with three tests. Firstly the patient is asked to move the eyes and head in the same direction

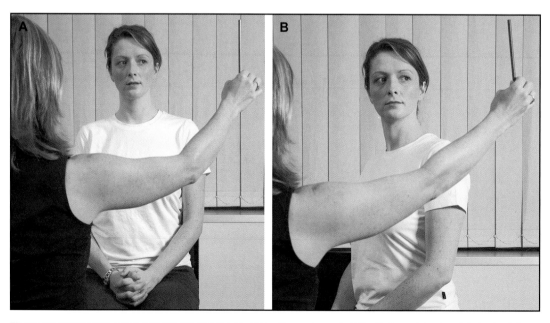

**Figure 12.13** Eye follow is tested (A) with the neck in a neutral position and repeated (B) with the neck torsioned via trunk rotation. Deterioration in eye follow in the neck torsion position when compared to the neutral position suggests a cervical origin of deficits in eye movement control.

to focus on a target, leading first with the eyes to the target and then the head, ensuring the eyes keep focused on the target. The test is performed to the left and right. Secondly the patient is asked to move the eyes and the head in opposite directions while maintaining focus on a predetermined point. Finally, the patient is asked to focus on two points and move the eyes first and then the head, to look between the two targets. The target points are positioned horizontally or vertically and the patient maintains focus between the two points (two-point focus).

## Other causes of disturbances to the postural control system

Primary vestibular pathology is possible following a whiplash injury and could be the origin of symptoms in these patients. However, more indirectly, there is some evidence that the neck may directly influence vestibular function[96] (Chapter 5). Altered neck input may give rise to a mismatch of sensory input from the cervical and vestibular systems and contribute to asymmetry of the vestibulo-ocular reflex (VOR).[97] Some patients with neck pain and previously normal vestibular function could feasibly have an asymmetry of the VOR of a cervical origin.[98] Therefore assessment in neck pain patients may need to address secondary vestibular influences on sensorimotor control.

There is overlap in responses between the vestibular and cervical musculoskeletal systems in a number of tests which have been described in this text. In some patients, additional tests may be necessary to look more closely at vestibular function. These could include tests of dynamic balance and functional ambulation as well as more specific tests of the VOR such as the dynamic visual acuity test[92] or the head impulse test.[99] In cases where benign paroxysmal positional vertigo is suspected, the Hallpike–Dix maneuver is included as a screening test.[92] For a more detailed review of vestibular evaluation the clinician should consult texts designed specifically for that purpose.[92] Referral for a more thorough investigation of the vestibular or central nervous systems may be warranted where cervical causes of dizziness or disturbances in the sensorimotor system cannot be substantiated.

There are other causes of disturbances to sensorimotor control which could be concomitant with neck pain. These include medical conditions such as diabetes and merely the factor of aging. Vestibular function deteriorates as a consequence of age.[100] In elders, neck pain may magnify the degree of disturbances in the postural control system.[101] Nevertheless such co-occurrences should not detract from the rehabilitation program but may influence speed of recovery or outcomes.

## Muscle strength and endurance

Deficits in strength, endurance, and fatigability have been demonstrated in the neck flexor and extensor muscles in association with neck pain as well as axioscapular muscles such as upper trapezius (Chapter 4). In the clinical setting, tests of strength are performed in subsequent assessments as early strength testing may aggravate symptoms or, conversely, pain inhibition may flaw test outcomes.

Strength and endurance measures of the cervical flexors and extensors may be tested using dynamometry measures (Figure 12.14),[102, 103] or by using graduated head load or free weights attached to the head when necessary. What is notable from studies utilizing dynamometry measurements is the discovery of impaired capacity of neck muscles over a spectrum of contraction intensities. Not only have cervical spine muscles demonstrated reduced maximal strength but also poorer endurance and fatigability at submaximal loads, 50% and

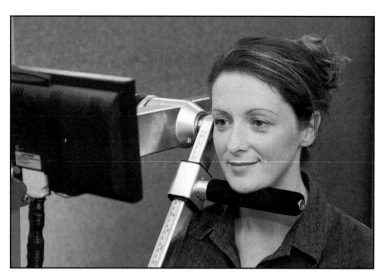

**Figure 12.14** Strength and endurance testing of the craniocervical flexor muscles with a dynamometer (Neckmetrix).

20–25% of maximum voluntary capacity.[104, 105] This directs testing of muscle performance towards these levels of contraction, as well as tests of maximum strength, as they are the functionally relevant loads for neck function for the average individual.

## Examination of work tasks

The way in which a person functions in activities of daily living, work, or sport can contribute to the development or perpetuation of neck pain. The best physical treatment will fail to have a lasting effect if provocative features or habits are not addressed. Tremendous advances have been made to workplace design and work practices by occupational health and ergonomic researchers and practitioners. Yet, even with appropriate workstations, the occurrence of neck pain in the workplace persists, especially with the increasing computer use both at work and at home.[106, 107] Multiple factors may contribute to this occurrence – physical, psychological, and social.[108, 109] The clinician must acquire an understanding of the patient's work situation and work practices from both the formal interview and casual conversation and understand what practices the patient perceives are provocative of neck pain.

There is increasing knowledge of the physical impact of work on the function of cervicobrachial neuromusculoskeletal structures and the disturbances associated with work. For example, those with neck pain may drift into a more forward head posture with computer work,[7, 8, 110] exhibit altered muscle recruitment patterns in the neck extensor, flexor, and upper trapezius muscles,[111, 112] demonstrate higher levels of fatigue in the upper trapezius[113] and an inability to relax their upper trapezius effectively during work tasks.[114, 115] The appreciation of the physical aspects of work practices is vital with the aim in management of optimizing the patient's posture and muscle recruitment patterns.

Assessment of the worker in the workplace is the preference, although the clinician may provide a work simulation to assess work practices. Key physical features to note in analysis of office or light industry work would include, for instance, the starting spinal posture and the changes in spinal orientation over time which seem to occur within a few minutes.[8] The orientation of the scapula is observed as it is loaded during small-range arm elevation such as computer work as well as many forms of bench work requiring prolonged periods of repetitive small-range upper-limb movements. Observations are made of the capacity of the axioscapular muscles to maintain steady control of the scapula, that is, the capacity to maintain upward rotation and avoid anterior tilt and internal rotation. Control can also be tested under increased load, speed, or range, as relevant to the patient's work tasks. The neck, upper trapezius, and levator scapulae muscles are observed or palpated for any abnormally increased activity.

Importantly, the patient must be given feedback and have a good understanding of any poor work practices and the implications for neck pain. This is essential to change habits and for the patient's active participation in the rehabilitation program.

## Conclusion

The findings from the patient interview, history, and physical examination are assimilated in the clinical reasoning process to provide the clinician with an understanding of the patient, the psychophysical processes underlying the neck disorder, and the impact of the disorder on the patient's working and social life as well as general well-being. Outcome measures must be established to measure treatment effects on pain, disability, functional recovery, and physical and any psychological impairment. Importantly, possession of knowledge of the interrelationships between symptoms, functional disturbances, and impairments within and between systems will direct the most appropriate management approach.

## References

1. *Maitland GD, Hengeveld E, Banks K, et al*. Maitland's Vertebral Manipulation. 7th edn. London: Butterworth, 2005.

2. *Dumas JP, Arsenault AB, Boudreau G, et al*. Physical impairments in cervicogenic headache: traumatic vs. nontraumatic onset. Cephalalgia 2001;21:884–893.

3. *Griegel-Morris P, Larson K, Mueller-Klaus K, et al*. Incidence of common postural abnormalities in the cervical, shoulder, and thoracic regions and their association with pain in two age groups of healthy subjects. Phys Ther 1992;72:425–431.

4. *Lee H, Nicholson LL, Adams RD*. Cervical range of motion associations with subclinical neck pain. Spine 2003;29:33–40.

5. *Treleaven J, Jull G, Atkinson L*. Cervical musculoskeletal dysfunction in post-concussional headache. Cephalalgia 1994;14:273–279.

6. *Watson DH, Trott PH*. Cervical headache: an investigation of natural head posture and upper cervical flexor muscle performance. Cephalalgia 1993;13:272–284.

7. *Szeto G, Straker L, Raine S*. A field comparison of neck and shoulder postures in symptomatic and asymptomatic office workers. Appl Ergon 2002;33:75–84.

8. *Falla D, Jull G, Russell T, et al*. The effect of neck exercise on sitting posture in patients with chronic neck pain. Phys Ther 2007;87:408–417.

9. *Szeto GP, Straker LM, O'Sullivan P*. The roles of upper trapezius and cervical erector spinae in controlling the neck–shoulder postures in symptomatic office workers performing continuous keyboard work: towards developing an etiological model for work-related neck and upper limb disorders. Seoul, Korea: IEA XVth Triennial Congress, 2003. Abstract no 1153.

10. *Richardson C, Hodges P, Hides J*. Therapeutic Exercise for Lumbopelvic Stabilization: A Motor Control Approach for the Treatment and Prevention of Low-back Pain, 2nd edn. Edinburgh: Churchill Livingstone, 2004.

11. *Falla D, O'Leary S, Fagan A, et al*. Recruitment of the deep cervical flexor muscles during a postural-correction exercise performed in sitting. Man Ther 2007;12:139–152.

12. *Moseley G*. Impaired trunk muscle function in sub-acute neck pain: etiologic in the subsequent development of low-back pain? Man Ther 2004;9:157–163.

13. *Sobush DC, Simoneau GG, Dietz KE, et al*. The Lennie test for measuring scapular position in healthy young adult females: a reliability and

validity study. J Orthop Sports Phys Ther 1996;23:39–50.

14. *Sahrmann SA*. Diagnosis and Treatment of Movement Impairment Syndromes. St. Louis: Mosby, 2002.

15. *Dall'Alba P, Sterling M, Treleaven J, et al*. Cervical range of motion discriminates between asymptomatic and whiplash subjects. Spine 2001;26:2090–2094.

16. *Sterling M, Jull G, Vicenzino B, et al*. Characterisation of acute whiplash associated disorders. Spine 2004;29:182–188.

17. *Zwart JA*. Neck mobility in different headache disorders. Headache 1997;37:6–11.

18. *Youdas J, Carey J, Garrett T*. Reliability of measurements of cervical spine range of motion – comparison of three methods. Phys Ther 1991;71: 98–104.

19. *Edwards BC*. Manual of Combined Movements, 2nd edn. Edinburgh: Churchill Livingstone, 1999.

20. *Grant R*. Clinics in Physical Therapy of the Cervical and Thoracic Spines, 3rd edn. St Louis: Churchill Livingstone, Elsevier Science, 2002.

21. *Berthoz A, Grantyn A*. Neuronal mechanisms underlying eye–head coordination. Prog Brain Res 1986;64:325–343.

22. *Vidal P, Roucoux A, Berthoz A*. Horizontal eye position-related activity in neck muscles of the alert cat. Exp Brain Res 1982;46:448–453.

23. *Vasavada AN, Li S, Delp SL*. Influence of muscle morphology and moment arms on moment-generating capacity of human neck muscles. Spine 1998;23:412–422.

24. *Amiri M, Jull G, Bullock-Saxton J*. Measuring range of active cervical rotation in a position of full head flexion using the 3D Fastrak measurement system: an intra-tester reliability study. Man Ther 2003;8:176–179.

25. *Hall T, Robinson K*. The flexion–rotation test and active cervical mobility – a comparative measurement study in cervicogenic headache. Man Ther 2004;9:197–202.

26. *Ogince M, Hall T, Robinson K, et al*. The diagnostic validity of the cervical flexion–rotation test in C1/2-related cervicogenic headache. Man Ther 2007;12:256–262.

27. *Falla D, Bilenkij G, Jull G*. Patients with chronic neck pain patients demonstrate altered patterns of muscle activation during performance of a functional upper limb task. Spine 2004;29:1436–1440.

28. *Jull G, Amiri M, Bullock-Saxton J, et al*. Cervical musculoskeletal impairment in frequent intermittent headache. Part 1: subjects with single headaches. Cephalalgia 2007;27:793–802.

29. *Crawford H, Jull GA*. The influence of thoracic posture and movement on range of arm elevation. Physiother Theory Pract 1993;9:143–148.

30. *Stewart S, Jull G, Willems J, et al*. An initial analysis of thoracic spine motion with unilateral

arm elevation in the scapular plane. J Manual Manipul Ther 1995;3:15–21.

31. *Rubinstein S, Pool J, van Tulder M, et al*. A systematic review of the diagnostic accuracy of provocative tests of the neck for diagnosing cervical radiculopathy. Eur Spine J 2007;16:307–319.

32. *Magarey M, Rebbeck T, Coughlan B, et al*. Pre-manipulative testing of the cervical spine review, revision and new clinical guidelines. Man Ther 2004;9:95–108.

33. *Thiel H, Rix G*. Is it time to stop functional pre-manipulation testing of the cervical spine? Man Ther 2005;10:154–158.

34. *Wainner R, Fritz J, Irrgang J, et al*. Reliability and diagnostic accuracy of the clinical examination and patient self report measures for cervical radiculopathy. Spine 2003;28:52–62.

35. *Butler D*. The Sensitive Nervous System. Adelaide: NOI Group Publications, 2000.

36. *Elvey R*. Physical evaluation of the peripheral nervous system in disorders of pain and dysfunction. J Hand Ther 1997;10:122–129.

37. *Balster S, Jull G*. Upper trapezius muscle activity in the brachial plexus tension test in asymptomatic individuals. Man Ther 1997;2:144–149.

38. *Coppieters M, Stappaerts K, Wouters L, et al*. Aberrant protective force generation during neural provocation testing and the effect of treatment in patients with neurogenic cervicobrachial pain. J Manipul Physiol Ther 2003;26:99–106.

39. *Coppieters M, Stappaerts K, Staes F, et al*. Shoulder girdle elevation during neurodynamic testing: an assessable sign? Man Ther 2001;6:88–96.

40. *van der Heide B, Allison GT, Zusman M*. Pain and muscular responses to a neural tissue provocation test in the upper limb. Man Ther 2001;6:154–162.

41. *Coppieters M, Stappaerts K, Janssens K, et al*. Reliability of detecting 'onset of pain' and 'submaximal pain' during neural provocation testing of the upper quadrant. Physiother Res Int 2002;7:146–156.

42. *Alix ME, Bates DK*. The proposed etiology of cervicogenic headache: the neurophysiologic basis and anatomical relationship between the dura mater and rectus posterior capitus minor muscle. J Manipul Physiol Ther 1999;22: 534–539.

43. *Hack GD, Koritzer RT, Robinson WL, et al*. Anatomic relation between the rectus capitis posterior minor muscle and the dura mater. Spine 1995;20:2484–2486.

44. *Jull G*. Management of cervical headache. Man Ther 1997;2:182–190.

45. *Sterling M, Treleaven J, Jull G*. Responses to a clinical test of nerve tissue provocation in whiplash associated disorders. Man Ther 2002;7:89–94.

46. *Jensen T, Baron R*. Translation of symptoms and signs into mechanisms in neuropathic pain. Pain 2003;102:1–8.

47. *Kaltenborn F, Evjenth O, Kaltenborn TB, et al.* Manual Mobilization of the Joints: The Spine, vol. 2, 4th edn. Oslo: Norli, 2003.

48. *Hollerwoger D.* Methodological quality and outcomes of studies addressing manual cervical spine examinations: a review. Man Ther 2006;11:93–98.

49. *Whiting P, Rutjes A, Reitsma J, et al.* The development of QUADAS: a tool for the quality assessment of studies of diagnostic accuracy included in systematic reviews. BMC Med Res Methodol 2003;3:25.

50. *Jull G, Bogduk N, Marsland A.* The accuracy of manual diagnosis for cervical zygapophysial joint pain syndromes. Med J Aust 1988;148:233–236.

51. *King W, Lau P, Lees R, et al.* The validity of manual examination in assessing patients with neck pain. Spine J 2007;7:22–26.

52. *Humphreys B, Delahaye M, Peterson C.* An investigation into the validity of cervical spine motion palpation using subjects with congenital block vertebrae as a 'gold standard'. BMC Musculoskel Disord 2004;5:19.

53. *Holden W, Taylor S, Stevens H, et al.* Neck pain is a major clinical problem in ankylosing spondylitis, and impacts on driving and safety. Scand J Rheumatol 2005;34:159–160.

54. *Kim D, Hilibrand A.* Rheumatoid arthritis in the cervical spine. J Am Acad Orthop Surg 2005;13: 463–474.

55. *Swinkels R, Beeton K, Alltree J.* Pathogenesis of upper cervical instability. Man Ther 1996;1: 127–132.

56. *Krakenes J, Kaale B, Moen G, et al.* MRI assessment of the alar ligaments in the late stage of whiplash – a study of structural abnormalities and observer agreement. Neuroradiol 2002;44:617–624.

57. *Taylor J, Taylor M.* Cervical spinal injuries: an autopsy study of 109 blunt injuries. J Musculoskel Pain 1996;4:61–79.

58. *Kaale B, Krakenes J, Albrektsen G, et al.* Whiplash-associated disorders impairment rating: neck disability index score according to severity of MRI findings of ligaments and membranes in the upper cervical spine. J Neurotrauma 2005;22:466–475.

59. *Krakenes J, Kaale B.* Magnetic resonance imaging assessment of craniovertebral ligaments and membranes after whiplash trauma. Spine 2006;31:2860–2826.

60. *Roy S, Hol P, Laerum L, et al.* Pitfalls of magnetic resonance imaging of alar ligament. Neuroradiol 2004;46:392–398.

61. *Volle E.* Functional magnetic resonance imaging – video diagnosis of soft-tissue trauma to the craniocervical joints and ligaments. Int Tinnitus J 2000;6:134–399.

62. *Aspinall W.* Clinical testing for craniovertebral hypermobility syndrome. J Orthop Sports Phys Ther 1990;12:47–53.

63. *Cattrysse E, Swinkels R, Oostendorp R, et al.* Upper cervical instability: are clinical tests reliable? Man Ther 1997;2:91–97.

64. *Swinkels R, Oostendorp R.* Upper cervical instability: fact or fiction? J Manipul Physiol Ther 1996;19:185–194.

65. *Hislop H, Montgomery J.* Daniels and Worthingham's Muscle Testing: Techniques of Manual Examination, 8th edn. Philadelphia: W.B. Saunders, 2002.

66. *Chiu T, Law E, Chiu T.* Performance of the craniocervical flexion test in subjects with and without chronic neck pain. J Orthop Sports Phys Ther 2005;35:567–571.

67. *Jull G, Barrett C, Magee R, et al.* Further characterisation of muscle dysfunction in cervical headache. Cephalalgia 1999;19:179–185.

68. *Jull G, Trott P, Potter H, et al.* A randomized controlled trial of exercise and manipulative therapy for cervicogenic headache. Spine 2002;27:1835–1843.

69. *Jull G, Sterling M, Kenardy J, et al.* Does the presence of sensory hypersensitivity influence outcomes of physical rehabilitation for chronic whiplash? A preliminary RCT. Pain 2007;129:28–34.

70. *Zito G, Jull G, Story I.* Clinical tests of musculoskeletal dysfunction in the diagnosis of cervicogenic headache. Man Ther 2006;11: 118–129.

71. *Mayoux-Benhamou MA, Revel M, Vallee C, et al.* Longus colli has a postural function on cervical curvature. Surg Radiol Anat 1994;16:367–371.

72. *Jull G, Falla D, Treleaven J, et al.* Retraining cervical joint position sense: the effect of two exercise regimes. J Orthop Res 2007;25:404–412.

73. *Falla D, Campbell C, Fagan A, et al.* Relationship between cranio-cervical flexion range of motion and pressure change during the craniocervical flexion test. Man Ther 2003;8:92–96.

74. *Falla D, Jull G, Hodges P.* Patients with neck pain demonstrate reduced electromyographic activity of the deep cervical flexor muscles during performance of the craniocervical flexion test. Spine 2004;29:2108–2114.

75. *Jull GA.* Deep cervical neck flexor dysfunction in whiplash. J Musculoskel Pain 2000;8:143–154.

76. *Jull G, Kristjansson E, Dall'Alba P.* Impairment in the cervical flexors: a comparison of whiplash and insidious onset neck pain patients. Man Ther 2004;9:89–94.

77. *Cagnie B, Danneels L, Cools A, et al.* The influence of breathing type, expiration and cervical posture on the performance of the craniocervical flexion test in healthy subjects. Man Ther 2008;in press.

78. *O'Leary S, Vicenzino B, Falla D, et al.* Specific therapeutic exercise of the neck induces immediate local hypoalgesia. J Pain 2008;in press.

79. *Evjenth O, Hamberg J.* Muscle Stretching in Manual Therapy. Alfta: Alfta Rehab Forlag, 1984.

80. *Janda V*. Muscles and motor control in cervicogenic disorders: assessment and management. In: Grant R (ed) Physical Therapy of the Cervical and Thoracic Spine. 2nd edn. New York: Churchill Livingstone, 1994:195–216.

81. *Elliott J, Jull G, Noteboom J, et al*. Fatty infiltration in the cervical extensor muscles in persistent whiplash associated disorders (WAD): an MRI analysis. Spine 2006;31:E847–E855.

82. *Elliott J, Jull G, Noteboom T, et al*. MRI study of the cross sectional area for the cervical extensor musculature in patients with persistent whiplash associated disorders (WAD). Man Ther 2008;in press.

83. *Revel M, Andre-Deshays C, Minguet M*. Cervicocephalic kinesthetic sensibility in patients with cervical pain. Arch Phys Med Rehabil 1991;72:288–291.

84. *Loudon JK, Ruhl M, Field E*. Ability to reproduce head position after whiplash injury. Spine 1997;22:865–868.

85. *Kristjansson E, Hardardottir L, Asmundardottir M, et al*. A new clinical test for cervicocephalic kinesthetic sensibility: "the fly". Arch Phys Med Rehabil 2004;85:490–495.

86. *Kristjansson E, Dall'Alba P, Jull G*. A study of five cervicocephalic relocation tests in three different subject groups. Clin Rehabil 2003;17:768–774.

87. *Treleaven J, Jull G, Sterling M*. Dizziness and unsteadiness following whiplash injury – characteristic features and relationship to cervical joint position error. J Rehabil Med 2003;35:36–43.

88. *Shumway-Cook A, Horak F*. Assessing the influence of sensory integration on balance. Phys Ther 1986;66:1548–1550.

89. *Treleaven J, Jull G, LowChoy N*. Standing balance in chronic whiplash – comparison between subjects with and without dizziness. J Rehabil Med 2005;37:219–223.

90. *Field S, Treleaven J, Jull G*. Standing balance: a comparison between idiopathic and whiplash induced neck pain. Man Ther 2008;in press.

91. *Hill K, Bernhardt J, McGann A, et al*. A new test of dynamic standing balance for stroke patients: reliability, validity and comparison with healthy elderly. Physiother Can 1996;48:257–262.

92. *Herdman S*. Vestibular Rehabilitation. Philadelphia: Davis, 2000.

93. *Shumway-Cook A, Baldwin M, Polissar N, et al*. Predicting the probability for falls in community-dwelling older adults. Phys Ther 1997;77:812–819.

94. *Fischer A, Huygen P, Folgering H, et al*. Vestibular hyperreactivity and hyperventilation after whiplash injury. J Neurol Sci 1995;132:35–43.

95. *Tjell C, Rosenhall U*. Smooth pursuit neck torsion test: a specific test for cervical dizziness. Am J Otol 1998;19:76–81.

96. *Hikosaka O, Maeda M*. Cervical effects on abducens motoneurons and their interaction with vestibulo-ocular reflex. Exp Brain Res 1973;18:512–530.

97. *Fischer A, Verhagen W, Huygen P*. Whiplash injury. A clinical review with emphasis on neurootological aspects. Clin Otolaryngol 1997;22:192–201.

98. *Padoan S, Karlberg M, Fransson P, et al*. Passive sustained turning of the head induces asymmetric gain of the vestibulo-ocular reflex in healthy subjects. Acta Otolaryngol 1998;118:778–782.

99. *Halmagyi G, Curthoys I*. Clinical testing of otolith function. Ann NY Acad Sci 1999;871:195–204.

100. *Speers R, Ashton-Miller J, Schultz A, et al*. Age differences in abilities to perform tandem stand and walk tasks of graded difficulty. Gait Posture 1998;7:207–213.

101. *Poole E, Treleaven J, Jull G*. The influence of neck pain on balance and gait parameters in community dwelling elders. Man Ther 2008;in press.

102. *O'Leary S, Falla D, Jull G, et al*. Muscle specificity in tests of cervical flexor muscle performance. J Electromyogr Kinesiol 2007;17:35–40.

103. *O'Leary S, Vicenzino B, Jull G*. A new method of isometric dynamometry for the craniocervical flexors. Phys Ther 2005;85:556–564.

104. *Falla D, Rainoldi A, Merletti R, et al*. Myoelectric manifestations of sternocleidomastoid and anterior scalene muscle fatigue in chronic neck pain patients. Clin Neurophysiol 2003;114:488–495.

105. *O'Leary S, Jull G, Kim M, et al*. Craniocervical flexor muscle impairment at maximal, moderate, and low loads is a feature of neck pain. Man Ther 2007;12:34–39.

106. *Jensen C*. Development of neck and hand–wrist symptoms in relation to duration of computer use at work. Scand J Work Environ Health 2003;29:197–205.

107. *Korhonen T, Ketola R, Toivonen R, et al*. Work related and individual predictors for incident neck pain among office employees working with video display units. Occup Environ Med 2003;60: 475–482.

108. *Johnston V, Jimmieson N, Souvlis T, et al*. Interaction of psychosocial risk factors explain increased neck problems among female office workers. Pain 2007;129:311–320.

109. *Ostergren P, Hanson B, Balogh I, et al*. Incidence of shoulder and neck pain in a working population: effect modification between mechanical and psychosocial exposures at work? Results from a one year follow up of the Malmo shoulder and neck study cohort. J Epidemiol Commun Health 2005;59:721–728.

110. *Szeto G, Straker L, O'Sullivan P*. A comparison of symptomatic and asymptomatic office workers performing monotonous keyboard work – 2: neck and shoulder kinematics. Man Ther 2005;10: 281–291.

111. *Johnston V, Jull G, Souvlis T, et al*. Neck movement and muscle activity characteristics in office workers with neck pain. 2008;in review.

112. *Szeto G, Straker L, O'Sullivan P*. A comparison of symptomatic and asymptomatic office workers performing monotonous keyboard work – 1: neck

and shoulder muscle recruitment patterns. Man Ther 2005;10:270–280.

113. *Falla D, Farina D*. Muscle fiber conduction velocity of the upper trapezius muscle during dynamic contraction of the upper limb in patients with chronic neck pain. Pain 2005;116:138–145.

114. *Fredin Y, Elert J, Britschgi N, et al*. A decreased ability to relax between repetitive contractions in patients with chronic symptoms after trauma of the neck. J Musculoskel Pain 1997;5:55–70.

115. *Veiersted K, Westgaard R, Andersen P*. Electromyographic evaluation of muscular work pattern as a predictor of trapezius myalgia. Scand J Work Environ Health 1993;19:284–290.

# 13

# Principles of Management of Cervical Disorders

## Introduction

The emphasis on evidence-based practice has brought rewards of intensive activity in the investigation of the efficacy of various methods and modalities of treatment for cervical disorders. There have been several systematic reviews within the structure of the pre-eminent Cochrane Collaboration, which have investigated modalities relevant to management of cervical disorders by physical therapies in various populations of neck pain patients. These include the effectiveness of manipulation and mobilization,[1] exercise,[2] cervical traction,[3] massage,[4] electrotherapy,[5] acupuncture,[6] multidisciplinary biopsychosocial management,[7] and conservative treatments for whiplash.[8] Furthermore, clinical practice guidelines have been published for the management of acute neck pain, both idiopathic and whiplash,[9] and chronic whiplash-associated disorders.[10]

Such systematic reviews and clinical practice guidelines provide the general evidence-based directions for management. Nevertheless, they reflect flaws in the randomized clinical trials (RCT) which are relevant to the clinical setting. The RCTs often do not consider the heterogeneity of neck disorders and thus assume a certain treatment will have responsiveness across the generic population studied. In the broadest context, RCTs may only have subclassified neck disorders by: time course – acute, subacute, and chronic disorders; pain area – neck pain, neck and arm pain, headache; pathoanatomically – nonspecific neck pain or cervical radiculopathy; or mode of onset – idiopathic or traumatic (e.g., whiplash). These subclassifications have inherent inadequacies and again do not reflect the variety of possible patient presentations even within these subclassifications, as demonstrated, for example, with both acute and chronic whiplash cohorts.[11, 12] Furthermore, while providing general evidence-based directions for management, they do not direct precise interventions for the presentation of an individual patient in the clinical setting. This has changed directions and stimulated research into new methods of classification for neck disorders. Physiotherapists have begun to investigate other ways that neck pain might be classified. These studies have been based largely on presenting clinical features and physical impairments either to determine better the types of interventions or to predict likely treatment outcomes.[13-17] Calls have been made for changes in future RCT designs to replicate better the clinical situation, taking into consideration the heterogeneity of the condition and the pragmatic nature of intervention prescription that occurs in "real-world" clinical practice.

In the clinical setting, treatment decisions are made in accordance with the principles of evidence-based practice, as ascribed by Sackett et al.[18] Treatment decisions represent an integration of three basic components: (1) the clinical expertise of the practitioner; (2) guidance from the best available evidence from systematic research; and, notably, (3) the individual patient's circumstances. The weight of evidence from systematic reviews favors multimodal management for the treatment of patients with neck disorders. This is not surprising given the evidence from an increasing volume of research into the nature and extent of the impairments in the various systems in cervical musculoskeletal disorders. It would be naive to believe that a single system or modality approach could be a "cure-all" and contemporary evidence has dismissed this notion.

Within an evidence-based framework in clinical practice, the precise management is guided by the presentation of the individual patient. This takes into consideration the specific impairments in the sensory, motor, and psychological systems gained from the history, interview, and physical examination. It also considers any relevant psychosocial circumstances as well as the patient's past experiences, attitudes, and beliefs. In line with the heterogeneous nature of neck disorders, patient presentations vary from uncomplicated neck pain disorders to complex and multifaceted pain syndromes. Management thus varies from being relatively straightforward, offered by a single practitioner, to being very challenging, often requiring a multiprofessional approach.

This chapter will address the management of cervical disorders by addressing principles of treatment based on current knowledge of the disorders in the various systems, rather than detail specific techniques. There are several manual therapy texts dedicated to describing treatment approaches to the articular and neural systems to which the reader is referred.[19-25] The clinical application of an exercise program for cervical disorders based on our and others' research into the impairments in the motor system and in sensorimotor control will be described in detail in the following chapter.

# The patient

The patient is the central figure in management. It is vital that patients understand their neck pain condition and participate in their recovery towards a normal, usual, or, in some circumstances, modified functional status as established mutually in the goals for their treatment. Thus explanations of the condition, assurance, and education are pivotal to good management. Such education and explanations are offered throughout the management period and rapport with the patient should encourage questions and, as is often needed, repetition of the education.

The advice, explanations, and education will vary from patient to patient depending on the type and nature of the presenting disorder. It is paramount that patients are provided with a general lay explanation of their condition in basic pathoanatomical terms. In cases of noncomplex neck disorders this could be as simple as an explanation of a neck joint strain. Understanding is often facilitated if an analogy with an extremity joint is used as patients can then visualize the condition more readily. Clinicians should steer away from discipline-specific terminology and especially jargon in providing this information; jargon may be more alarming to the patient than educative. Viewing and explaining the significance of X-ray findings can be reassuring, in either the presence or absence of imageable changes. Assuring the patient that the condition is not sinister, that it is musculoskeletal in origin, and that neck pain in general has a good prognosis for recovery will often help allay anxieties.

At the other extreme, patients may present with a more complex pain syndrome in either the acute or chronic state. Education about pain physiology is warranted in association with other advice. Moseley et al.[26] have shown, albeit in patients with low-back pain, that such education is more beneficial than traditional anatomy and physiology education in outcome measures of pain attitudes and catastrophizing as well as physical performance tasks. Of note from the rehabilitation perspective, such education did not result in meaningful change in self-reported disability. Understanding the possible mechanisms of pain, both peripheral and central, the role of augmented central pain processing, and the influence of the several levels of the central nervous system on the perception and control of pain can not only assure the patient, but can also assist in providing the rationale for treatment methods as well as the rationale for patient's conduct of

self-management strategies and activities of daily living.

It is quite reasonable and normal, although not inevitable, for a patient to have some level of anxiety, depression, or frustration in association with neck pain. The presence and magnitude of these reactions often relate to the magnitude of the disorder, its acuteness or chronicity, and the impact that the neck pain is having on work and quality of life (Chapter 7). In the case of a whiplash injury, there is also the element of blame if the patient was not at fault in the car crash. Patients may exhibit other psychological features in association with general distress, such as fear avoidance behaviors or posttraumatic stress symptoms in the case of whiplash. The clinician is well placed in a physical therapy environment to recognize these features and to provide assurance and education to lessen these anxieties and modify behaviors. In addition, many of these features will lessen or resolve as pain is relieved and function restored.[11, 27, 28] The exception could be posttraumatic stress symptoms associated with a whiplash injury. As shown by Sterling et al.,[29, 30] there is not always resolution of these symptoms with time and they are one of the collection of features predictive of a poorer long-term prognosis. Questionnaires can be used to gain some quantification of this and other behaviors. If any such psychological features do not change in line with decreasing symptoms or their presence is not facilitating recovery, then referral to a health psychologist may be needed for expert assistance in a multiprofessional approach to the management plan.

## Management of pain

Pain is usually the main reason that patients seek assistance for the management of their neck disorders. Current knowledge of pain processes (Chapter 2) and particularly those inherent in the patient's presentation influence the application of all interventions. As an overall guiding principle, no physical therapy intervention should provoke neck pain or any other symptoms. This is absolutely essential in the suspected presence of augmented processing of nociceptive information. Further provocation will aggravate the pain syndrome. This does not mean that treatment is necessarily withheld or minimized, but it does mean that appropriate interventions have to be applied in a manner that does not provoke pain. Any prescribed self-management programs should likewise not provoke pain.

It is essential that the patient has adequate pharmaceutical pain management. Medication may not be required in more minor pain syndromes. However, medication should be considered in acute pain states, in syndromes with moderate or severe pain, and particularly in syndromes where a neuropathic pain state is suspected. Pain management should be discussed with the patient's medical practitioner. Rehabilitation may proceed more effectively if the patient has effective pain management.

Many of the physical therapy methods used in the rehabilitation process have a proven pain-relieving effect. The evidence for these modalities should be discussed with the patient in management planning.

## Manipulative therapy

Possibly the major benefit derived from manipulative therapy procedures is their effect on pain. Clinical trials have demonstrated that manipulative therapy can decrease neck pain, albeit a better effect is achieved when therapy is combined with exercise.[1] There has also been increasing research into the physiological mechanisms of the effect of manipulative therapy. It is likely that manipulative therapy procedures act on multiple levels of the central nervous system to effect changes in several systems

(sensory, motor, and sympathetic nervous systems) to achieve their analgesic effects.[31-35]

Historically there have been various manipulative therapy approaches but the results from recent clinical trials which tested manipulative therapy for neck disorders would suggest that the various methods achieve comparable outcomes.[36-38] In tandem, laboratory studies, which have in common investigated sympathoexcitatory effect, have shown a similarity in effect of various mobilization techniques.[35, 39, 40] Thus it would seem that the critical variable may be the local movement applied to the symptomatic segment and surrounding structures to achieve the effect, rather than necessarily the particular technique itself. Nevertheless Bolton and Budgell[41] have recently proposed a hypothesis which suggests that there could be differences in neural mechanisms of effect of joint manipulation and mobilization, with manipulation more likely stimulating receptors in the deep segmental muscles and mobilization the more superficial axial muscles. Further research will uphold or reject this hypothesis, but at present, there is no convincing evidence of any difference in effect of the two treatment technique categories.[42]

## Exercise

Therapeutic exercise has likewise been shown to have a pain-relieving effect for neck pain in both the short and long term, especially in combination with manipulative therapy. In a systematic review of Kay et al.,[2] the evidence for relief of neck pain with exercise was derived from studies of programs using low-load exercises directed at improvement in motor control, strengthening programs, as well as those addressing sensorimotor function. Thus all exercise programs may have beneficial effects on pain, but other circumstances may dictate the suitability of different modes of exercise at various stages of the patient's cervical disorder. In prescribing exercise, the clinician must consider the patient's pain levels and mechanisms, as premature introduction of high-load strengthening exercise may be pain-provocative rather than relieving. In addition, some exercises appear to have some specificity of effect. A recent study found that specific low-load training of the deep craniocervical flexors had an immediate local mechanical hypoalgesic effect on the painful zygapophyseal joint in patients with neck pain, an effect not achieved with a higher-load head lift exercise.[43] Furthermore, a 6-week program with a focus on low-load training of the craniocervical flexors for cervicogenic headache patients demonstrated a postintervention as well as a long-term (12-month follow-up) reduction in palpable tenderness of symptomatic upper cervical joints, indicating a positive cumulative local response to this exercise regime which also translated to a reduction of neck pain and headache.[37] Interestingly, O'Leary et al.[43] found that, whereas the specific low-load training of the deep craniocervical flexors had mechanical hypoalgesic effects, it had no sympathoexcitatory effect. This may reflect some differences in mechanisms of effect of manipulative therapies and specific low-load exercise, which may be one of the reasons for their complementarity.

It has also been shown that general modes of exercise, including aerobic exercise, have a systemic analgesic effect.[44] Thus neck pain patients should be encouraged to undertake general activity such as a walking program which would be nonprovocative of neck pain. This is beneficial not only for their general well-being, but also in its overall contribution to pain management. There is certainly evidence that maintaining activity rather than resting is more beneficial for neck pain disorders.[9] Thus exercise should

be prescribed and encouraged at local, regional, and general levels.

## Electrophysical agents

There is no convincing evidence for the effect of electrophysical agents for the management of neck pain,[5] although there is some evidence for pain relief with acupuncture when measured in the short term.[6] This directs against an electrotherapy-focused management program for neck pain. Nevertheless, clinical experience would support the judicious use of a thermal or electrophysical agent as an adjunct therapy in a multimodal management plan. However, there is clearly a need for more carefully planned research to assess the use of electrophysical agents in this adjunct role in the management of neck pain.

# Management of the articular system

Regional movement loss and locally painful segmental movement abnormalities are characteristic of mechanical neck disorders,[45-51] and are sequelae of injury, adverse strain, or degenerative disease.[46, 51-53] Both manipulative therapy and active exercise are management strategies used to address these movement impairments. They are applied with the dual purpose of improving the range of movement and function as well as improving the pain state. As the evidence indicates, it is the use of manipulative therapy in conjunction with therapeutic exercise that has most effectiveness for the management of neck pain.[1]

## Manipulative therapy

The selection of a manipulative therapy technique evolves from the information gained about the nature and direction of the movement dysfunction in the physical examination, taking equally into consideration the nature, behavior, and severity of the patient's pain. Technique modification and progression are guided by the process of constant evaluation of effect as well as the change in the patient's pain and movement signs.[23] As mentioned previously, history has seen the development of various manipulative therapy approaches,[20-24] most of which have been used in various RCTs contributing to the evidence of effectiveness of manipulative therapy as part of a multimodal program. Treatment movements may be performed passively by the clinician or passively with an active contribution from the patient. Contemporary practice takes advantages of knowledge and skills from all approaches and selects the most appropriate techniques for the presenting patient.

Treatment is applied to the local region of segmental dysfunction and to other regions that may have a contributory role. For instance, segmental hypomobility is not uncommonly found in the cervicothoracic region, whose movement normally contributes to total head excursion (Figure 13.1). Repeated and skilled examination of the cervical and upper thoracic spinal segments and ribs should be conducted during the treatment process. Muscle guarding in the initial assessment may augment or mask segmental dysfunction and there will be changes in response to treatment which need to be monitored consistently for efficient application and progression of technique.

Due care is taken not to provoke the patient's symptoms, especially in cases of acute or moderate to severe pain. We would signal particular care and caution with all whiplash patients, but especially those with generalized hypersensitivity, which can be present in both the acute and chronic state. Pain of a confirmed or suspected neuropathic origin or symptoms of paresthesia or anesthesia, whether of traumatic or insidious

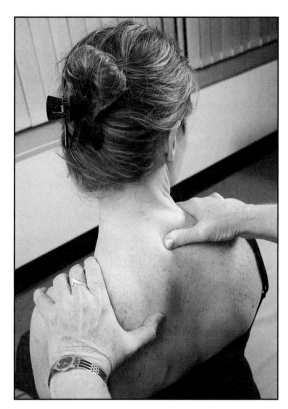

**Figure 13.1** Mobilization of the upper thoracic joints with a transverse glide to the thoracic spinous process while the patient actively rotates the cervical spine to augment the effect of the glide to restore thoracic segmental rotation.

onset, should not be reproduced by any treatment technique. Likewise provocation of cervicogenic headache with treatment to the upper cervical region should be avoided, as should any symptoms of dizziness.

In cases of trauma-induced neck pain, due care should be taken with the type of manipulative therapy technique from a pathoanatomical perspective. There is no certainty of the nature and extent of the underlying structural damage and little assistance is gained from results of radiological imaging or clinical tests of ligamentous instability (Chapters 3 and 12). The term "clinical instability," as proposed by Panjabi et al.,[54] reflects a broader definition than osseoligamentous instability, and encompasses insufficiencies in the articular and muscle systems and their neural control. The theory is well understood and is supported by a large volume of biomechanical and neurophysiological research. In relation to the articular system, minor segmental instabilities may occur with loss of control or increased neutral-zone movements. Consensus-based studies have been undertaken to provide groupings of symptoms and signs potentially indicative of a cervical clinical instability syndrome.[55, 56] However, in the absence of any gold-standard diagnostic method, it is difficult to determine the sensitivity and specificity of these proposed clinical patterns. Cases of suspected compromise of the ligamentous integrity of a cervical segment joint complex would direct the clinician's attention to rehabilitation of motor control.

The contemporary debate is the use or not of high-velocity manipulative thrust techniques in the cervical region where there are risks, albeit probably small, of serious or dire adverse events. Most notable among these is trauma to the vertebral artery with the risk of stroke or even death.[57] Incidences of rupture of cervical disks have also been reported with cervical manipulation.[58] Protagonists for the continued use of high-velocity thrust techniques strongly argue the relative risk of cervical manipulation[59, 60] but equally as strongly, others can find no justification for their use.[61] The true risk rate is uncertain.[42] Although there has been little comparative research of the relative clinical effectiveness of cervical mobilization versus manipulation, the available evidence suggests that both techniques seem to have similar effects.[42] Practice trends point to a preference, although not exclusive use, of cervical joint mobilization by Australian physiotherapists at least. In a clinical trial of the management of cervicogenic headache, practitioners were free to choose to use either mobilization or manipulation techniques.[62] In offering 1090 treatments to 100 subjects, clinicians chose to use cervical joint mobilization only, in 77.6% of treatments. In recognition of the risk of cervical manipulation, Cleland et al.[63] in the USA undertook preliminary investigations of the effect of the safer option of thoracic manipulation for neck pain. They demonstrated immediate effects on the perceived pain level in the cervical region. Thus the need for and use of cervical manipulation in the future is somewhat uncertain and will not be resolved until there is more dedicated comparative research. Certainly the use of cervical manipulation in practice should be guided by definitive indications, patient consent, coupled with the absence of any symptoms and signs suggestive of the presence of any contraindications. Regarding the necessity for an X-ray prior to performing a manipulation, Maigne et al.[64] found a lack of data in a literature review to link radiological signs with complications following cervical manipulation, but suggested it was wise for a patient to have premanipulative X-rays on the basis of due care and medicolegal issues.

## Active exercise for range of movement

Active exercise is an essential element of rehabilitation to restore regional and segmental range of cervical movement. Considering regional exercise, range-of-movement exercises can be preformed in sitting or, in cases when acute pain is limiting movement, exercises may be performed in the four-point kneeling position. This latter position appears to allow more comfortable performance of flexion/extension and rotation ranges of motion. The reason for this difference in performance in the sitting and four-point kneeling positions is not certain. Logic could point to the relative relief of the compressive axial loads of gravity and head weight on the joints in conjunction with the support afforded by the stronger extensor muscle group during their concentric and eccentric actions in the sagittal plane in the four-point kneeling position. Again, advantage should be taken of the central and reflex connections between the visual system and neck muscles[65, 66] and all exercises should be performed with the patient looking first in the direction of the movement.

Studies have shown that a gain in range of movement occurs immediately after a manipulative therapy procedure,[67, 68] but Nansel et al.[68] showed that the gain can be lost within 48 hours. Rather than view this occurrence negatively, the clinician should capitalize on the increased motion gained immediately after manipulative therapy procedures, with reinforcement through active exercise. Indeed, Dishman and Bourke[31] found that a manipulation led to transient suppression of motor neuron excitability, which from a clinical perspective would facilitate active range-of-movement exercise in the presence of muscle relaxation immediately following the procedure.

Active movement exercises should be focused to the segmental level and direction of movement restriction. This precision in active mobilization reinforces that used in applying segmental manipulative therapy techniques. Patients can be taught to palpate a segmental level with their finger tips to localize the movement (Figure 13.2) or alternately assistive straps can be used to apply a self-assisted mobilization with movement technique, as described by Mulligan (Figure 13.3).[24, 69] Active exercise can be focused on cervical regions. Craniocervical flexion and extension are mobilized with a chin lift and nodding exercise in sitting or four-point kneeling position. Craniocervical rotation (C1–2) is emphasized by rotating the head in a preflexed position of the cervicothoracic spine in sitting or supine lying.[70, 71] Full rotation of the head induces an ipsilateral rotation down to the T2–3 segments and full arm elevation in the scapular plane has been

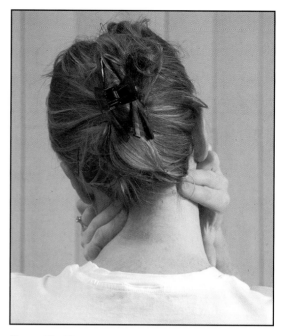

**Figure 13.2** The patient localizes a lateral flexion self-mobilization technique to the C2–3 level by palpating/fixing the C3 segment.

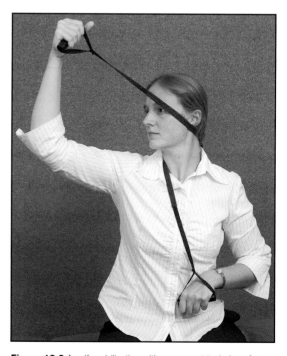

**Figure 13.3** A self-mobilization with movement technique for the C1–2 segment.[69]

shown to induce ipsilateral rotation and lateral flexion in the upper thoracic segments.[72] Thus a suitable active exercise for this often hypomobile cervicothoracic region combines head rotation and arm elevation. As a principle, the clinician should design the active exercise to replicate the segmental precision used in joint positioning and movement in the passive mobilization technique. If, for instance, the clinician has progressed a lateral flexion segmental passive mobilization technique by prepositioning the joint in some extension towards achieving a full range of extension and medial facet glide, the active segmental lateral flexion technique for home practice is similarly progressed and performed with the joint preplaced in some extension.

## Management of the neural system

Involvement of the nervous system in presentation of cervicobrachial pain may present as an overt cervical radiculopathy, more covertly as possible minor nerve injury or as irritated or sensitized nerve tissue (Chapter 10). The C2 nerve or greater occipital nerve may exhibit allodynia in cases of cervicogenic headache. One overriding principle is that treatment applied should be nonprovocative of pain or any other symptoms, not only with respect to the nerve tissue itself but with respect to the possible sensory hyperalgesia and allodynia that may be present in the patient's pain syndrome. In instances of neuropathic pain, it is likely that the patient requires adequate pharmacological management in addition to any physical therapy intervention. Furthermore, in cases of cervical radiculopathy, neurological signs must be carefully monitored and any deterioration in signs or symptoms or nonresponsiveness to management may warrant a surgical review.

There are several passive mobilization techniques that can potentially be used in the management of cervicobrachial pain of a known or suspected neuropathic origin. From an anatomical perspective, the historic rule that any technique selected should not compromise the size of the intervertebral foramen in treating a patient with a cervical radiculopathy still has merit. A specific technique for the management of cervicobrachial pain, the cervical lateral glide technique, has been described.[73, 74] There have been some initial clinical studies showing positive results into the effectiveness of the cervical lateral glide technique (Figure 13.4) for cervicobrachial pain.[75-78] However, there is an urgent need for full-scale clinical trials before its effectiveness can be truly evaluated.

Cervical traction has been used historically in cases of cervical radiculopathy. However a recent systematic review[3] found it was difficult to provide definitive evidence for the use of cervical traction due to the low quality of the trials. There were suggestions of benefit for intermittent cervical traction. Low-quality case series propose the benefits of cervical traction for acute cases of cervical radiculopathy (< 12 weeks).[79-81] It is clear that there is a need for clinical trials of

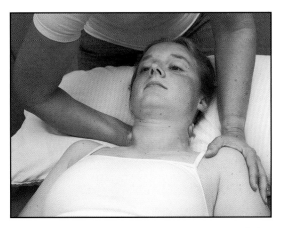

**Figure 13.4** The cervical contralateral glide technique applied to the C5–6 segment. The position of shoulder girdle is supported. The glide is performed contralaterally to the side of pain.

management methods specifically for patients with cervical radiculopathy to support (or not) the use of cervical traction.

Nerve tissues may exhibit mechano-sensitivity – local tenderness over nerve trunks and pain in response to neck or limb movements that cause nerve stretch, which is deduced from a pattern of clinical signs and responses to the brachial plexus provocation test (Chapter 10). Clinicians within physiotherapy have introduced systems of movement-based treatment that have been evolving over the past two to three decades, to address neural tissue mechanosensitivity, and the reader is referred to such sources.[19, 25, 82, 83] Movement combinations and sequences of upper-limb and neck movement are used to move or slide the nerve and nerve bed gently. The physiological effects of these techniques have been promoted and there is evidence emerging that sliding techniques induce more movement but less strain on the nerve than movement sequences which tension the nerve.[84] This would indicate their use rather than any tensioning technique in states of nerve mechanosensitivity to avert the risk of spontaneous ectopic activity from a nerve trunk which may be affected by inflammation and worsening of symptoms (Chapter 10). Highly responsive inflamed nerve fibers have been shown to fire with as little as 3% stretch, which is within the range of nerve stretch seen during normal limb movements.[85] Movement sequencing techniques can be used as primary treatments or they may be used in conjunction with passive mobilization techniques. Use of, and purported success with, these techniques in clinical practice for cervicobrachial pain far outstrips their evidence base, again pointing to the need for more dedicated clinical trials to establish their role and efficacy.

Nevertheless, there is no question that the nerve tissues can become mechanosensitive and contribute in greater or lesser part to a cervical pain syndrome. Care must be taken with all joint and nerve tissue mobilization and other exercise techniques in their presence. For example, scapular muscle and craniocervical flexor training may have to be modified in the presence of mechanosensitive nerve tissues as these techniques may place undue strain on mechanosensitive neural structures and be pain-provocative. Equally important is to recognize a potentially false-positive brachial plexus provocation test, as was observed in our study of chronic whiplash.[86] Here these subjects demonstrated a bilateral loss of elbow extension irrespective of whether they reported the presence or not of arm pain. Such nonspecific responses may reflect hypersensitive flexor withdrawal responses as a consequence of central nervous system sensitization (Chapter 10), in which case nerve tissue mobilization techniques would not be indicated.

## Management of the muscle system

Impairment in cervical muscle function is an inevitable consequence of pain and joint injury/pathology, as is readily observed in extremity joints. Furthermore, there is no evidence that there is spontaneous recovery of normal function with alleviation of pain. Quite the converse, we have shown that impairment in cervical muscle function can persist despite the alleviation of symptoms.[37, 87] It is known that neck pain tends to be a persistent and recurrent disorder and up to 60% of persons can expect some degree of ongoing pain for many years after their first episode.[88] The challenge for those involved in rehabilitation is to lessen this transition to recurrent or persistent pain to allow people who have had an episode of neck pain to resume their normal activities and enjoy quality of life. Rehabilitation of muscle system to restore adequate support and control to the cervical spine can logically make a significant contribution to this aim.

Muscles react immediately to pain and injury. Thus rehabilitation of the muscle system assumes a prominent place from the outset in the management of patients with neck disorders. The impairments in cervical muscle function are diverse and wide-ranging and there is evidence for specificity in exercise prescription to address the precise impairments (Chapter 4). As indicated, a full description of the clinical application of an exercise approach for cervical disorders, which aims to address the impairments identified in research in association with neck pain, will be presented in the following chapter.

## Management of disturbances in sensorimotor control

Disturbances in cervical kinesthetic awareness, eye movement control, and balance can occur in association with cervical disorders and can contribute to, or be the basis for, a myriad of symptoms (Chapter 6). There is again some evidence from studies of whiplash indicating that disturbances occur early after the onset of neck pain (Chapter 6), warranting early consideration in a rehabilitation program. It has been proposed that these changes reflect disturbances in afferent signals emanating from cervical mechanoreceptors. Thus management of these changes in sensorimotor control may need to address not only the possible causes of abnormal cervical afferent input and their effects on the visual and vestibular systems, but also any secondary adaptive changes in, for example, the vestibular system. A combination of therapies that address the pain and enhance muscle function as well as specific exercises for sensorimotor control is likely to be most beneficial in management due to their overlapping benefits.

Improvements, for example, in joint position sense and pain have been demonstrated with manipulative therapy,[89-91] specific muscle training,[92] as well as the more traditional programs that have trained cervical joint position sense, eye–head coordination and gaze stability.[92, 93] Collectively these treatment methods could address changes in sensorimotor control as well as the underlying cause of these disturbances when abnormal cervical afferent input is in conflict with vestibular and ocular input. However, more extensive research is needed to determine the most effective methods of management of these disturbances in patients with neck pain. The rehabilitation approach will likewise be discussed in the following chapter.

## Work and lifestyle practices

Prevention of adverse strain to the neck inherent in work or lifestyle practices and optimization of the work or home environment are very vital components of management of neck disorders. Clinicians are well versed in fundamental ergonomic principles and can advise patients on such aspects as office design, workstation set-ups, optimal chair configurations, bench heights, or other factors as relevant to the patient's work or lifestyle practices. It may be appropriate to recommend a formal worksite assessment from those specialized in the field. There is also the human factor and how the person functions even within the best-designed workplace. Discussion here will focus on rehabilitation and preventive strategies that are focused on the patient's contribution to better work and lifestyle practices.

Education is of paramount importance in changing or modifying work or lifestyle habits and practices. The evidence should be clearly provided and, when possible, a practical demonstration provided of the relationship between a certain activity, strain on cervical structures, and pain. Patients must be encouraged to recognize provocative work or lifestyle practices and, importantly, those that they can perform comfortably without neck pain. They are helped to recognize the poor and good elements of these practices in relation to strain or symptom provocation in the learning process. The clinician should be alert to discrepancies between what patients believe is supposed to be a good posture, good exercise, good pillow or sleeping position and what in reality might be more beneficial for their condition. Patients must gain a good understanding of the consequences of repeated adverse and unnecessary strain on neck structures for current and long-term prognoses. They must understand their role and responsibilities in training new work or lifestyle habits in the management of their condition and prevention of any future recurrence.

Several physical features have been associated with the report of neck, neck and arm pain, or cervicogenic headache with computer use both at work and at home, for example, the tendency for those with neck pain to drift into a more forward head posture with computer work.[94–96] Hence patients should be taught to position themselves well in the chair to limit this occurrence but at regular intervals actively to assume an upright neutral spinal posture which they initiate from the pelvis (Chapter 14). They should aim to hold this position for at least 10–15 seconds either while continuing to work or in a mini-pause break. This change in position not only relieves structures from static strain but will also activate the deep flexor supporting musculature of the cervical curve.[97] The postural correction exercise should be performed approximately every 15 minutes, as it is known that it only takes a few minutes of work for the posture to begin to slump.[94] We find repetitive practice throughout the

day is better tolerated by patients rather than asking them to try to hold a neutral posture permanently, which results in fatigue and quick abandonment of the exercise. With repetitive practice, patients usually develop a new sense of a better working posture as well as developing postural holding endurance.

Improvement of the control of head postural position also occurs as the activation capacity and tonic endurance capacity of deep neck flexors are trained with more formal therapeutic exercise.[94] Patients need reminders to assume the neutral upright postural position in the initial stages of training. The cue could be in the form of an alarm preset into the computer or watch, or the correction exercise could be performed in conjunction with a repetitive activity in the day, for example, answering the telephone. A flexed or forward-head working posture is not restricted to computer workers, but occurs with many occupations. The principles of repeatedly relieving static strain and activating postural supporting muscles are applied in a way relevant to the patient's occupation or activity. This is an important principle as it has been shown that force variations (that is, variability in task performance) result in less muscle fatigue and redistribution of muscle activity compared to a static task/contraction.[98]

It is also known that computer or desk workers with neck pain exhibit altered activation of the superficial neck extensor, flexor and upper trapezius muscles.[99, 100] An altered motor pattern between the deep and superficial cervical flexors has been demonstrated in the craniocervical flexion test[101] and formal training of the deep neck flexors results in a desired reduction in activity of the superficial flexors.[11] However this reduction in activity does not appear to translate automatically to functional tasks in sitting.[102] This would reinforce the need for task-specific training of the deep cervical muscles. It is possible that this could be achieved with repeated activation of deep neck flexors in the frequent correction to the upright neutral spinal postural position during the working day. However it is yet to be shown if this postural correction exercise decreases the activity of the superficial flexors during functional tasks such as typing.

Pain in the regions of the upper trapezius and insertion of the levator scapulae is commonly reported in association with office work and other process workers. Szeto et al.[96] showed that there was a subtle change in scapular position to a more protracted position during computer work in those with neck pain. There has been extensive study of the myoelectric activity of upper trapezius in association with office work and computer use. For example, it has been shown that the upper trapezius exhibits a decreased ability to relax, reduced muscle rest periods during repetitive tasks, and is susceptible to increased activity during tasks involving mental demand (Chapter 4). There are several therapeutic strategies that can be employed in an effort to address the problem in scapular control and upper trapezius function. Scapular muscles and postural positioning of the scapulae need to be trained for functional demands. Exercise also includes specific task-based training so that patients can maintain postures and function with muscle patterns comparable to their asymptomatic counterparts (Chapter 14). The task-specific training is incorporated in the workplace. For example, the patient is taught to activate scapular muscles and correct scapular posture in association with the repeated corrections to the upright neutral spinal postural position during the working day. This positioning often leads to a palpable reduction in tenderness and relaxation of the levator scapulae and/or upper trapezius.

There are many other workplace variables, both physical and psychosocial, which may contribute to the development of neck pain in the workplace. The clinician must work with patients to identify these and help them to modify how they may perform functional tasks to avoid unnecessary strain or aggravation of their neck or cervicobrachial pain. This also applies to recreational and household activities. Much of the advice is seemingly common sense, but strategies might not have occurred to patients and should be reinforced. Such strategies can assist patients to continue their normal activities with simple adaptations. For instance, they should be advised to choose a center seat at theaters or at dinner parties to avoid prolonged sustained rotation positions and taught good lifting and carrying practices, including limiting the weight carried. This applies to the weight of shopping bags, handbags, briefcases, or hand luggage. Household activities such as cleaning tasks or gardening can be spread out over days or tasks rotated frequently between lighter and heavier ones. Patients' individual circumstances need to be understood and identified to assist them to develop strategies that allow them to maintain their functional activities without unnecessarily adversely straining their necks.

## Self-management strategies

Successful long-term outcomes rely on active participation of the patient in their management. As discussed in the various sections of this chapter, all aspects of treatment are complemented with a home program of exercise. This is essential to achieve treatment aims of pain relief, improvement in segmental and regional movement, muscle performance and, most importantly, enhanced function. Exercises and advice with regard to modifications to work or lifestyle activities should be given to the patient in writing as accurate recall of specifics of exercise or advice cannot be relied upon. Preferably a personally written exercise program should be provided to patients as words or descriptions that they understand will better cue them to the exercise. Home programs must be reviewed and progressed regularly in line with the change in the patient's condition and the progression of exercise and manual therapy procedures. At discharge, the patient should have a realistic program to continue with in the long term for maintenance, as well as self-management strategies in the event of any sign of renewed onset of neck pain.

Compliance with exercise programs as well as with modifications to work and lifestyle practices depends on the patient having a full understanding of their relevance and need in the rehabilitation process. In cases of noncompliance, a change in teaching and communication strategies may reverse this undesirable situation.

## Outcome evaluation

Evaluation of outcomes is a continuous process throughout the management period and it directs treatment and its progression. Several outcomes are monitored. The first is the change in the functional status and reported pain levels which is important to the patient, and indeed the clinician, for it justifies the continuance of the management approach or points to the need for reflection, re-evaluation, and modification of the management program. The second is the patient's compliance with the self-management program. Priority in questioning about the self-management strategies in follow-up treatments transmits to the patient the importance the clinician places on them in the overall management plan. The inclusion early in follow-up interviews of questions such as "what cues are you using for the postural correction at work?" or "when in the day has been the better time for the formal exercises?" inform both the clinician and patient. The third is the assessment of the change in the measures of physical impairments in the sensory, articular, muscle, and nervous systems as relevant to the patient's presenting condition. Such re-evaluations inform the clinician in continuous planning for their outcomes and direct changes in or progression of specific treatment components. Positive relationships have been shown between self-reported pain and disability levels and magnitude of physical impairments in neck pain disorders.[12, 99, 103] This is regardless of its traumatic or insidious onset or the involvement or not of third-party payers. Thus there should be some consistency between changes in self-reports and physical signs. Appropriate outcome tools have been discussed (Chapter 11) and formal questionnaires should be used at a frequency appropriate to the acuteness or chronicity of the patient's condition.

Considering outcomes raises questions regarding what outcomes should be expected and how long treatment should be provided by the practitioner. These are difficult questions to answer on an evidence base, for there has been little research which has examined treatment "dosage" in any depth in the management of neck disorders. As a consequence, many clinical trials have arbitrarily chosen a length of intervention which can vary from 2 to 10–12 weeks, which does not inform clinical practice for individual patients. In addition, patient response rates can be expected to vary according to the time course of the disorder, the likely magnitude of the pathology/injury, the underlying mechanism of pain, as well as other physical and psychosocial issues.

Rules of thumb for the clinic would suggest that treatment should cease once self-reported pain and disability scores are within normal limits, or when such scores have failed to change, indicating no further beneficial effect of management. However, while these rules are acceptable, especially on a cost basis, they could be challenged from various perspectives, especially if a rehabilitation aim is to prevent further recurrence of pain, the source of the major financial burden of musculoskeletal pain. For example, how long does it take to effect change or reversal of the neuromuscular adaptations found in association with neck pain to restore normal muscle function and support to the spine? There are many such questions that cannot be answered at this time. Pain may be alleviated relatively quickly, but it would seem reasonable that a rehabilitation process would take 6–8 weeks for many and up to 12 weeks or longer for some. Treatment dosage with current knowledge must be guided by the changes in outcome measures of functional and physical impairment, respecting cost.

Resolution of pain and physical impairments is an ideal. Resolution of pain but persistence of some physical impairment signals the need for the patient to continue to progress exercise with possible intermittent follow-up with the clinician. Lack of change or lack of further change in pain and physical function may signal that the practitioner's skills have been exhausted and it is timely to refer the patient to a more specialist clinician in the field or another clinician of a different discipline. Conversely, it may signal the need for the patient to accept some pain and modification of lifestyle and this should be thoroughly discussed with and acknowledged by the patient, to prevent the patient boarding the very costly traditional or complementary medical merry-go-round.

# References

1. *Gross A, Hoving J, Haines T, et al.* A Cochrane review of manipulation and mobilization for mechanical neck disorders. Spine 2004;29: 1541–1548.

2. *Kay T, Gross A, Goldsmith C, et al.* Exercises for mechanical neck disorders. Cochrane Database Syst Rev 2005;3:CD004250.

3. *Graham N, Gross A, Goldsmith C.* Mechanical traction for mechanical neck disorders: a systematic review. J Rehabil Med 2006;38:145–152.

4. *Haraldsson B, Gross A, Myers C, et al.* Massage for mechanical neck disorders. Cochrane Database Syst Rev 2006;3:CD004871.

5. *Kroeling P, Gross A, Goldsmith C.* A Cochrane review of electrotherapy for mechanical neck disorders. Spine 2005;30:E641–E648.

6. *Trinh K, Gross A, Goldsmith C, et al.* Acupuncture for neck disorders. Cochrane Database Syst Rev 2006;3:CD004870.

7. *Karjalainen K, Malmivaara A, van Tulder M, et al.* Multidisciplinary biopsychosocial rehabilitation for neck and shoulder pain among working age adults. Cochrane Database Syst Rev 2003;2:CD002194.

8. *Verhagen A, Peeters G, de Bie R, et al.* Conservative treatments for whiplash. Cochrane Database Syst Rev 2004;1:CD003338.

9. *Australian Acute Musculoskeletal Pain Guidelines Group.* Evidence Based Management of Acute Musculoskeletal Pain. Brisbane: Australian Academic Press, 2004.

10. *Scholten-Peeters G, Bekkering G, Verhagen A, et al.* Clinical practice guideline for the physiotherapy of patients with whiplash-associated disorders. Spine 2002;27:412–422.

11. *Jull G, Sterling M, Kenardy J, et al.* Does the presence of sensory hypersensitivity influence outcomes of physical rehabilitation for chronic whiplash? A preliminary RCT. Pain 2007; 129:28–34.

12. *Sterling M, Jull G, Vicenzino B, et al.* Characterisation of acute whiplash associated disorders. Spine 2004;29:182–188.

13. *Childs J, Fritz J, Piva S, et al.* Proposal of a classification system for patients with neck pain. J Orthop Sports Phys Ther 2004;34: 686–696.

14. *Clair D, Edmondston S, Allison G.* Physical therapy treatment dose for nontraumatic neck pain: a comparison between 2 patient groups. J Orthop Sports Phys Ther 2006;36:867–875.

15. *Clare H, Adams R, Maher C.* Reliability of McKenzie classification of patients with cervical or lumbar pain. J Manipul Physiol Ther 2005;28: 122–127.

16. *Jull G, Stanton W.* Predictors of responsiveness to physiotherapy treatment of cervicogenic headache. Cephalalgia 2005;25:101–108.

17. *Sterling M.* A proposed new classification system for whiplash associated disorders. Man Ther 2004;9:60–70.

18. *Sackett D, Richardson W, Rosenberg W, et al.* Evidence-based Medicine. How to Practice and Teach EBM. London: Churchill Livingstone, 1997.

19. *Butler D.* The Sensitive Nervous System. Adelaide: NOI Group Publications, 2000.

20. *Edwards BC.* Manual of Combined Movements, 2nd edn. Edinburgh: Churchill Livingstone, 1999.

21. *Grieve GP.* Common Vertebral Joint Problems. Edinburgh: Churchill Livingstone, 1988.

22. *Kaltenborn F, Evjenth O, Kaltenborn TB, et al.* Manual Mobilization of the Joints: The Spine, vol. 2, 4th edn. Oslo: Norli, 2003.

23. *Maitland GD, Hengeveld E, Banks K, et al.* Maitland's Vertebral Manipulation, 7th edn. London: Butterworth, 2005.

24. *Mulligan B.* Manual Therapy 'NAGS', 'SNAGS', 'MWMS', 5th edn. Wellington: Plane View Press, 1995.

25. *Shacklock M.* Clinical Neurodynamics. Edinburgh: Elsevier, 2005.

26. *Moseley G, Nicholas M, Hodges P.* A randomized controlled trial of intensive neurophysiology education in chronic low-back pain. Clin J Pain 2004;20:324–330.

27. *Sterling M, Kenardy J, Jull G, et al.* The development of psychological changes following whiplash injury. Pain 2003;106:481–489.

28. *Wallis B, Lord S, Bogduk N.* Resolution of psychological distress of whiplash patients following treatment by radiofrequency neurotomy: a randomised, double-blind, placebo controlled trial. Pain 1997;73:15–22.

29. *Sterling M, Jull G, Kenardy J.* Physical and psychological factors maintain long term predictive capacity following whiplash injury. Pain 2006;122:102–108.

30. *Sterling M, Jull G, Vicenzino B, et al.* Physical and psychological predictors of outcome following whiplash injury. Pain 2005;114:141–148.

31. *Dishman J, Burke J.* Spinal reflex excitability changes after cervical and lumbar spinal manipulation: a comparative study. Spine J 2003;3:204–212.

32. *Haavik-Taylor H, Murphy B.* Cervical spine manipulation alters sensorimotor integration: a somatosensory evoked potential study. Clin Neurophysiol 2007;118:391–402.

33. *Skyba D, Radhakrishnan R, Rohlwing J, et al.* Joint manipulation reduces hyperalgesia by activation of monoamine receptors but not opioid or GABA receptors in the spinal cord. Pain 2003;106:159–168.

34. *Sterling M, Jull G, Wright A.* Cervical mobilisation: concurrent effects on pain, motor function and sympathetic nervous system activity. Man Ther 2001;6:72–81.

35. *Vicenzino B, Collins D, Benson H, et al.* An investigation of the interrelationship between manipulative therapy-induced hypoalgesia and sympathoexcitation. J Manipul Physiol Ther 1998;21:448–453.

36. *Hoving JL, Koes BW, deVet HC, et al.* Manual therapy, physical therapy or continued care by a general practitioner for patients with neck pain. Ann Intern Med 2002;136:713–722.

37. *Jull G, Trott P, Potter H, et al.* A randomized controlled trial of exercise and manipulative therapy for cervicogenic headache. Spine 2002;27:1835–1843.

38. *Rosenfeld M, Gunnarsson R, Borenstein P, et al.* Early intervention in whiplash associated disorders: a comparison of two treatment protocols. Spine 2000;25:1782–1787.

39. *Moulson A, Watson T.* A preliminary investigation into the relationship between cervical snags and sympathetic nervous system activity in the upper limbs of an asymptomatic population. Man Ther 2006;11:214–224.

40. *Sterling M, Jull G, Wright A.* The effect of musculoskeletal muscle pain on motor activity and control. J Pain 2001;2:135–145.

41. *Bolton P, Budgell B.* Spinal manipulation and spinal mobilization influence different axial sensory beds. Med Hypotheses 2006;66:258–262.

42. *Gross A, Kay T, Kennedy C, et al.* Clinical practice guideline on the use of manipulation or mobilization in the treatment of adults with mechanical neck disorders. Man Ther 2002;7: 193–205.

43. *O'Leary S, Vicenzino B, Falla D, et al.* Specific therapeutic exercise of the neck induces immediate local hypoalgesia. J Pain 2008; in press.

44. *Hoffman M, Shepanski M, Mackenzie S, et al.* Experimentally induced pain perception is acutely reduced by aerobic exercise in people with chronic low-back pain. J Rehabil Res Dev 2005;42:183–190.

45. *Amevo B, Aprill C, Bogduk N.* Abnormal instantaneous axes of rotation in patients with neck pain. Spine 1992;17:748–756.

46. *Dall'Alba P, Sterling M, Treleaven J, et al.* Cervical range of motion discriminates between asymptomatic and whiplash subjects. Spine 2001;26:2090–2094.

47. *Dvorak J, Froehlich D, Penning L, et al.* Functional radiographic diagnosis of the cervical spine. Flexion/extension. Spine 1988;13:748–755.

48. *Jull G, Amiri M, Bullock-Saxton J, et al.* Cervical musculoskeletal impairment in frequent intermittent headache. Part 1: Subjects with single headaches. Cephalalgia 2007;27:793–802.

49. *Jull G, Zito G, Trott P, et al.* Inter-examiner reliability to detect painful upper cervical joint dysfunction. Aust J Physiother 1997;43: 125–129.

50. *Kristjansson E, Leivseth G, Brinckmann P, et al.* Increased sagittal plane segmental motion in the lower cervical spine in women with chronic whiplash-associated disorders, grades I–II: a

case-control study using a new measurement protocol. Spine 2003;28:2215–2221.

51. *Zwart JA*. Neck mobility in different headache disorders. Headache 1997;37:6–11.

52. *Hagen K, Harms-Ringdahl K, Enger N, et al*. Relationship between subjective neck disorders and cervical spine mobility and motion-related pain in male machine operators. Spine 1997;22:1501–1507.

53. *Reading I, Walker-Bone K, Palmer K, et al*. Utility of restricted neck movement as a diagnostic criterion in case definition for neck disorders. Scand J Work Environ Health 2005;31:387–393.

54. *Panjabi MM, Lyndon C, Vasavada A, et al*. On the understanding of clinical instability. Spine 1994;19:2642–2650.

55. *Cook C, Brismee J, Fleming R, et al*. Identifiers suggestive of clinical cervical spine instability: a Delphi study of physical therapists. Phys Ther 2005;85:895–906.

56. *Niere K, Torney S*. Clinicians' perceptions of minor cervical instability. Man Ther 2004;9:144–150.

57. *Ernst E*. Manipulation of the cervical spine: a systematic review of case reports of serious adverse events, 1995–2001. Med J Aust 2002;176:376–380.

58. *Tseng S, Lin S, Chen Y, et al*. Ruptured cervical disc after spinal manipulation therapy: report of two cases. Spine 2002;27:80–82.

59. *Dabbs V, Lauretti WJ*. A risk assessment of cervical manipulation vs NSAIDs for the treatment of neck pain. J Manipul Physiol Ther 1995;18:530–536.

60. *Haldeman S, Kohlbeck FJ, McGregor M*. Risk factors and precipitating neck movements causing vertebrobasilar artery dissection after cervical trauma and cervical manipulation. Spine 1999;24:785–794.

61. *Ernst E, Canter P*. A systematic review of systematic reviews of spinal manipulation. J R Soc Med 2006;99:192–196.

62. *Jull G*. The use of high and low velocity cervical manipulative therapy procedures by Australian manipulative physiotherapists. Aust J Physiother 2002;48:189–193.

63. *Cleland J, Childs J, McRae M, et al*. Immediate effects of thoracic manipulation in patients with neck pain: a randomized clinical trial. Man Ther 2005;10:127–135.

64. *Maigne J, Goussard J, Dumont F, et al*. Is systematic radiography needed before spinal manipulation? Recommendations of the SOFMMOO. Ann Readapt Med Phys 2007;50:111–116.

65. *Berthoz A, Grantyn A*. Neuronal mechanisms underlying eye–head coordination. Prog Brain Res 1986;64:325–343.

66. *Vidal P, Roucoux A, Berthoz A*. Horizontal eye position-related activity in neck muscles of the alert cat. Exp Brain Res 1982;46:448–453.

67. *Martinez-Segura R, Fernandez-de-las-Penas C, Ruiz-Saez M, et al*. Immediate effects on neck pain and active range of motion after a single cervical high-velocity low-amplitude manipulation in subjects presenting with mechanical neck pain: a randomized controlled trial. J Manipul Physiol Ther 2006;29:511–517.

68. *Nansel D, Peneff A, Cremata E, et al*. Time course considerations for the effects of unilateral lower cervical adjustments with respect to the amelioration of cervical lateral-flexion passive end-range asymmetry. J Manipul Physiol Ther 1990;13:297–304.

69. *Mulligan B*. Self Treatments for Back, Neck, and Limbs, A New Approach. Wellington: Plane View Press, 2003.

70. *Amiri M, Jull G, Bullock-Saxton J*. Measuring range of active cervical rotation in a position of full head flexion using the 3D Fastrak measurement system: an intra-tester reliability study. Man Ther 2003;8:176–179.

71. *Hall T, Robinson K*. The flexion–rotation test and active cervical mobility – a comparative measurement study in cervicogenic headache. Man Ther 2004;9:197–202.

72. *Stewart S, Jull G, Willems J, et al*. An initial analysis of thoracic spine motion with unilateral arm elevation in the scapular plane. J Manual Manipul Ther 1995;3:15–21.

73. *Elvey R*. Treatment of arm pain associated with abnormal brachial plexus tension. Aust J Physiother 1986;32:225–233.

74. *Hall T, Elvey R*. Nerve trunk pain: physical diagnosis and treatment. Manual Ther 1999;4:63–73.

75. *Allison G, Nagy B, Hall T*. A randomized clinical trial of manual therapy for cervicobrachial pain syndrome – a pilot study. Man Ther 2002;7:95–102.

76. *Cowell I, Phillips D*. Effectiveness of manipulative physiotherapy for the treatment of a neurogenic cervicobrachial pain syndrome: a single case study – experimental design. Man Ther 2002;7:31–38.

77. *Coppieters M, Stappaerts K, Wouters L, et al*. The immediate effects of a cervical lateral glide treatment technique in patients with neurogenic cervicobrachial pain. J Orthop Sports Phys Ther 2003;33:369–378.

78. *Hall T, Elvey R, Davies N et al*. Efficacy of manipulative physiotherapy for the treatment of cervicobrachial pain. Tenth Biennial Conference of the MPAA. Melbourne: MPAA, 1997. Bartram (ed) pp 73–74.

79. *Constantoyannis C, Konstantinou D, Kourtopoulos H, et al*. Intermittent cervical traction for cervical radiculopathy caused by large-volume herniated disks. J Manipul Physiol Ther 2002;25:188–192.

80. *Moeti P, Marchetti G*. Clinical outcome from mechanical intermittent cervical traction for the treatment of cervical radiculopathy: a case series. J Orthop Sports Phys Ther 2001;31:207–213.

81. *Olivero W, Dulebohn S*. Results of halter cervical traction for the treatment of cervical radiculopathy: retrospective review of 81 patients. Neurosurg Focus 2002;12:ECP1.

82. *Elvey R*. Brachial plexus tension test and the pathoanatomical origin of arm pain. In: Glasgow E, Twomey L (eds) Aspects of Manipulative Therapy. Lincoln: Institute of Health Sciences, 1979:105–110.

83. *Elvey R*. Physical evaluation of the peripheral nervous system in disorders of pain and dysfunction. J Hand Ther 1997;10:122–129.

84. *Coppieters M, Butler D*. Do 'sliders' slide and 'tensioners' tension? An analysis of neurodynamic techniques and considerations regarding their application. Man Ther 2008: in press.

85. *Dilley A, Lynn B, Pang S*. Pressure and stretch mechanosensitivity of peripheral nerve fibres following local inflammation of the nerve trunk. Pain 2005;117:462–472.

86. *Sterling M, Treleaven J, Jull G*. Responses to a clinical test of nerve tissue provocation in whiplash associated disorders. Manual Ther 2002;7:89–94.

87. *Sterling M, Jull G, Vicenzino B, et al*. Development of motor system dysfunction following whiplash injury. Pain 2003;103:65–73.

88. *Gore D, Sepic S, Gardner G, et al*. Neck pain: a long-term follow-up of 205 patients. Spine 1987;12:1–5.

89. *Heikkila H, Johansson M, Wenngren B-I*. Effect of acupuncture, cervical manipulation and NSAID therapy on dizziness and impaired head repositioning of suspected cervical origin: a pilot study. Manual Ther 2000;5:151–157.

90. *Palmgren P, Sandstrom P, Lundqvist F, et al*. Improvement after chiropractic care in cervicocephalic kinesthetic sensibility and subjective pain intensity in patients with nontraumatic chronic neck pain. J Manipul Physiol Ther 2006;29:100–106.

91. *Reid S, Rivett D, Katekar M, et al*. Sustained natural apophyseal glides (SNAGs) are an effective treatment for cervicogenic dizziness. Man Ther 2008: in press.

92. *Jull G, Falla D, Treleaven J, et al*. Retraining cervical joint position sense: the effect of two exercise regimes. J Orthop Res 2007;25:404–412.

93. *Revel M, Minguet M, Gergoy P, et al*. Changes in cervicocephalic kinesthesia after a proprioceptive

rehabilitation program in patients with neck pain: a randomized controlled study. Arch Phys Med Rehabil 1994;75:895–899.

94. *Falla D, Jull G, Russell T, et al*. The effect of different neck exercise regimes on control of sitting posture in patients with chronic neck pain. Phys Ther 2007;87:408–417.

95. *Szeto G, Straker L, O'Sullivan P*. A comparison of symptomatic and asymptomatic office workers performing monotonous keyboard work – 2: neck and shoulder kinematics. Man Ther 2005;10:281–291.

96. *Szeto G, Straker L, Raine S*. A field comparison of neck and shoulder postures in symptomatic and asymptomatic office workers. Appl Ergon 2002;33:75–84.

97. *Falla D, O'Leary S, Fagan A, et al*. Recruitment of the deep cervical flexor muscles during a postural correction exercise performed in sitting. Man Ther 2007;12:139–152.

98. *Falla D, Farina D*. Periodic increases in force during sustained contraction reduce fatigue and facilitate spatial redistribution of trapezius muscle activity. Exp Brain Res 2007;182:99–107.

99. *Johnston V, Jull G, Souvlis T, et al*. Neck movement and muscle activity characteristics in office workers with neck pain. Spine 2008; in press.

100. *Szeto G, Straker L, O'Sullivan P*. A comparison of symptomatic and asymptomatic office workers performing monotonous keyboard work – 1: neck and shoulder muscle recruitment patterns. Man Ther 2005;10:270–280.

101. *Falla D, Jull G, Hodges P*. Neck pain patients demonstrate reduced activity of the deep neck flexor muscles during performance of the craniocervical flexion test. Spine 2004;29:2108–2114.

102. *Falla D, Jull G, Hodges P*. Training the cervical muscles with prescribed motor tasks does not change muscle activation during a functional activity. Man Ther 2008; in press.

103. *Hermann K, Reese C*. Relationships among selected measures of impairment, functional limitation, and disability in patients with cervical spine disorders. Phys Ther 2001;81:903–914.

# 14

# Therapeutic Exercise for Cervical Disorders: Practice Pointers

## Introduction

Evidence has been presented of the possible impairments in the cervical muscles and in sensorimotor control that can present in patients with cervical disorders (Chapters 4 and 6). The assessment of these features (Chapter 12) guides the prescription of exercise. In clinical practice, exercises to address the various changes are performed concurrently and as well, are integrated with pain management strategies, manipulative therapy, active range-of-motion exercise, and self-management programs in the multimodal approach to the management of cervical disorders. Constant evaluation of the interplay between effects of each component of the multimodal program on the different features helps practitioners understand the interactions of their effects and assists in decisions for the possible need for priority or more emphasis on one or more systems at different stages of the patient's rehabilitation.

Several principles underlie the exercise approach:
- Therapeutic exercise commences early in the rehabilitation process, usually within the patient's initial presentation
- Exercises should not provoke neck pain
- Exercises are designed to address the specific changes identified in the muscle system and in sensorimotor function
- Precision in exercise is emphasized in the motor relearning process
- Muscles are trained specifically and within a functional and task-specific context

- Repetition is essential in the learning process to establish or re-establish appropriate movement and muscle control
- Patients must understand the rationale underpinning the various components and phases of the exercise approach. Their contribution to, and compliance with, the exercise program is critical to the learning process

These principles are derived from the evidence of the rapidity of onset of changes in sensorimotor function, the changes in muscle activity in response to pain, the specific changes in the muscles' properties in association with neck pain, as well as the evidence for specificity in exercise to address the often complex and various impairments that may be present in a patient's presenting disorder (Chapters 4 and 6). In addition, evidence has been presented throughout this text that indicates that there cannot be an expectation of automatic reversal of these changes in motor control in all patients on alleviation of symptoms. Changes are present in the acute state as well as those with recurrent or chronic pain states.

An appropriate well-constructed exercise program is mandatory in rehabilitation of patients with cervical disorders to assist optimal recovery as well as attempt to intervene into the transition to recurrent or chronic pain. This chapter will present an exercise approach based on the research evidence to date. For clarity of presentation, the exercise approaches for rehabilitation of the muscle system and of sensorimotor control related to changes in kinesthetic sense, eye movement control, and balance will be presented separately.

## Muscle system

There are changes in motor control of cervical and axioscapular muscles as well as peripheral adaptations in the muscles themselves in cervical musculoskeletal disorders. Evidence has been provided for the presence of a collection of changes in neuromuscular function, including: changes in control strategies of the neck and axioscapular muscles, insufficiency in the preprogrammed activation of cervical muscles, greater fatigability, decreased maximum strength and endurance, as well as reduced endurance at low and moderate loads (Chapter 4).

The exercise program aims to address these neuromuscular impairments through a progressive motor learning and training program consisting of three phases, containing both formal and functional exercises. Phase 1 focuses on low-load precision exercise to activate the deep cervical and axioscapular muscles and train basic patterns of movement of the cervical and axioscapular regions. Low-load endurance exercise is used to train the deep neck and axioscapular muscles in their functional role and frequent activation is promoted in a posture correction exercise. Phase 2 continues muscle re-education by training muscle coordination and movement patterns of the neck and girdle, coactivation of the deep postural muscles in posture, as well as task-specific exercise. This phase gradually introduces load to the exercises. Phase 3 addresses strength and endurance of the muscles and training is progressed to the level required to meet the patient's work, recreational, or sporting requirements. It is noted that the boundaries between these phases will blur.

## Phase 1

The first phase of the exercise program, as indicated, aims to activate and train the deep cervical and axioscapular muscles with precise exercises and to integrate their actions into their functional supporting role in upright posture. Low-load endurance exercises are introduced to train the deep muscles in line with their functional supporting role. The initial and progressive exercise program will be presented separately for each muscle group, noting that exercises for each group are performed concurrently. From the outset and in tandem with formal training, the muscles are trained functionally in the re-education of upright postures.

## Training the craniocervical flexors

Initial training of the craniocervical flexor muscles, the longus capitis and longus colli, is performed in the supine lying position. This removes head load and allows a focus on these target muscles. The ultimate aim is to improve endurance for their postural supporting function. However in the first instance the patient must be able to activate the longus capitis and longus colli appropriately to perform craniocervical flexion in a correct manner, that is, as a rotation of the cranium without unwanted excessive activation of the superficial cervical flexors, the sternocleidomastoid and scalene muscles. The common fault in training is that a substitution strategy for their contraction is not recognized (Chapter 12), and in effect the patient trains to hold an inappropriate substitution pattern. The movement pattern must be correct before training endurance of the longus capitis and longus colli muscles.

### Re-education of the craniocervical flexion movement

Craniocervical flexion is practiced as an active movement at a slow speed with an essential emphasis on precision and control (Figure 14.1). The craniocervical flexion test undertaken in the physical examination often reveals that, in the presence of weakness or poor control of the deep neck flexors, the patient may use one or more of several substitution strategies in attempts to achieve the task. The common faults as

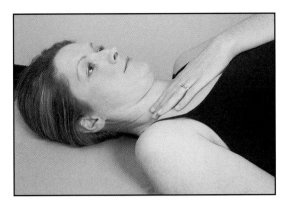

**Figure 14.1** The patient trains the craniocervical flexion movement while self-monitoring unwanted activity in the sternocleidomastoid and anterior scalene muscles.

well as remedial strategies are presented in Table 14.1. Importantly, practice of the craniocervical flexion movement should be painfree in all circumstances of acute or chronic neck pain and this is possible in most cases. There may be reservations about introducing the exercise in the presence of acute pain or injury because of its potential effect on the pain or pathology. If there were risks that the exercise could exacerbate pathology, then it would be consistent that the patient is unable to perform a gentle nodding movement to answer yes without pain – a rare occurrence. If pain is produced with practice of this gentle exercise, it signals either that the patient has been practicing the movement too vigorously or is performing the movement with a shearing, push-back action of the upper cervical region. The movement needs to be retaught with the emphasis on precision and the rotation of the cranium inherent in the movement. Alternate facilitation strategies may be required. However, pain with the exercise may indicate that mechanosensitive nerve tissue has not been identified in the pretest screening in the physical examination. In these latter circumstances, the patient is positioned in crook lying with the arms resting across the abdomen to minimize any tension on the nerve tissues. If this strategy does not permit painfree

**Table 14.1** Craniocervical flexion training: correction of muscle and movement faults

| Fault | Remedial strategies |
| --- | --- |
| The patient performs a neck retraction movement rather than the correct rotation action of craniocervical flexion | This may reflect either poor kinesthetic sense or weakness in the craniocervical flexors. Facilitation is required. |
| | 1.  Make the patient aware of the sliding of the back of the head on the bed when performing the correct craniocervical flexion movement. Encourage slow and large-range movements, moving from some craniocervical extension into flexion to improve movement awareness |
| | 2.  Teach the patient to initiate the movement with the eyes. Look down with the eyes and follow with a slow and controlled chin nod. Look up to the ceiling with the eyes only and follow with the chin to resume the neutral position. The exercise may be progressed into extension for more movement awareness in the early stages. This is a preferable strategy to facilitate the deep flexors and can be a progression of strategy 1 |
| The pressure change is achieved using excessive superficial cervical muscle activity | Teach the patient to palpate the sternocleidomastoid and scalene muscles during the movement, to give an awareness of the onset of superficial muscle contraction. Limit the range of craniocervical flexion to the point just short of palpating the contraction of superficial muscle activity. Initially encourage movement into extension to allow a sufficient excursion for the patient to gain a sense of the movement |
| The patient has an upper costal breathing pattern or is holding the breath | Teach the patient to perform the craniocervical flexion action during relaxed expiration[30] |
| | Teach the patient a basal breathing pattern |
| There is evident jaw clenching and/or the patient depresses the jaw (hyoids) to assist the craniocervical action | Teach the patient a relaxed position of the mandible; the anterior one-third of the tongue rests on the roof of the mouth, the lips are together, but teeth remain apart |
| The patient rests in slight craniocervical flexion or cannot return to the neutral position after the action and maintains the craniocervical region in slight flexion | Educate the awareness of the neutral posture. The patient focuses the eyes to the ceiling above the head and then lifts the chin to attain a neutral craniocervical position. The patient simultaneously palpates the sternomastoid and scalene muscles to appreciate the difference in tension between the flexed and neutral positions. Repetition is required so that the patient develops a new sense of the neutral position |
| Tension will be palpated in the scalene muscles | |
| | In cases where the patient has an upper costal breathing pattern, teach a basal breathing pattern to help relax respiratory accessory muscles |
| The patient overshoots the neutral position and returns to a slight extension position of the craniocervical region, suggesting an impairment in cervical kinesthetic sense | Educate the awareness of the neutral posture. Repetition is required so that the patient develops a new sense of the neutral position |

performance of craniocervical flexion, then the rotation of the cranium is practiced from outer range (i.e., craniocervical extension) to a neutral or nonprovocative flexion position in the first instance.

The pressure biofeedback is not used in initial training of the craniocervical movement. Rather, the patient uses other feedback and strategies to facilitate the movement (Table 14.1). It has been found clinically that the feedback from the pressure sensor often dominates the patient's attention, whereas at this early stage concentration should be on the actual movement and its quality. Formal practice of the movement should be undertaken two to three times a day, for example before the patient gets out of bed in the morning and on retiring at night. Arbitrarily, approximately 10 repetitions on each occasion seem sufficient. Most patients achieve a correct movement pattern with a few days of practice.

## Training the endurance of the deep neck flexors

Training the holding capacity or low-level endurance of the deep neck flexors is commenced as soon as the patient can perform the craniocervical flexion movement correctly. The pressure biofeedback is used to guide training. Without this feedback, it is difficult for the clinician or patient to know if the contraction is being maintained. The feedback signals a loss of longus capitis/ colli contraction with a drop in pressure from the target. It also displays the poorer accuracy in sustaining the contraction at the target level that has been demonstrated in neck pain patients.[1] The constant fluctuation of the needle on the dial may reflect the muscle tremor of fatigue.[2] The feedback is also motivational for the patient and assists compliance. It allows the clinician to gain some quantification of improvement to guide progression of the exercise. Training is commenced at the pressure level that the patient has been assessed to be able to achieve and hold steadily with a good movement pattern, without dominant use or substitution by the superficial flexor muscles. This is often at the lowest levels of the test (22 or 24 mmHg). The movement is facilitated with eye movement into the flexion direction and emphasis is always on precision and control. Any fast or jerky movements are discouraged as they often mask inadequacies in activation of the deep neck flexors. The patient continues to monitor any unwanted activity of the superficial flexors by self-palpation of the muscles. Some patients who present with a poor pattern of craniocervical flexion revert to this pattern when given the feedback to train endurance. In this instance, such patients should first focus on the action of craniocervical flexion and then look at the

pressure dial and maintain the pressure level that they have achieved. In all circumstances, training should be short of fatigue, so that an incorrect pattern is not encouraged.

Home practice is encouraged at least twice daily, continuing the pattern of practice before rising in the morning and when retiring at night. This means that the exercise is not too intrusive on patients' daily activities. For each pressure level, the holding time is built up to 10 seconds, and 10 repetitions are performed. Once the holding contractions at a certain pressure level are achieved, the exercise is progressed to train endurance at the next pressure level. Studies have shown that most asymptomatic subjects can achieve pressure levels between 26 and 30 mmHg[3–6] and can hold the pressure steady for 10 seconds with 10 repetitions. The aim for neck pain patients is to train the muscles towards an optimal performance (30 mmHg) and most neck pain patients are capable of achieving these higher levels.[7]

Training with feedback from the pressure sensor is generally conducted in the clinical setting. In preparation for training at home, patients can practice by visually targeting the pressure level and holding the position steadily. Once they are familiar with the exercise and with the feedback, they are encouraged to concentrate and feel the movement and the nature of the deep neck flexor contraction in the sustained hold of the position. They practice the craniocervical flexion movement and holding action with the visual feedback, and then close their eyes and attempt to relocate the position. Patients obtain feedback of their accuracy by rechecking the dial and can also recheck after 10 seconds to determine if they have maintained the position. This provides a deeper understanding of the exercise and prepares them for effective home practice. They practice to progressive levels as their skill improves. They also train to locate any of the five pressure levels in random order.

There are other benefits of this specific mode of training. It has been shown to improve cervical kinesthetic sense, as measured by a reduction in joint position error.[8] This improvement probably relates to both the improvement in muscle function as well as the relocation practice inherent in the training protocol.

The time taken to achieve and hold the five levels of the craniocervical test is variable but can usually be achieved in 4–6 weeks. Some patients with more complex neck conditions may require longer whereas, in others, it may be achieved in a shorter time. A clinical point of importance arose from a recent randomized controlled trial of chronic whiplash. Patients who were randomized to the self-management group were given a full written description of the training protocol for the craniocervical flexors and practiced the protocol for 10 weeks in an unsupervised manner. Unlike the intervention group who received supervised training, the self-management group showed no improvement on follow-up evaluation of the craniocervical flexion test.[9] This points to the need for the clinician to supervise carefully and monitor training through the stages to achieve the desired outcomes, which are unlikely to be obtained if the training is just relegated to a home program for expediency.

## Training the neck extensors

The initial training protocol for the suboccipital and neck extensor muscles replicates the movements and tests used in the assessment of these muscles in the physical examination. The exercises are performed in the four-point kneeling position or can be performed in a prone-on-elbows position in instances of wrist discomfort in four-point kneeling. Attention must first be given to the spinal and scapular postures in the four-point kneeling position. Trunk weight should be squarely over the

upper limbs with the hip and thighs at right angles to the trunk. The clinician may need to facilitate trunk posture to ensure the curves of the lumbar, thoracic, and cervical spines are in a "neutral" position with the patient's head parallel to the treatment couch. Scapular muscles such as the serratus anterior may need to be facilitated to ensure that the scapulae are well positioned on the chest wall. The four-point kneeling position will potentially work all cervical extensor muscles to hold the head weight against gravity. Thus the exercises are designed in line with the muscles' anatomical actions to target particular muscles within the neck extensor group.

The first exercise is biased towards the rectus capitis posterior major and minor muscles in recognition of their key proprioceptive function, their role in supporting and controlling the upper cervical joints, and evidence of the changes that can occur in these muscles with neck pain (Chapters 3–5). The patient performs a craniocervical extension and flexion (head-nodding) exercise whilst maintaining the cervical spine proper in its neutral position. This action is usually instantly learnt by the patient as the familiar function of saying "yes." The second exercise facilitates the obliquus capitis superior and inferior and again in a familiar movement of saying "no." Rotation movement of less than 40° is required to focus rotation to the craniocervical region. Some patients have a little difficulty in performing well-coordinated C1–2 rotation. The clinician may use tactile cues by manually stabilizing the C2 vertebra to give the patient the sense of the local head movement, use verbal terms such as "gently shake the head," or utilize gaze fixation to assist the movement. The patient fixes the gaze on a spot on the supporting surface and rotates the head, maintaining the gaze fixed on the spot. As will be discussed in the section on exercises for oculomotor control, this exercise can be practiced in various positions.

The third exercise is biased towards training the deep cervical extensors, the semispinalis cervicis/multifidus group. The exercise consists of extension of the typical cervical spine while keeping the craniocervical region in a neutral position (Figure 14.2). Thus the exercise does not bias action towards the more powerful torque-producing extensors of the head, such as splenius and semispinalis capitis. Even at this early stage of the exercise, the deeper extensor muscles are worked in coactivation with the deep cervical flexor muscles which control the craniocervical neutral position, not permitting it to move into craniocervical extension, which would occur if the superficial cranial extensors dominated the exercise.

This exercise can be a more difficult one for the patient to grasp and perform in the first instance. Several strategies can be used to facilitate the action. Explanation of the caudad location of the axis of motion in the lower cervical region in tandem with a comparative demonstration by the clinician of craniocervical extension and extension of the typical cervical region can enhance the patient's understanding. The clinician may gently grasp the C2 spinous process and neck to provide the patient with the sense of from where to initiate the movement. Using the instructions of curving or curling the neck may avoid the patient's temptation to retract the neck. In the first instance, this neck extension exercise may be limited to curling the neck into flexion and returning to the neutral position. This avoids full cervical extension, which is often a tentative movement for patients in an acute state. More importantly, patients not uncommonly fatigue quite quickly with the exercise. Limiting exercise to the extensor's outer to middle range in the first instance accounts for this fatigability and weakness. Patients can also self-check the precision of their exercise for the cervical extensors.

On return of the neck to the neutral position, patients' gaze should be on the surface of the bed between their hands (rather than well in front of their hands) if they have successfully maintained the neutral craniocervical position. A dominant craniocervical extension action is also signaled if prominent ridges of the semispinalis capitis muscle are evident. Once patients have achieved this exercise from the outer range to the neutral position, it is progressed towards inner-range extension. Again the emphasis should be placed on minimizing craniocervical

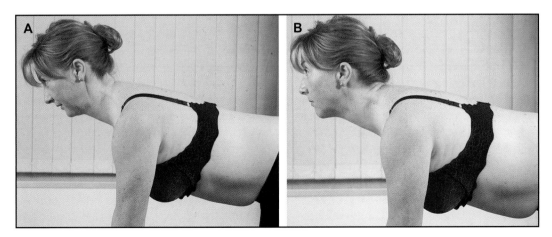

**Figure 14.2** The exercise for the extensors of the typical cervical region. (A) The exercise is performed correctly and the craniocervical region remains in a mid-position while the cervical region extends. (B) The exercise is performed incorrectly with inclusion of craniocervical extension in the exercise: this will encourage activity of muscles such as splenius and semispinalis capitis.

extension to avoid overactivity of the superficial extensor muscles but some craniocervical extension should be expected at inner-range extension. The instruction is to lift (curl) the head and neck backwards without lifting the chin. The range of cervical extension through which the extensor muscles are trained is progressively increased in this phase of the exercise program. As an exercise set, training of the craniocervical and cervical extensors is integrated in the self-management exercise program. For example, a set of five repetitions of each of craniocervical extension, rotation, and cervical extension may be the initial exercise dose. This can be progressed to three sets of five repetitions and ultimately three sets of 10 repetitions.

Training of the extensor muscles of the typical cervical spine may be commenced with gentle isometric exercises in the supine position as an alternative for patients who find the exercise too difficult in four-point kneeling or prone on elbows. The head and neck are positioned in a neutral position, as for craniocervical flexion training. The patient is instructed to exert pressure gently on to the supporting surface with the back of the head, visualizing a curling-back action. The patient is specifically instructed to avoid either a primary lift of the chin, which would encourage craniocervical extension and superficial extensor muscle activity, or conversely craniocervical flexion, which would encourage a retraction movement. The exercise is performed at an intensity of less than 20% of maximum effort. The clinician can palpate bilaterally over the lamina of the relevant cervical motion segment for the desired contraction of the deep cervical multifidus/semispinalis muscle group during the exercise, as well as palpating for the undesired contraction of the superficial semispinalis capitis muscles. Often a poorer contraction response is detected from the deeper muscles on the side of dysfunction associated with

asymmetrical action of the superficial extensor muscles. Tactile facilitation can be applied gently (and without pain) to the deep muscles at the relevant segments to address this imbalance. Attention is given firstly to the correct muscle contraction and effort. The exercise is progressed to practicing repeated sustained contractions to encourage low-load endurance of these deep cervical extensor muscles. The exercise is subsequently progressed to the through-range movement in four-point kneeling.

## Training the scapular muscles

Training appropriate scapular orientation and control in posture and during upper-limb activities is believed clinically to be a vital aspect of the rehabilitation program for neck disorders. Nevertheless even a casual review of the literature reveals that most research into scapular motion, muscle dysfunction, and pathomechanics has been in conjunction with shoulder disorders (Chapter 3). Little research at this time has formally and specifically investigated scapular muscle impairment in relation to cervical spine disorders. However, its identification and rehabilitation have long been emphasized in clinical texts[10, 11] and its training has been incorporated into successful interventions in clinical trials and case studies of the management of neck pain patients.[7, 12, 13] There is initial evidence emerging of the link between scapular posture and movement and neck pain. For example, it has been shown that the scapular posture changes (drifts into protraction in association with a forward drift of the head) during typing tasks in persons with neck pain[14] and the predominant use of levator scapulae to move or stabilize the scapula may produce adverse compressive strain on the cervical structures,[15] and that the upper trapezius fatigues during repetitive arm raising in persons with neck pain.[16] More dedicated research is required to understand fully the impact of scapular pathomechanics and muscle load specifically on neck pain as well as the effect of their management on neck pain. At this time, clinical evaluation and re-evaluation of the effect of scapular muscle training on neck pain direct the management of the individual patient.

## Training scapular orientation in an upright posture

Training of scapular orientation in upright postures is conducted in conjunction with the training of spinal posture, which will be discussed in the next section. It is usually introduced in the first treatment session, and at the latest, delayed to the second session. In the first instance, patients should understand the connection and potential impact of abnormal scapular orientation and control on their neck pain. The most potent teaching tool is a reduction in palpable tenderness in the levator scapulae/upper trapezius region or an increase in cervical rotation range that occurs when the scapula is supported or held in the appropriate position. A degree of skill is required by both the patient and clinician in re-education of scapular orientation and movement. The scapula is out of the patient's direct sight and subtle and sometimes multiplanar changes may be required to improve scapular posture. One or more of a variety of facilitation techniques can be used, including visual feedback with two mirrors, tactile feedback, subtle resistance to the desired corrective action, and, importantly, increasing the patient's awareness of scapular movement across the chest wall. The corrective movement may have to be broken into components or movements exaggerated in the initial learning process until the patient develops the sense of the movement.

When a positional fault of the scapula is observed, the scapula is first manually assisted to the desired orientation on the chest wall and this is usually repeated several times to assist the patient to learn the movement and the position. Assisted active facilitated movements may then be used (Figure 14.3). The patient then attempts an active repositioning of the scapulae and the clinician evaluates the patient's level of skill. Some patients gain the sense of the movement quite quickly. Others may require other learning strategies. For example, a not uncommonly observed postural fault in the neck pain patient is a downwardly rotated, anteriorly tilted, and protracted position of the scapula in association with evident overuse of the levator scapulae and pectoralis minor muscles. A cue that may assist correction is to have patients place their opposite hand along the line of pectoralis minor with the index finger on the coracoid process. They move the coracoid process up and away from the fingertip along the line of the hand.[17] It is a subtle action which aims to facilitate the coordinated action of all parts of trapezius and serratus anterior to correct the rotation and reposition the scapular on the chest wall. It may be necessary to place emphasis on a certain muscle. For example,

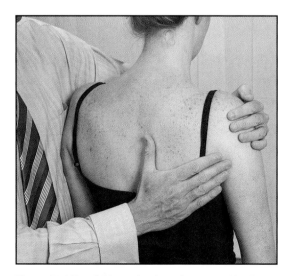

**Figure 14.3** The clinician assists the patient to reposition the scapula: the left hand controls the upward rotation and retraction, and the right hand controls the inferior angle into upward and external rotation and posterior tilt.

to encourage the contribution of serratus anterior, the patient maintains the corrected scapular position while gently pushing on to the thigh with the heel of the hand. This appears to facilitate the serratus anterior in fixating the scapular flush to the thorax and has a relaxation effect on the levator scapulae muscle. Alternately the scapulae may be protracted. A simple corrective instruction to open or spread the anterior chest wall can appropriately activate the middle and lower fibers of the trapezius muscle.

The patient's scapular correction strategy needs to be reassessed regularly in subsequent treatments. The need to reteach the correction exercise is often required. In the learning phase, patients may overcorrect the position or use excessive muscle activity and in time they need to be encouraged to use less muscle activity. They may have adopted poor techniques such as fixing the scapula to the humerus, which encourages scapular motion by the scapulohumeral rather than the scapulothoracic muscles, or substituting thoracic extension for scapulothoracic movement. These faults need to be corrected. Taping may be used if patients cannot grasp the sense of orientation of their scapula.

Once the patient learns the correct scapular orientation, the focus shifts to training the new postural habit. This requires frequent and repeated practice throughout the day for the learning and skill acquisition process. Practice is incorporated with that for the correction of spinal posture.

There is one time for caution and that is when scapular orientation (subtle elevation) is a protective response to mechanosensitive nerve tissues. Any mechanosensitivity of the nerve tissues needs to be addressed before scapular retraining is commenced, otherwise symptoms may be aggravated. Once mechanosensitivity has decreased, the residual position of the scapula is assessed and corrected as required.

## Training endurance of the scapular stabilizers

Scapular muscle endurance is trained formally in association with the training of scapular postural orientation in upright postures. This training is low-load in line with the tonic holding required of these muscles functionally in control of scapular posture. Training is usually commenced in side lying with the arm elevated to approximately 140° (Figure 14.4). The advantage of this position is that it deters the unwanted use of latissimus dorsi and presets the scapular in some upward rotation. A large excursion of scapular movement from protraction to retraction and depression of the medial scapular border is used initially to enhance the patient's awareness of scapular movement over the chest wall. Again a holding contraction is emphasized for lower trapezius in this exercise.

For home practice, the patient's arm is supported by two pillows. Patients are instructed to concentrate on movement of the scapula over the chest wall (rather than any focus on the arm). They perform the scapular action and hold the position for 10 seconds, then slide the arm back up the

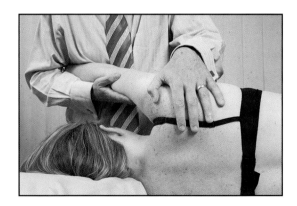

**Figure 14.4** Facilitation of the scapular muscles in the side-lying position. Emphasis is placed on the patient feeling the movement of the scapula across and slightly down the chest wall, a sensation that the patient replicates in training scapular orientation in upright postures.

pillows using serratus anterior. The exercise is repeated 10 times. It is performed twice per day in conjunction with the craniocervical flexion training, that is, before the patient arises in the morning and retires in the evening. The exercise can be subsequently progressed to a prone lying position, arm by the side as per the scapular holding test, to add the load of gravity. The 10 × 10-seconds hold protocol is followed. The exercise can be further progressed by placing the arm in elevation, as per the grade 3 muscle test for lower trapezius. This exercise with arm load trains the control and coordination between all muscles, although this final progression should not be rushed in this stage of training endurance at low levels of maximum force.

## Re-education of the neutral spinal posture

There are many positive benefits and outcomes for the patient in actively assuming a neutral upright spinal posture at regular intervals throughout the day. From a mechanical perspective, the upright neutral posture is likely to relieve passive load on cervical structures and any resultant pain. The need for the exercise is evident in those with a tendency to drift into a forward head posture, with an increasing thoracic kyphosis and protraction of the shoulder girdle during computer or any other bench work.[14, 18] Furthermore it is a key activity that allows time-efficient repeated practice of activation of the deep cervical flexors in their functional role throughout the day, which reinforces the formal training of this muscle group.[19]

Re-education of control of spinal and pelvic posture begins from the first treatment. It is a painfree and in fact a pain-relieving exercise. The upright neutral spine posture is trained initially in sitting. Correction is initiated from the lumbopelvic region. Precision is required as it has been shown that the instruction merely to sit up straight produces lesser activation of the longus capitis/colli and lumbar multifidus muscles,[19] muscles important for support of the postural curves. Posture is corrected by first drawing the pelvis up to an upright neutral position with the formation of a normal lumbar lordosis. There are many ways by which this posture can be facilitated. One way which we have found to be relatively simple and quickly learnt by the patient is to facilitate the position with pressure on the L5 spinous process (Figure 14.5). This emphasizes the restoration of the lumbar lordosis with use of multifidus rather than the patient dominating the correction with use of the long thoracolumbar extensors which attach to the pelvis and may result in formation of the lordosis in the thoracolumbar region.

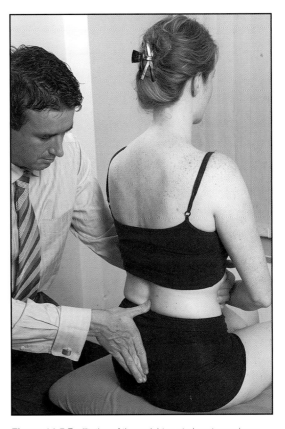

**Figure 14.5** Facilitation of the upright neutral posture using a pressure stimulus through the spinous process of L5.

The thoracic and cervical postures are often automatically corrected with the correction of the lumbopelvic position. An instruction subtly to lift the sternum may correct any residual thoracic kyphosis or, conversely, the patient can be encouraged to relax and subtly depress the sternum if the thorax is being rigidly held in too much extension. Additional visual feedback with a set of mirrors may be helpful for those patients for whom the position feels quite foreign. Patients are taught self-facilitation for the initial periods of posture training. They replicate the clinician's facilitation by placing their own thumb or fingers on the L5 spinous process. The correction is undertaken with the facilitation until they gain an awareness of the position and the muscles used for the correction.

Patients are advised to practice the posture correction exercise at least every 15 minutes during the day and hold the position for at least 10 seconds while they continue their activity. This practice can be undertaken in sitting or standing according to the patient's activity of the time. The patient requires cues or memory joggers, especially in the early stages, until the active correction of posture becomes a habit. It is a time-efficient and nonintrusive exercise for activating the deep muscles and repetitive practice will develop good postural skills with the aim of achieving automatic postural habits over time.

The second phase of re-education of posture adds correction of scapular orientation with strategies previously discussed. This is sometimes delayed until the second treatment in patients who are having some difficulty in learning the spinal postural position. Care needs to taken that, with the addition of this second scapular element, the patient does not revert to a poor spinal posture. Breaking down the skill into the component parts and concentrating on single elements at a time with staged additions to the task may be necessary in some cases. A final element of the posture correction exercise is to ask the patient to add a gentle occipital lift (imagine lifting the occiput 1 mm off the atlas). This subtle craniocervical flexion action or gentle lengthening of the neck has been shown to activate the longus colli[20] and reinforces the automatic contraction of the muscle achieved with the active spinal postural correction exercise.

## Summary

A particular emphasis is placed on phase 1 of the exercise program. It focuses on motor learning and specificity of exercise to address the impaired muscle function in those with neck pain. The ability of these exercises to change these impairments has been researched using the cervical flexors as the model (Chapter 4). This low-load motor relearning approach has been shown to increase the activation of the deep cervical flexor muscles in the craniocervical flexion test,[7, 9, 21] and reduce unwanted activity in the superficial neck flexors.[9, 21] The training enhanced the speed of deep flexor activation when challenged by a postural perturbation, a feature not generally observed with the comparison neck flexor strength-training regime.[21] Nevertheless the 6-week training program did not change the timing of the deep neck flexor muscles during a perturbation task to values comparable to persons without neck pain. Further research is required to determine whether this is possible or not with a longer training program. Specific training of the craniocervical flexors was also shown to improve the ability to maintain an upright posture of the cervical spine during prolonged sitting. Similar benefits were not achieved following 6 weeks of higher-load strength and endurance training for the cervical muscles.[18, 21] In addition, improvements in cervical kinesthetic sense occurred with this specific training.[8]

Somewhat surprisingly, improvements also occurred in craniocervical flexor muscle strength as well as endurance at 50% of maximal force following a 6-week training period.[22] These improvements may be associated with neuromuscular adaptations such as greater synchronization of motor units.[23] Such gains were made without risk of provoking pain, which can occur with high-load exercise in the patient presenting with moderate or severe levels of pain.

Thus the evidence of benefit of the motor learning approach for the first phase of rehabilitation is emerging. Changes in the muscle system and its neuromotor control occur rapidly with neck pain (Chapter 4) and need to be addressed early in the patient's management. The exercises in this phase are unlikely to strain injured cervical structures. To the contrary, this training program has been shown to reduce pain.[7, 9] Importantly, the exercises are low-load and nonprovocative in nature and can be immediately introduced in management, even with patients with a notable cervical pain syndrome.

# Phase 2

The exercise program in phase 2 continues to have a focus on motor learning but also begins to add load in both the formal and functional exercises of this stage.

## Rhythmical stabilization exercises

Mayoux-Benhamou et al.[24] aptly described the deep neck flexor and extensor muscles as a muscle sleeve which supports the cervical spine and joints, a good description to use in patient education. Coactivation of these muscles is observed during movements of the neck in healthy subjects.[25] Self-resisted rhythmical stabilization or alternating isometric exercises, particularly in axial rotation, are added to the exercise program in this phase as a further method to train the coactivation of the deep flexors and extensors.

The exercise is performed in sitting and the patient first assumes an upright neutral spinal posture. The occipital lift is added to the correct postural position to prefacilitate the activation of the longus colli/capitis before adding the gentle resistance. The rotation movement is resisted by the palm of the patient's hand, placed on the side of the face, and the exercise is prefaced with eye movement in the direction of the movement. The patient performs the alternating isometric contractions with an emphasis on slow-onset and slow-release holding contractions, using resistance to match about a 10% effort to avoid coactivation of the more superficial muscles. This exercise is performed twice a day and can easily be incorporated into a daily work routine.

## Training control of cervical spine extension

Cervical extension is a common movement in daily activities requiring looking or reaching upwards and is often painful and a poorly controlled movement in neck pain patients. Cervical extension in sitting or standing is initiated by the extensors but quickly requires eccentric control of the cervical flexors and, in particular, the craniocervical flexors (Chapter 3). It would be expected that the patient is starting to achieve the higher levels of cranioflexion endurance training (28–30 mmHg) prior to commencing this exercise.

The patient looks to the ceiling and eyes follow the ceiling backwards so that the head is slowly extended past the frontal plane of the shoulders, remaining within a range that is painfree and able to be controlled. The return to the upright position trains concentric control and is initiated by craniocervical flexion in order to facilitate activation of the deep cervical flexors. A dominant action of sternocleidomastoid in the presence of weakness of the deep neck flexors encourages extension in the upper cervical region, a pattern to be avoided. The range to which the head is moved into extension is gradually increased as control is improved and any pain permits.

The second stage of the exercise adds isometric holds in positions through range and begins the strength and endurance training of the cervical flexor synergy. The patient extends the head and neck to a predetermined position in range that is able to be controlled and is painfree. The clinician supports the head in this position and the patient relaxes. The holding contraction is initiated by looking down together with a slight craniocervical flexion action. Controlling this position, the patient then initiates a head lift, just taking the weight of the head off the clinician's hand (Figure 14.6). The position is held for

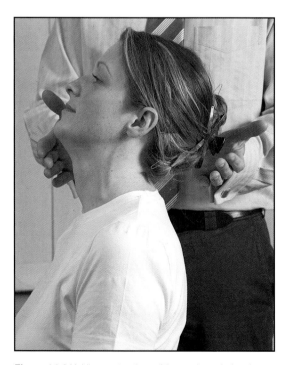

**Figure 14.6** Holding contractions of the craniocervical and cervical flexors are trained against the load of gravity and head weight. The craniocervical flexion position must be maintained throughout the exercise.

5 seconds prior to curling the neck back up to the neutral upright position. The exercise is repeated five times, or a number up to the patient's ability. For home practice, the support of the clinician's hand is replaced by that of the patient. The exercise is progressed by progressively increasing the range of extension in which the exercise is performed. These latter positions are relatively high-load and should be progressed with care so as not to provoke the patient's neck pain.

## Training scapular control with arm movement and load

The control of scapular orientation in posture is progressed to train it under movement or loaded conditions of the upper limb as required in the patient's functional or work activities. These work activities often provoke pain. In addition, altered muscle control has been demonstrated in axioscapular muscles and in scapular orientation in these tasks in persons with neck pain (Chapter 4).

There is only a small change in scapular orientation in the initial phases of upper-limb elevation; circumstances which replicate work activities such as keyboard or mouse use, benchtop light processing work, and many home activities (Chapter 3). In the first instance, the control of scapular orientation is challenged with arm movements of less than 40° of elevation, which requires the axioscapular muscles to provide a static, stable base of support for the arm activities. The patient maintains correct scapular orientation while performing small-range arm elevation and/or rotation movements, and while performing a previously aggravating activity such as mouse operation (Figure 14.7). Electromyography biofeedback may be used over the levator scapulae/upper trapezius muscles or the clinician may observe scapular orientation and palpate

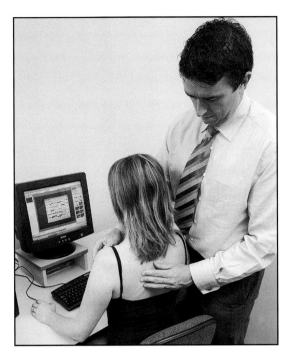

**Figure 14.7** Training the control of scapular orientation and spinal posture during functional activities such as mouse use.

the muscles to assess performance. At the same time, the head and neck posture is monitored, as is any unwanted activity in the superficial neck flexors (Chapter 4). The task-specific exercise can be progressed by time to improve endurance. The axioscapular muscles' control of scapular position can be challenged with the addition of faster arm movement or light load provided by a resistive strap such as Theraband (Pro-Med Products) or hand weights, as replicates the patient's functional needs.

The scapular orientation and control by the axioscapular muscles may also need to be trained through full elevation of the arm with the use of facilitation strategies. Additionally greater fatigue of the upper trapezius has been found in persons with neck pain during a repetitive arm elevation task.[16] Thus both the pattern of axioscapular muscle control as well as the endurance of these muscles may need attention, especially for those patients whose work requires such repetitive arm action. Progressive load should be added to the arm movement as pertains to the functional demands of the patient. Control of craniocervicothoracic posture must be monitored and maintained with all such exercises.

## Muscle length

Clinical tests have revealed an incidence of muscle tightness associated with cervical disorders.[4, 26, 27] Altered scapular orientation may be accompanied by changes in muscle length, for instance, levator scapulae tightness or overactivity may be present in association with a downwardly rotated scapular position. Our preference as the first approach to management of muscle length changes is to facilitate the correct scapular position which, in the example of the downwardly rotated scapula, will lengthen the levator scapulae in association with the re-education of the three divisions of the trapezius and serratus anterior. Similarly, any shortness in the suboccipital extensors is first addressed by training the craniocervical flexors, which promotes reciprocal relaxation and lengthening of the suboccipital extensors.

Stretching is often prescribed for the upper trapezius muscle in general exercise programs and exercise handouts. The upper trapezius region is a frequent site of pain but care should be taken in prescribing stretching. For example, in the presentation of a downwardly rotated scapula, the upper trapezius is more likely to be weak and resting in a lengthened position. Further stretching is not indicated. Furthermore slight elevation of the scapula suggesting some subtle shortness in the upper trapezius may be a protective response for mechanosensitive nerve tissues. Nerve tissues must also be considered in cases of apparent scalene muscle shortness. Stretching is contraindicated in these circumstances.

We are not trying to suggest that there is no indication for muscle stretching in patients with neck pain. That would be inaccurate. There are indications for muscles such as the pectoralis minor, whose shortness may not permit effective training of scapular orientation. Rather we are suggesting that there are alternatives to address problems of muscle shortness in many instances that may be more successful in addressing the impairments in the long term.

# Phase 3

This phase focuses on strength and endurance training. This phase should be approached with some caution from both muscle control and symptom perspectives. As the program progressively adds more load to the muscle system, the performance of the deep muscles should be continually re-evaluated with tests such as the craniocervical test to ensure that their performance is maintained. Muscle performance in the control of spinal and scapular orientation should likewise be repeatedly checked. Exercise that exceeds their control has been progressed too quickly. From the symptom perspective, the patient's pain should have reduced to the mild status and the condition should be stable to begin this third phase. Pain and other symptoms that are still fluctuant may indicate that either the pathology or pathophysiology has not settled sufficiently for this stage which loads the musculoskeletal structures. Care must be taken that strength training is not introduced too early, thus provoking symptoms. Furthermore the level of strength training should take into consideration the functional requirements of the patient as well as patient age and gender. High levels of strength training may be required for some but not necessarily for all patients.

Modalities used for strength training may vary depending on the clinician and patient's circumstances and available equipment. To provide the resistance, use may be made of gravity and head load, resistive elastic straps or weights or formal neck muscle training machines may be used for cervical[28] or specific craniocervical muscle training.[29] Whatever the medium, training should commence well within the patient's capacity and be progressed conservatively. For example, when using head weight and gravity for training cervical flexor strength, the exercise is commenced with the head supported on two pillows or sufficient towels to reduce the load of gravity. The head lift must be preceded by craniocervical flexion followed by cervical flexion to clear the head from the supporting surface and the craniocervical flexion position must be maintained throughout the exercise (Figure 14.8). Patients may begin by performing one set of 5 repetitions with a 1–2-second holding time, gradually increasing the repetitions as the patient improves. Depending on the desired training effect, the number of repetitions and sets may be increased as permitted by the patient's response to the exercise, or

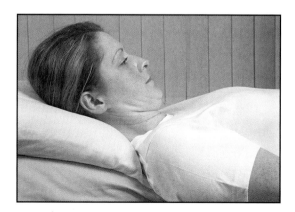

**Figure 14.8** Strength training for the cervical flexors is begun with the support of two pillows. Care must be taken to ensure that the craniocervical region does not extend with dominant action by the sternocleidomastoid muscles.

an endurance element can be incorporated by increasing the time the position is held. Ultimately the exercise can be progressed to the use of one pillow. This is usually sufficient for many patients as lifting the head from a flat surface is often too difficult.

Extension strength may be trained in standing, or alternately, in the four-point kneel/prone-on-elbows position against a weight or a resistive strap such as Theraband (Figure 14.9). Here the cervical extension exercise previously performed as an active free movement in the earlier phase of training can be progressed with resistance. Again, the strength and endurance training is taken to the level required by the patient for recreational, work, or sporting endeavors.

Some patients also participate in gym programs for general fitness. It is important that patients are questioned about the type of exercises that they are performing in aerobic or weight-training programs. Exercises should be analyzed for the effect that they are having on the neck and axioscapular regions from postural position, movement, and load perspectives. Advice and modifications are frequently required to ensure exercises are beneficial rather than detrimental for the cervicobrachial region.

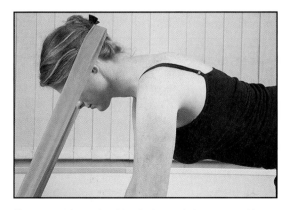

**Figure 14.9** Strength training for the cervical extensors with the use of a Theraband. The exercise can be progressed using increasing densities of the band as required.

# Rehabilitation of disturbed sensorimotor control

Proprioceptive deficits, disturbances in eye movement control, and disturbances in control of posture have been observed in patients with neck pain (Chapter 6). The following exercise regime is based on the knowledge and evidence available to date which describe impairment in sensorimotor control (Chapters 5 and 6). Exercises consist of relocation practice, gaze stability, eye follow, eye–head coordination, and balance exercises. The tasks can be introduced early into the rehabilitation program in the first or second treatment sessions. Exercises should be performed such that they do not produce or exacerbate pain or other symptoms, although a temporary exacerbation of dizziness may need to be accepted. As a point of interest, clinicians will encounter occasional patients with severe neck pain syndromes, as can occur in acute whiplash. Here because of their pain state, therapeutic exercise for the articular and muscle systems may be severely curtailed in the initial stages of management. However exercises such as eye follow or balance which do not move the neck can be used to commence the active rehabilitation program.

The elements of the exercise program are introduced at the clinically assessed level of impairment. The clinician determines which exercises are of most benefit in improving impairments based on the symptoms and the physical findings in each of the tests for cervical kinesthetic sense, eye movement control, and balance (Chapter 12). If the patient demonstrates disturbed sensorimotor control in each area, one or two exercises for each area may be most appropriate in the first instance. Exercises should be performed two to three times per day, gradually increasing the degree of difficulty and duration of the activity.

## Training cervical joint position sense

Cervical joint position sense is trained by the patient practicing to relocate the head back to the natural head posture and to predetermined positions in range. All movement directions, cervical flexion, extension, rotation, and lateral flexion are trained with particular emphasis in some tasks on the craniocervical region. Patients practice first with the eyes open and then with eyes closed, always ensuring that they are sitting in a good postural position. Feedback on performance is essential to improve accuracy. This may be done by patients lining up their natural head posture and target positions with points on the wall and visually checking their accuracy on return to these positions. However, feedback is far more precise and potent with the use of a laser pointer or pencil torch to display accuracy. The laser or pencil torch attached to a headband which was used for assessment purposes is used in training and is easily built for home use. Patients position themselves within 1 meter of a wall and line up the point of the laser or the center of the torch beam with a point on the wall or mark this point indicating their natural head posture position. As mentioned, relocating this point after a movement is first practiced with the eyes open and then is progressed to practice with eyes closed. Patients monitor their accuracy in relocation. This is simple and nonexpensive apparatus for home use and has major benefits in improving the precision of training. The feedback provides major incentive to the patient and improves compliance.

Joint position sense is trained to higher levels of skill. Tasks could include following a moving target at a set speed and distance with the eyes open and then replicating the same speed and distance with the eyes closed. Confirmation of the performance by opening the eyes again provides feedback. The laser or torch beam can be used to trace intricate patterns such as a figure of eight placed on the wall. This exercise particularly emphasizes craniocervical movement. The task can be progressed by altering the speed and excursion of movement. The future may provide opportunities for even more potent visual and auditory feedback on performance with the advances in virtual reality technology and with the general public's access to them improving daily.

Kinesthetic training may be incorporated into other exercises. The example of practicing targeting to the different pressure levels with and without visual feedback while training the craniocervical flexors has already been mentioned. There are other options. The headband with the laser or torch could be worn whilst performing active range-of-motion and neuromuscular control exercises to provide feedback about patterns of movement. For example, when training the craniocervical flexion action, an arc of light occurs if the correct nodding action is performed. If the patient were inappropriately substituting a retraction action, little movement of the light would be seen, alerting the patient to this incorrect movement strategy. Similarly, when practicing craniocervical rotation in the four-point kneeling position, a straight line of light backwards and forwards would signal that rotation was being achieved whilst maintaining a neutral cervical spine. If patients were unable to maintain the correct movement and cervical position, they would see the light deviating off the line and be able to correct and fine-tune the exercise.

## Oculomotor training

The exercise program for eye movement control is developed for the individual patient and is based on the level of patient performance in the oculomotor assessment in the physical examination. The exercises appear to be quite simple, but they can be quite provocative of symptoms, such as dizziness, headache, and neck pain. Exercises may be practiced to the point of onset of dizziness, but they should not provoke pain. They may need to be commenced in lying for some patients with severe symptoms of dizziness, unsteadiness, or pain and subsequently progressed to sitting and standing positions. Conversely, if certain exercises exacerbate symptoms, the patient's position should be changed to a more supported position such as from sitting to lying or the number or speed of repetitions reduced.

## Eye follow with a stationary head

The retraining of eye follow usually commences with the patient in a sitting position, although some patients with marked symptoms may commence the exercises in a supine lying position. They maintain their head still for all exercises, moving only their eyes to follow the target. The clinician (or the patient for home practice) holds a pen or other suitable object and moves it from side to side and upwards and downwards (Figure 14.10). Eye follow is initially performed at a comfortable speed at which patients can concentrate and control their gaze on the object without pain or lasting symptoms of dizziness. It is often wise to commence these exercises with, for example, merely 10-second bursts of practice 5 times per day to assess initial reactions to the exercise. The time can be quickly built up as tolerated to a target of 30 seconds of sustained practice.

There are several ways that the exercises are progressed as the initial task becomes easy and symptoms permit. The eye-follow exercises can be performed with the trunk in a prerotated position (up to 45°) akin to the principle of the smooth-pursuit neck torsion test (Chapter 6). In addition, the speed of

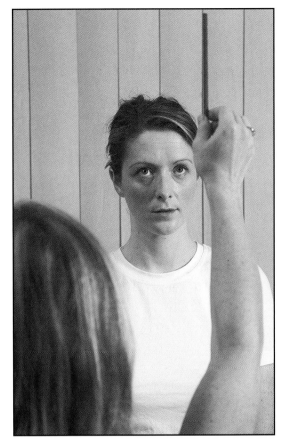

**Figure 14.10** The patient practices eye follow in an upwards and downwards direction.

eye follow can be increased and the position in which the exercises are undertaken progressed to standing. As the patient improves, further challenges can be introduced such as saccadic or sudden deviations in the movements of the object at random eye positions. The exercises can be combined with balance exercises to challenge sensorimotor control further.

## Gaze fixation with head movement

The patient concentrates on fixing the gaze on a stationary point while the head is moved in these exercises. The training may be commenced in a supine lying position in patients whose symptoms warrant a conservative start to these exercises. In this instance, the head movement may be performed passively by the clinician or actively by the patient while fixing the gaze on a point on the ceiling. Such initial training can easily be integrated with manual therapy treatment or training the craniocervical flexion movement.

Gaze fixation exercises are usually commenced in a sitting position or quickly progressed to this position and then to a standing position. The patient visually fixes on a target while moving the head through all active movement directions. The clinician can also passively move the trunk while the patient maintains gaze on a target. Any gaze fixation task may be made more challenging by restricting peripheral vision. Peripheral vision can be restricted with the use of a pair of swimming goggles that have been blackened out, leaving a small clear area in the center of each side.

There are several other strategies that can be used to progress gaze fixation exercises. These include increasing the speed and range of head movements, adding busy patterns (e.g., stripes or checks) to the background of the visual target or making the target a word to keep in focus rather than just a spot. These latter conditions can easily be established by the patient for home use using a computer (e.g., Powerpoint presentation) or printed pages can be provided which the patient can attach to a notice board or the fridge at home.

In functional activities patients must be able to fix their gaze while moving, for example, watching another car ahead while they approach an intersection, searching for a certain item on a supermarket shelf while walking down a shopping aisle. Thus gaze fixation can be practiced under a variety of conditions, for instance, while sitting on an unstable surface such as a therapy ball or wobble board or while standing with feet in an unstable base of support as in a tandem, heel–toe position. Ultimately gaze fixation can be practiced while walking and turning the head (Figure 14.11).

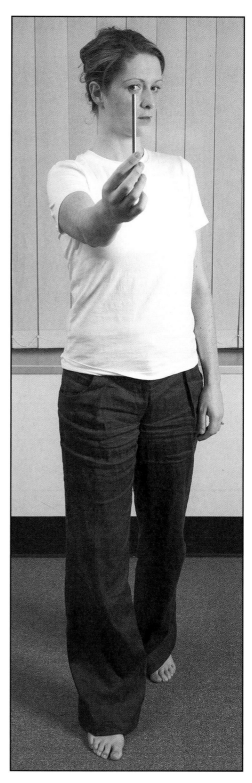

**Figure 14.11** Gaze fixation practice while walking.

## Eye–head coordination exercises

The exercises for eye–head coordination are performed in the sitting or standing positions. They commence with the patient rotating the eyes and head to the same side to both the left and the right as well as in upwards and downwards directions. This eye–head coordination has been emphasized in all practice of active movement in examination and treatment. In the second exercise, the patient practices leading with the eyes first to a target, followed by the head, ensuring the eyes keep focused on the target. In a further progression, the eyes are moved first, followed by the head, to look between two targets positioned horizontally or vertically. The patient could also practice active neck rotation to follow a slowly moving target with peripheral vision restricted. Finally the patient practices rotating the eyes and head to the opposite side, in both the left and right directions.

As with other oculomotor exercises, the eye–head coordination exercises can be progressed by increasing the speed and range of movements, adding busy patterns to the background of the visual target or making the target a word to keep in focus rather than just a spot. Exercises can be performed in tandem with balance exercises to challenge sensorimotor coordination further.

## Balance training

Balance training is the third component of the sensorimotor control program for the neck pain patient. Once again, the tasks for training balance commence at the level at which the patient failed or had difficulty. This could be comfortable, narrow-base, tandem, or single-leg stance. Patients train at the relevant level until they can maintain their balance steadily for a period of 30 seconds. The conditions for training balance in the neck pain patient are similar to those for other musculoskeletal or neurological conditions and progress from eyes open, eyes closed to different supporting surfaces, for example standing on foam or an unstable surface. Progression to trampolines or wobble boards may also be appropriate for selected patients.

Patient safety must be of concern for home practice, especially for those who have quite marked disturbances in balance which can be observed in some whiplash patients or the older person with a cervical disorder. Patients may practice balance exercises at home in a corner area, such that they are able to regain balance easily if necessary.

Challenges to balance can be further increased by adding a variety of conditions or tasks in the final stages of rehabilitation. Relocation practice or oculomotor exercises can be superimposed on balance exercises. More functional tasks such as reach or stepping can be added and the limits of stability can be challenged with external perturbations. The patient can be further challenged by tasks such as walking forwards, backwards, and sideways whilst actively moving the head into different directions and while maintaining direction and velocity of gait. Progression could include decreasing the confinement of the walking area and increasing the speed of both neck movements and walking.

## General remarks

Exercise is a vital part of the management of patients with cervical disorders and is integrated with other components of the multimodal management approach, as outlined in Chapter 13. The exercise program described is a staged program which progresses through three basic phases. Clinicians must "sell" the program to patients, demonstrate the impairments and, importantly, provide feedback of their improving performance in order to gain the necessary compliance. Furthermore, initiating a treatment session with exercise not only demonstrates the beneficial effects that the exercise may have on pain, but it informs the patient of the priority that is being placed on exercise. The exercise program must be continually progressed in line with changes shown in the continuous evaluation process and the home program regularly reviewed and modified.

A question regularly posed by patients and clinicians alike is for how long the exercises should be performed. This is a difficult question and impossible to answer scientifically at this point. One would hope that if muscle and sensorimotor control are adequately rehabilitated then resumption of normal activities would sustain their appropriate function and no further formal exercise is required. Indeed, this may happen in the 40% of people who sustain a single episode of neck pain and have no recurrence. Hopefully this percentage may increase with the better foundation for therapeutic exercise that research is now providing. However, it is likely in cases, for example, of an active degenerative process, a primary osteoarthrosis of a zygapophyseal joint, when there has been marked trauma or when a patient is in a working environment that constantly strains the cervical musculoskeletal system, that exercise needs to be continued to counter any inhibitory or facilitatory effects that underlying pathology may have on the muscle system and its neural control.

Such programs should be realistic if the patient is to continue exercise in the long term and exercises should be tagged to a regular habit or activity. For example, continuance of the posture correction exercise which facilitates the deep neck and girdle muscle at work is a good habit to adopt. A selected few neck exercises included in a gym program or a warmdown program after a patient has returned from a walk might suit some patients. Weekly self-checking of performance in key exercises that the patient has performed in rehabilitation might indicate the need to resume the program for a week or two to keep muscles at a desired performance level. Importantly, any hint of neck stiffness, aching, or pain should prompt the immediate return to an exercise program. Such strategies should be discussed with patients and patients nominate the time or activity that would be most conducive to them following a maintenance program in efforts to curtail recurrent episodes of neck pain.

## References

1. *O'Leary S, Jull G, Kim M, et al.* Craniocervical flexor muscle impairment at maximal, moderate, and low loads is a feature of neck pain. Man Ther 2007;12:34–39.

2. *Gandevia SC.* Spinal and supraspinal factors in human muscle fatigue. Physiol Rev 2001;81:1725–1789.

3. *Chiu T, Law E, Chiu T.* Performance of the craniocervical flexion test in subjects with and without chronic neck pain. J Orthop Sports Phys Ther 2005;35:567–571.

4. *Jull G, Barrett C, Magee R, et al.* Further characterisation of muscle dysfunction in cervical headache. Cephalalgia 1999;19:179–185.

5. *Jull GA.* Deep cervical neck flexor dysfunction in whiplash. J Musculoskel Pain 2000;8:143–154.

6. *Jull G, Kristjansson E, Dall'Alba P.* Impairment in the cervical flexors: a comparison of whiplash and insidious onset neck pain patients. Man Ther 2004;9:89–94.

7. *Jull G, Trott P, Potter H, et al.* A randomized controlled trial of exercise and manipulative therapy for cervicogenic headache. Spine 2002;27:1835–1843.

8. *Jull G, Falla D, Treleaven J, et al.* Retraining cervical joint position sense: the effect of two exercise regimes. J Orthop Res 2007;25:404–412.

9. *Jull G, Sterling M, Kenardy J, et al.* Does the presence of sensory hypersensitivity influence outcomes of physical rehabilitation for chronic whiplash? A preliminary RCT. Pain 2007;129:28–34.

10. *Janda V*. Muscle and cervicogenic pain syndromes. In: Grant RE (ed) Physical Therapy for the Cervical and the Thoracic Spine. New York: Churchill Livingstone, 1988:153–166.

11. *Janda V*. Muscles and motor control in cervicogenic disorders: assessment and management. In: Grant R (ed) Physical Therapy of the Cervical and Thoracic Spine, 2nd edn. New York: Churchill Livingstone, 1994:195–216.

12. *McDonnell M, Sahrmann S, Dillen LV*. A specific exercise program and modification of postural alignment for treatment of cervicogenic headache: a case report. J Orthop Sports Phys Ther 2005;35: 3–15.

13. *Petersen S*. Articular and muscular impairments in cervicogenic headache: a case report. J Orthop Sports Phys Ther 2003;33:21–30.

14. *Szeto G, Straker L, Raine S*. A field comparison of neck and shoulder postures in symptomatic and asymptomatic office workers. Appl Ergon 2002;33:75–84.

15. *Behrsin JF, Maguire K*. Levator scapulae action during shoulder movement. A possible mechanism of shoulder pain of cervical origin. Aust J Physiother 1986;32:101–106.

16. *Falla D, Farina D*. Muscle fiber conduction velocity of the upper trapezius muscle during dynamic contraction of the upper limb in patients with chronic neck pain. Pain 2005;116:138–145.

17. *Mottram S*. Dynamic stability of the scapula. Man Ther 1997;2:123–131.

18. *Falla D, Jull G, Russell T, et al*. Effect of neck exercise on sitting posture in patients with chronic neck pain. Phys Ther 2007;84:408–417.

19. *Falla D, O'Leary S, Fagan A, et al*. Recruitment of the deep cervical flexor muscles during a postural correction exercise performed in sitting. Man Ther 2007;12:139–152.

20. *Fountain FP, Minear WL, Allison PD*. Function of longus colli and longissimus cervicis muscles in man. Arch Phys Med Rehabil 1966;47:665–669.

21. *Jull G*. Cervical flexor muscle retraining: physiological mechanisms of efficacy. In: Cairns M, Comerford M, Gibbons S et al (eds). Kinetic Control and Manipulation Association of Charted Physiotherapists: pp L01.

22. *O'Leary S, Jull G, Kim M, et al*. Specificity in retraining craniocervical flexor muscle performance. J Sports Phys Ther 2007;37:3–9.

23. *Conley MS, Stone MH, Nimmons M, et al*. Resistance training and human cervical muscle recruitment plasticity. J Appl Physiol 1997;83: 2105–2111.

24. *Mayoux-Benhamou MA, Revel M, Vallee C*. Selective electromyography of dorsal neck muscles in humans. Exp Brain Res 1997;113:353–360.

25. *Conley MS, Meyer RA, Bloomberg JJ, et al*. Noninvasive analysis of human neck muscle function. Spine 1995;20:2505–2512.

26. *Treleaven J, Jull G, Atkinson L*. Cervical musculoskeletal dysfunction in post-concussional headache. Cephalalgia 1994;14:273–279.

27. *Zito G, Jull G, Story I*. Clinical tests of musculoskeletal dysfunction in the diagnosis of cervicogenic headache. Man Ther 2006;11: 118–129.

28. *Burnett A, Naumann F, Price R, et al*. A comparison of training methods to increase neck muscle strength. Work 2005;25:205–210.

29. *O'Leary S, Vicenzino B, Jull G*. A new method of isometric dynamometry for the craniocervical flexors. Phys Ther 2005;85:556–564.

30. *Cagnie B, Danneels L, Cools A, et al*. The influence of breathing type, expiration and cervical posture on the performance of the craniocervical flexion test in healthy subjects. Man Ther 2008; in press.

CHAPTER

# 15

# Future Directions

The past 10–20 years in particular have seen rapid growth in research and consequently knowledge of cervical spine disorders. As a result, clinicians are now better placed to make more informed decisions in their clinical reasoning process, based on the evidence currently available, for both diagnosis and selection of management approaches for patients with a variety of cervical disorders. Importantly, there has been a change in health care ethos and health care generally has become more patient-centered. The patient has become an active participant in management and in goal-setting for outcomes.

There is no doubt that conservative approaches to management of cervical disorders are advancing and have a more rational basis, as we trust has been demonstrated in this text. Nevertheless the next decade will doubtlessly see more advancement in knowledge in the musculoskeletal field, in both the clinical and basic sciences, which will further enhance the management of cervical musculoskeletal disorders. An ultimate aim is for neck pain to be prevented or at least managed optimally, with the endeavor of preventing the transition to chronicity or to recurrent episodes of pain. It is thus fitting to conclude this text with some examples of the many fields of work requiring future attention by clinicians and researchers alike.

# Identification of responders and nonresponders to physical therapies

An urgent area for future research is to identify those with neck disorders who are likely responders, partial responders, and nonresponders to conservative physical therapies. This is in fairness to the patient and the clinician, as well as the payer of such services. Recognition of responders and nonresponders is intimately linked with possession of suitable classification and subclassification systems for neck disorders as well as prognostic indicators for recovery. One feature that has become eminently clear is that there is heterogeneity in the presentation of persons with neck disorders, even within the current broad classifications, such as cervicogenic headache, whiplash-associated disorders, cervicobrachial pain, work-related neck pain, and nonspecific neck pain. This heterogeneity is likely to reflect differences in underlying pathology, pain mechanisms, pathophysiological processes of altered sensorimotor function, and associated psychosocial influences. It could be expected that any subclassification system which is to inform of the need or not for physical therapy treatments and likely outcomes will have to consider a combination of these factors in a management algorithm. Such an algorithm would necessarily include the roles and input from other health disciplines, the workplace, health insurers, and other personnel as required in a patient-centered management plan.

Physiotherapists have undertaken studies that have investigated aspects such as presenting clinical symptoms and movement features, pathophysiological processes in the sensory, motor, and psychological systems as well as responses to certain treatment approaches to determine better the types of interventions which may be suitable for a certain patient or to predict prognosis and likely treatment outcomes.[1–6] Significant progress is being made in whiplash-associated disorders when pathophysiological processes are considered.[5,6] However, meager progress has been made from a physical therapy perspective in other conditions such as cervicogenic headache, nonspecific neck pain, or cervicobrachial disorders. Current knowledge will help to direct the necessary future work.

Areas of challenge where more work is urgently needed include, for example, the role of physical therapies in the presence of overt or even more subtle neuropathic pain states and states where there are alterations in the neurobiological processing of pain. There is little hard evidence for the efficacy of physical therapies for cervical radiculopathies, let alone clear characteristics of those who may respond to physical therapies. There is some very preliminary evidence in relation to the influence of the presence of certain patterns of sensory disturbances, at least in the management of patients with chronic whiplash-associated disorders. Patients with widespread mechanical as well as cold hyperalgesia were less responsive to multimodal physiotherapy, although those with mechanical hyperalgesia only responded reasonably well.[7] It would seem that pain relief which can be afforded by physical therapies such as manipulative therapy or specific exercise as a sole therapy may not be able to address successfully the neurobiological processes in the pain syndromes of particular patients with widespread and multiple sensory abnormalities. The influence of the presence of augmented pain processing in the central nervous system on the outcomes of physical therapies needs further exploration to validate these preliminary findings and to understand better the role of physical therapies in the rehabilitation of such patients. Certainly there are pointers to the need for multidisciplinary management with a particular emphasis on adequate medical pain management in the first instance to provide a better environment for rehabilitation of musculoskeletal function.

There is probably better support for a future direction of research to investigate and understand pain processes rather than other characteristics of pain such as its acuteness or chronicity or even its intensity in seeking to identify responders or nonresponders to physical therapies. For example, in a clinical trial of the management of persons with cervicogenic headache of an age span of 18–60 years, it was found that the patient's age, the intensity of headache, and its chronicity were not predictors of outcome and they did not prevent relief of headache with physical therapy interventions.[4] Nevertheless, Hoving et al.,[8] in studying a group of neck pain patients of 18–70 years attending general medical practices found that older age, and especially concomitant back pain, were predictors of prognosis but their predictive capacity was weak. In tandem with our findings in cervicogenic headache, they found that history, levels of neck pain and disability, and routine and somewhat cursory physical examination did not assist in predicting prognosis.

These few examples, we consider, point to the need for deeper investigations of pathophysiological processes in the sensory, motor, and psychological systems as well as their possible interactions in neck pain disorders to better gain prognostic indicators. This will also better inform on relevant treatment options which in turn will give a better indication of potential responders and nonresponders to conservative physical therapies.

## Physiological effects of interventions

We have demonstrated in this text some of the pathophysiological changes that can be present in cervical musculoskeletal disorders, particularly in the motor control and sensorimotor function. We have undertaken and reported some initial research into the physiological effectiveness of exercise using the cervical flexors as the model (Chapter 4) and indeed have presented a case for the need for specificity of exercise when addressing the physiological changes in sensorimotor function. However, this type of research, investigating the physiological effects of particularly low-load training on the cervical neuromuscular system, is in its infancy. There are many questions to answer and muscles and functions to be examined. For example, we know that we can improve the speed of activation of the deep cervical flexors in response to a perturbation with specific low-load training of craniocervical flexion in many patients, but do not know the characteristics of the patients in whom there was no change.[9] We do not know as yet if the feedforward activation of the deep neck flexors can be re-established to mirror that observed in nonneck pain subjects and what dosage is required in this type of exercise to effect such change. We also do not know how relevant improving or re-establishing feedforward control of the neck muscles is to an overarching aim of preventing recurrent episodes of pain.

As with the muscle system, there is also a need to have a deeper understanding of the physiological effects of manipulative therapy and indeed what we are capable of achieving with manual spinal examination of the cervical region. The literature abounds with examiner reliability studies on perceived motion and pain responses with manual examination with very equivocal results. Yet this examination method persists in clinical practice despite evidence which could suggest that it be abandoned as an examination technique. Practitioners skilled in the art of manual examination contend that they gain valuable information from the manual examination of the cervical joints for both segmental diagnosis and for treatment directions. But what exactly is that information? Outcomes based on segmental compliance and motion, as primary features of manual examination, are difficult to defend scientifically. Is it more what a local provocative manual force does to the sensory (pain) system and central nervous system in reflex muscle activity that informs the practitioner? There needs to be more carefully planned research into the art of manual examination to understand its diagnostic parameters.

There has been quite a volume of research into the physiological effects of manipulative therapy. It is known, for example, that manipulative therapy techniques have effects on neuromuscular control,[10-12] and induce transient plastic cortical changes[13] and changes in the sympathetic nervous system as well as the sensory system.[12, 14-17] Effects, measured in the sensory and sympathetic nervous systems, are repeatedly produced with applications of a manipulative therapy technique in progressive treatments.[18] Of interest, while there is some evidence that manual therapy has an effect on mechanical hyperalgesia, it does not appear to have an effect on thermal hyperalgesia (at least in the case of heat hyperalgesia).[12, 16] The effect of manual therapies on cold hyperalgesia is unknown but it is tempting to speculate that it would be similar to heat hyperalgesia. This may in part explain why the chronic whiplash patients with widespread mechanical hyperalgesia were responsive to physical therapies, whereas those with widespread mechanical and cold hyperalgesia were not so responsive.[7] Further research into the physiological effects of manipulative therapy will bring us closer to understanding its mechanisms of action.

## Intervention techniques

The growing evidence of the nature of impairments in the various systems in cervical musculoskeletal disorders as well as the physiological effects of various techniques is directing the development of new physical therapy interventions or, at least, modifications, adaptations, and refinements of existing techniques. This evolution must continue with research informing practice and, equally, practice informing research. The future must see the development and validation of new techniques for assessment and intervention based on emerging evidence to keep physical therapy practices contemporary as well as forward-thinking.

The evidence points to the greater benefit of multimodal treatment. It is believed that further research may enhance the benefits of a multimodal approach. As can be readily observed, there is overlap in some of the physiological effects of the various techniques used to treat cervical disorders. A better understanding of the interaction of these techniques may assist in treatment prescription and provide information as to how best to utilize their complementary effects to maximize the benefits of a multimodal approach and deliver treatment expediently and cost-efficiently. Cervicogenic dizziness and the impairment in cervical joint position sense can be used as an example. We know that manipulative therapy can improve symptoms of dizziness, pain, and joint position sense[19, 20] and an initial study has shown improvements in balance.[21] Likewise specific protocols of relocation practice, eye–head coordination, and gaze stability[22, 23] as well as specific retraining of the craniocervical flexors[22] can improve symptoms and joint position sense. We advocate in this text simultaneous application of all three interventions for their specific effects on a primary impairment in the relevant system, which, in a de facto manner, also utilizes the possible benefits of their concurrent effects on the other systems. However it is not known if there is a true additive effect of the three interventions when used in this way, or indeed use of one or two of the three interventions may be equally effective. We do know, nevertheless, that a protocol of relocation practice, eye–head coordination, and gaze stability better improved joint position error from rotation than did craniocervical flexion training[22] and, interestingly, the only predictor of a poorer response to manipulative therapy and specific exercise in a cervicogenic headache treatment trial was the presence of dizziness or light-headedness.[4] No dedicated program of relocation practice, eye–head coordination, or gaze stability exercises were incorporated into the trial interventions so it is tempting to speculate that results may have been different with this more specific training. Nevertheless we do not know and more research needs to be undertaken to understand fully the need for and benefits of a multimodal approach for cervicogenic dizziness.

A final point in consideration of cervicogenic dizziness relates back to the development of new physical therapy interventions. Current protocols of eye–head coordination and gaze stability exercises have been taken from training regimes for other disorders such as vestibular dysfunction. While their appropriateness for cervical disorders can be well argued on a physiological basis and indeed the benefits for cervicogenic dizziness have been demonstrated, it could be questioned whether there are other exercises or strategies which could be designed or adapted to be more specific for the cervical somatosensory system.

## Multidisciplinary management

The many patients who present with noncomplex cervical disorders can usually be managed quite adequately by a single practitioner. However, when patients present with more complicated disorders which may involve, for instance, significant pain syndromes, marked pathology, marked psychological reactions, or significant psychosocial issues, there is an evident need for multidisciplinary management. There is not a wealth of research investigating

the potential benefits of multidisciplinary management of the more difficult cervical disorders or those recalcitrant to conservative physical therapies when used as a single management approach.

There is at present equivocal evidence of benefit for standard multidisciplinary biopsychosocial rehabilitation programs for patients with chronic neck pain.[24, 25] Many of the principles and practices of these programs have been transferred from those used in the management of chronic low-back pain and applied to chronic neck pain and this may be a fundamental flaw. There are differences in the nature and incidence of many of the physical, psychological, and psychosocial features of neck pain disorders, which suggests that these programs may achieve more if the problems presenting in neck disorders are addressed more specifically (Chapter 7). In whiplash, for example, it has been found that posttraumatic stress symptoms is one of the features that predicts a poorer prognosis.[5, 6] Thus it could be suggested that specific health psychological interventions are in order when the condition has been formally diagnosed[26] in tandem with physical rehabilitation. Furthermore, the reactions appear soon after injury,[27] which suggests that this multidisciplinary management may be more effective if introduced in the acute or subacute stage of the disorder, rather than be relegated to times when the whiplash disorder has become chronic.

More specific areas of multidisciplinary management should also be explored. For example, is there benefit in adding an active rehabilitation program following the pain relief afforded by the surgical procedure of cervical radiofrequency neurotomy of the medial branch of the dorsal ramus? This surgical technique is being used particularly in the management of recalcitrant cases of whiplash-associated disorders and cervicogenic headache in whom there is a significant pain problem arising from a cervical zygapophyseal joint. Often such patients have failed to respond to conservative medical or physical therapies. There are several studies which, in the main, support the effectiveness of cervical radiofrequency neurotomy in relieving pain.[28–32] However pain relief is usually not permanent – the nerve will regenerate. The period of pain relief is variable and in most cases will last from a few months to a year and the neurotomy is often repeated. It is most probable that the underlying impairments and disordered afferent input from the sensory and motor systems persist. A trial investigating the addition of specific but nonaggressive rehabilitation of the muscle function and sensorimotor control in the period of pain relief following the neurotomy could reveal whether more permanent pain relief is achievable with this combined multidisciplinary management. There are many such examples where the potential benefits of multidisciplinary management need to be examined.

## Cost-effectiveness

The call for proof of cost-effectiveness of interventions is growing louder as health insurance companies and governments face the challenges of higher health costs coupled with an aging population who place higher demands on the health system. Cost of care as well as attendant costs such as those of work time lost need to be evaluated in all future clinical trials. Already studies are evaluating costs of different treatment approaches, frequency of treatment, as well as costs of different practitioner disciplines.[33–35] In relation to costs, it is important that research is conducted which gives a clearer indication of treatment dosages required to achieve the desirable outcomes. This is not only in terms of pain relief and functional outcomes but, importantly, in terms of adequate rehabilitation of the sensorimotor function. The amount and time required for therapeutic exercise to achieve the changes in cervical motor control and other impairments of sensorimotor function must be broadly established. It is possible that extra costs in the short term may prevent the greater costs of prolonged, recurrent, or chronic pain.

## Conclusion

Management of patients with cervical disorders has become a very satisfying field of practice as research is increasingly informing and directing practice. The future will see further evolution in assessment and intervention strategies for the clinician to embrace in the management of the individual patient. It is important that a monitor is kept on quality, especially in these times of fiscal pressures on health care delivery. The evidence is assisting practitioners to be able to provide relevant and quality interventions in a variety of practice settings.

## References

1. *Childs J, Fritz J, Piva S, et al*. Proposal of a classification system for patients with neck pain. J Orthop Sports Phys Ther 2004;34:686–696.

2. *Clair D, Edmondston S, Allison G*. Physical therapy treatment dose for nontraumatic neck pain: a comparison between 2 patient groups. J Orthop Sports Phys Ther 2006;36:867–875.

3. *Clare H, Adams R, Maher C*. Reliability of McKenzie classification of patients with cervical or lumbar pain. J Manipul Physiol Ther 2005;28:122–127.

4. *Jull G, Stanton W*. Predictors of responsiveness to physiotherapy treatment of cervicogenic headache. Cephalalgia 2005;25:101–108.

5. *Sterling M, Jull G, Kenardy J*. Physical and psychological factors maintain long term predictive capacity following whiplash injury. Pain 2006;122:102–108.

6. *Sterling M, Jull G, Vicenzino B, et al*. Physical and psychological predictors of outcome following whiplash injury. Pain 2005;114:141–148.

7. *Jull G, Sterling M, Kenardy J, et al.* Does the presence of sensory hypersensitivity influence outcomes of physical rehabilitation for chronic whiplash? A preliminary RCT. Pain 2007;129:28–34.

8. *Hoving J, de Vet H, Twisk J, et al.* Prognostic factors for neck pain in general practice. Pain 2004;110:639–645.

9. *Jull G.* Cervical flexor muscle retraining: physiological mechanisms of efficacy. 2nd International Conference on Movement Dysfunction. Edinburgh, Scotland: 2005.

10. *Dishman J, Cunningham B, Burke J.* Comparison of tibial nerve H-reflex excitability after cervical and lumbar spine manipulation. J Manipul Physiol Ther 2002;25:318–325.

11. *Dishman J, Burke J.* Spinal reflex excitability changes after cervical and lumbar spinal manipulation: a comparative study. Spine J 2003;3:204–212.

12. *Sterling M, Jull G, Wright A.* Cervical mobilisation: concurrent effects on pain, motor function and sympathetic nervous system activity. Man Ther 2001;6:72–81.

13. *Haavik-Taylor H, Murphy B.* Cervical spine manipulation alters sensorimotor integration: a somatosensory evoked potential study. Clin Neurophysiol 2007;118:391–402.

14. *Skyba D, Radhakrishnan R, Rohlwing J, et al.* Joint manipulation reduces hyperalgesia by activation of monoamine receptors but not opioid or GABA receptors in the spinal cord. Pain 2003;106:159–168.

15. *Sluka K, Wright A.* Knee joint mobilization reduces secondary mechanical hyperalgesia induced by capsaicin injection into the ankle joint. Eur J Pain 2001;5:81–87.

16. *Vicenzino B, Collins D, Benson H, et al.* An investigation of the interrelationship between manipulative therapy-induced hypoalgesia and sympathoexcitation. J Manipul Physiol Ther 1998;21:448–453.

17. *Vicenzino B, Paungmali A, Buratowski S, et al.* Specific manipulative therapy treatment for chronic lateral epicondylalgia produces uniquely characteristic hypoalgesia. Man Ther 2001;6:205–212.

18. *Souvlis T, Wright A.* The tolerance effect: its relevance to analgesia produced by physiotherapy interventions. Phys Ther Rev 1997;2:227–237.

19. *Heikkila H, Johansson M, Wenngren B-I.* Effect of acupuncture, cervical manipulation and NSAID therapy on dizziness and impaired head repositioning of suspected cervical origin: a pilot study. Man Ther 2000;5:151–157.

20. *Palmgren P, Sandstrom P, Lundqvist F, et al.* Improvement after chiropractic care in cervicocephalic kinesthetic sensibility and subjective pain intensity in patients with nontraumatic chronic neck pain. J Manipul Physiol Ther 2006;29:100–106.

21. *Reid S, Rivett D, Katekar M, et al.* Sustained natural apophyseal glides (SNAGs) are an effective treatment for cervicogenic dizziness. Man Ther 2008;in press.

22. *Jull G, Falla D, Treleaven J, et al.* Retraining cervical joint position sense: the effect of two exercise regimes. J Orthop Res 2007;25:404–412.

23. *Revel M, Minguet M, Gregoy P, et al.* Changes in cervicocephalic kinesthesia after a proprioceptive rehabilitation program in patients with neck pain: a randomized controlled study. Arch Phys Med Rehabil 1994;75:895–899.

24. *Buchner M, Zahlten-Hinguranage A, Schiltenwolf M, et al.* Therapy outcome after multidisciplinary treatment for chronic neck and chronic low back pain: a prospective clinical study in 365 patients. Scand J Rheumatol 2006;35:363–367.

25. *Karjalainen K, Malmivaara A, van Tulder M et al.* Multidisciplinary biopsychosocial rehabilitation for neck and shoulder pain among working age adults. Cochrane Database Syst Rev 2003;2:CD002194.

26. *Bryant R, Harvey A, Dang S, et al.* Treatment of acute stress disorder. J Consult Clin Psychol 1998;66:862–866.

27. *Sterling M, Kenardy J, Jull G, et al.* The development of psychological changes following whiplash injury. Pain 2003;106:481–489.

28. *Govind J, King W, Bailey B, et al.* Radiofrequency neurotomy for the treatment of third occipital headache. J Neurol Neurosurg Psychiatry 2003;74:88–93.

29. *Haspeslagh S, van Suijlekom H, Lame I, et al.* Randomised controlled trial of cervical radiofrequency lesions as a treatment for cervicogenic headache. BMC Anesthesiol 2006;16:1.

30. *Manchikanti L, Damron K, Cash K, et al.* Therapeutic cervical medial branch blocks in managing chronic neck pain: a preliminary report of a randomized, double-blind, controlled trial: clinical trial NCT0033272. Pain Phys 2006;9:279–281.

31. *McDonald GJ, Lord SM, Bogduk N.* Long-term follow-up of patients treated with cervical radiofequency neurotomy for chronic neck pain. Neurosurgery 1999;45:61–67.

32. *Prushansky T, Pevzner E, Gordon C, et al.* Cervical radiofrequency neurotomy in patients with chronic whiplash: a study of multiple outcome measures. J Neurosurg Spine 2006;4:365–373.

33. *Korthals-de-Bos I, Hoving J, van-Tulder M, et al.* Cost effectiveness of physiotherapy, manual therapy, and general practitioner care for neck pain: economic evaluation alongside a randomised controlled trial. Br Med J 2003;326: 911.

34. *Rainville J, Jouve C, Hartigan C, et al.* Comparison of short- and long-term outcomes for aggressive spine rehabilitation delivered two versus three times per week. Spine J 2002;2:402–407.

35. *Scholten-Peeters G, Neeleman-van der Steen CW, van der Windt DA, et al.* Education by general practitioners or education and exercises by physiotherapists for patients with whiplash-associated disorders? A randomized clinical trial. Spine 2006;31:723–731.

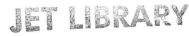

# Index

---

*Note*: Page numbers in italics represent figures or tables.